AF348878

Personalized Care and Treatment Compliance in Chronic Conditions

Personalized Care and Treatment Compliance in Chronic Conditions

Editors

Fábio G. Teixeira
Catarina Godinho
Júlio Belo Fernandes

MDPI • Basel • Beijing • Wuhan • Barcelona • Belgrade • Manchester • Tokyo • Cluj • Tianjin

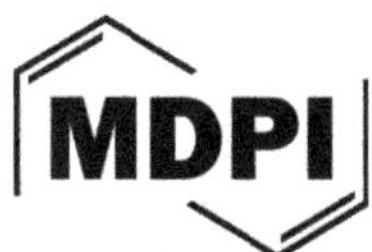

Editors

Fábio G. Teixeira
Life and Health Sciences
Research Institute
School of Medicine
University of Minho
Braga
Portugal

Catarina Godinho
Fisiologia
Egas Moniz Higher School
of Health
Almada
Portugal

Júlio Belo Fernandes
Nursing
Egas Moniz Higher School
of Health
Almada
Portugal

Editorial Office
MDPI
St. Alban-Anlage 66
4052 Basel, Switzerland

This is a reprint of articles from the Special Issue published online in the open access journal *Journal of Personalized Medicine* (ISSN 2075-4426) (available at: www.mdpi.com/journal/jpm/special_issues/treatment_compliance).

For citation purposes, cite each article independently as indicated on the article page online and as indicated below:

LastName, A.A.; LastName, B.B.; LastName, C.C. Article Title. *Journal Name* **Year**, *Volume Number*, Page Range.

ISBN 978-3-0365-4242-3 (Hbk)
ISBN 978-3-0365-4241-6 (PDF)

Contents

Journal of
Personalized
Medicine

MDPI

Editorial

Personalized Care and Treatment Compliance in Chronic Conditions

Júlio Belo Fernandes [1,2,*], Fábio Teixeira [3,4,5,6] and Catarina Godinho [1,2]

[1] Escola Superior de Saúde Egas Moniz, 2829-511 Almada, Portugal; cgodinho@egasmoniz.edu.pt
[2] Grupo de Patologia Médica, Nutrição e Exercício Clínico (PaMNEC), Centro de Investigação Interdisciplinar Egas Moniz (CiiEM), 2829-511 Almada, Portugal
[3] Life and Health Sciences Research Institute (ICVS), School of Medicine, University of Minho, 4710-057 Braga, Portugal; fabiogrodri@gmail.com
[4] ICVS/3B's Associate Lab, PT Government Associated Laboratory, 4710-057 Braga, Portugal
[5] Medical and Industrial Biotechnology Laboratory (LABMI), Porto Research, Technology, and Innovation Center (PORTIC), Porto Polytechnic Institute, 4200-465 Porto, Portugal
[6] I3S—Instituto de Investigação e Inovação em Saúde, Universidade do Porto, 4200-135 Porto, Portugal
* Correspondence: juliobelo01@gmail.com

Citation: Fernandes, J.B.; Teixeira, F.; Godinho, C. Personalized Care and Treatment Compliance in Chronic Conditions. *J. Pers. Med.* **2022**, *12*, 737. https://doi.org/10.3390/jpm12050737

Received: 28 April 2022
Accepted: 29 April 2022
Published: 1 May 2022

Publisher's Note: MDPI stays neutral with regard to jurisdictional claims in published maps and institutional affiliations.

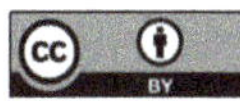

Chronic diseases are commonly defined as conditions that last one year or more and require ongoing medical attention, limit activities of daily living, or both [1]. These include, for example, diabetes, cancer, and cardiovascular and neurodegenerative disorders. Such diseases are growing at an alarming rate, especially in the aging population, and are the leading causes of death and disability for adults in developed countries [2].

Living with a chronic condition can be stressful because it changes patients' lives, distressing their physical or/and mental health or threatening their survival [3]. Nevertheless, people are able to take steps to cope with these new situations, manage their condition, and maintain a good quality of life.

People who have chronic diseases spend a significant amount of time in self-management in out-of-hospital environments, in their homes, and in their community settings. These patients have different disease statuses and management requirements.

Medicine and healthcare have been profoundly transformed as a result of technological progress along with clinical research achievements, resulting in an increased disease-management capacity [4].

Over time, medicine and healthcare models have evolved towards a practice that is technically feasible, economically valuable [4,5], and culturally, ethically, and socially accepted. In this evolution, personalized care could be the key. It represents an opportunity to improve care for all individuals from a singular or collective point of view that holds promise for the prevention and treatment of diseases.

The development of personalized care implies strong involvement and commitment from society. Researchers and policymakers must analyze the potential effect of personalized care approaches within healthcare and recommend reorganization of services, infrastructures, regulations, and policies for personalized care to become truly embedded/implemented in healthcare systems [4]. Additionally, patients, caregivers, family, and healthcare providers identify and discuss problems caused by or related to the patient's condition and then develop plans and goals to empower patients and their families.

A personalized care approach could greatly benefit patients with chronic conditions given its impact on aspects of physical health, mental health, and the ability to self-manage conditions. New approaches that allow for the development of personalized care and improvement of overall treatment adherence should be strongly encouraged by healthcare providers.

With this editorial and Special Issue focusing on personalized care and treatment compliance in chronic conditions, we aimed to stimulate the research community to continue producing evidence that supports the positive effects of a personalized care approach on the diagnosis and treatment of chronically ill patients.

The accepted topics included a variety of research studies, from study protocols [6] to original qualitative [7–9] and quantitative studies [10–17]. Additionally, review protocols [18,19] and literature reviews [20–23] were included, covering different areas of care, from studies addressing ageism [6] or stigma [17] to a personalized approach to diagnosing and managing ischemic stroke [16]. We highlighted the importance of recognizing that in order to enhance healthcare delivery, all stakeholders involved in providing care must actively partner with patients and families to enable changes in the care process, obtaining higher patient satisfaction and better health outcomes. Therefore, studies involving family caregivers, which are central to delivering better healthcare, were also considered and published in the Special Issue.

Several internationally renowned research groups contributed with research. We highlight two studies in particular. The first study reported on a novel boot-camp program to help guide personalized exercise in people with Parkinson's disease. This study shows the program's acceptability and usefulness regarding participation in a PD-personalized educational and exercise boot-camp program. This program was considered a valuable example of personalized care used to better influence patients' exercise habits [15]. Second, we highlight a study aiming to assess the effect of virtual-reality-based therapy to reduce the impact of fibromyalgia syndrome in outcomes such as pain, dynamic balance, aerobic capacity, fatigue, quality of life, anxiety, and depression. The findings demonstrated that virtual-reality-based therapy can effectively reduce pain, fatigue, anxiety, and depression and increase dynamic balance, aerobic capacity, and quality of life in women with fibromyalgia syndrome [21].

Overall, 19 articles were published, all with a common aim of increasing knowledge in the field of personalized care.

Funding: This research received no external funding.

Acknowledgments: The authors would like to thank the support of Santa Casa Neurociências Prize Mantero Belard for Neurodegenerative Diseases Research (MB-28-2019), and Prize BPI Fundação "la Caixa" Seniores 2021 and Fundação para a Ciência e Tecnologia (FCT-EXPL/SAL-SER/0761/2021).

Conflicts of Interest: The authors declare no conflict of interest.

References

1. Centers for Disease Control and Prevention: About Chronic Diseases. Available online: https://www.cdc.gov/chronicdisease/about/index.htm#:~{}:text=Chronic%20diseases%20are%20defined%20broadly,disability%20in%20the%20United%20States (accessed on 31 March 2022).
2. World Health Organization. Facts and Figures. Available online: https://www.who.int/whr/2003/en/Facts_and_Figures-en.pdf (accessed on 31 March 2022).
3. Benkel, I.; Arnby, M.; Molander, U. Living with a chronic disease: A quantitative study of the views of patients with a chronic disease on the change in their life situation. *SAGE Open Med.* **2020**, *8*, 2050312120910350. [CrossRef] [PubMed]
4. Nardini, C.; Osmani, V.; Cormio, P.G.; Frosini, A.; Turrini, M.; Lionis, C.; Neumuth, T.; Ballensiefen, W.; Borgonovi, E.; D'Errico, G. The evolution of personalized healthcare and the pivotal role of European regions in its implementation. *Per. Med.* **2021**, *18*, 283–294. [CrossRef] [PubMed]
5. Doble, B.; Lorgelly, P. Clinical players and healthcare payers: Aligning perspectives on the cost-effectiveness of next-generation sequencing in oncology. *Per. Med.* **2015**, *12*, 9–12. [CrossRef]
6. Fernandes, J.B.; Ramos, C.; Domingos, J.; Castro, C.; Simões, A.; Bernardes, C.; Fonseca, J.; Proença, L.; Grunho, M.; Moleirinho-Alves, P.; et al. Addressing Ageism—Be Active in Aging: Study Protocol. *J. Pers. Med.* **2022**, *12*, 354. [CrossRef]
7. Ferreira, R.; Baixinho, C.L.; Ferreira, Ó.R.; Nunes, A.C.; Mestre, T.; Sousa, L. Health Promotion and Disease Prevention in the Elderly: The Perspective of Nursing Students. *J. Pers. Med.* **2022**, *12*, 306. [CrossRef] [PubMed]
8. Tu, P.; Smith, D.; Clark, R.; Bayzle, L.; Tu, R.; Lin, C. Patients' Characterization of Medication, Emotions, and Incongruent Perceptions around Adherence. *J. Pers. Med.* **2021**, *11*, 975. [CrossRef] [PubMed]
9. Pedrosa, R.; Ferreira, Ó.; Baixinho, C.L. Rehabilitation Nurse's Perspective on Transitional Care: An Online Focus Group. *J. Pers. Med.* **2022**, *12*, 582. [CrossRef] [PubMed]
10. Ferreira, B.; Diz, A.; Silva, P.; Sousa, L.; Pinho, L.; Fonseca, C.; Lopes, M. Bibliometric Analysis of the Informal Caregiver's Scientific Production. *J. Pers. Med.* **2022**, *12*, 61. [CrossRef]

11. Plotogea, O.-M.; Gheorghe, G.; Stan-Ilie, M.; Constantinescu, G.; Bacalbasa, N.; Bungau, S.; Diaconu, C.C. Assessment of Sleep among Patients with Chronic Liver Disease: Association with Quality of Life. *J. Pers. Med.* **2021**, *11*, 1387. [CrossRef]
12. Moleirinho-Alves, P.M.M.; Cebola, P.M.T.C.; dos Santos, P.D.G.; Correia, J.P.; Godinho, C.; Oliveira, R.A.N.d.S.; Pezarat-Correia, P.L.C. Effects of Therapeutic and Aerobic Exercise Programs on Pain, Neuromuscular Activation, and Bite Force in Patients with Temporomandibular Disorders. *J. Pers. Med.* **2021**, *11*, 1170. [CrossRef]
13. De Barros, G.M.; Melo, F.; Domingos, J.; Oliveira, R.; Silva, L.; Fernandes, J.B.; Godinho, C. The Effects of Different Types of Dual Tasking on Balance in Healthy Older Adults. *J. Pers. Med.* **2021**, *11*, 933. [CrossRef] [PubMed]
14. Varallo, G.; Scarpina, F.; Giusti, E.M.; Suso-Ribera, C.; Cattivelli, R.; Guerrini Usubini, A.; Capodaglio, P.; Castelnuovo, G. The Role of Pain Catastrophizing and Pain Acceptance in Performance-Based and Self-Reported Physical Functioning in Individuals with Fibromyalgia and Obesity. *J. Pers. Med.* **2021**, *11*, 810. [CrossRef] [PubMed]
15. Domingos, J.; Dean, J.; Cruickshank, T.M.; Śmiłowska, K.; Fernandes, J.B.; Godinho, C. A Novel Boot Camp Program to Help Guide Personalized Exercise in People with Parkinson Disease. *J. Pers. Med.* **2021**, *11*, 938. [CrossRef] [PubMed]
16. Śmiłowska, K.; Śmiłowski, M.; Partyka, R.; Kokocińska, D.; Jałowiecki, P. Personalised Approach to Diagnosing and Managing Ischemic Stroke with a Plasma-Soluble Urokinase-Type Plasminogen Activator Receptor. *J. Pers. Med.* **2022**, *12*, 457. [CrossRef]
17. Fernandes, J.B.; Família, C.; Castro, C.; Simões, A. Stigma towards People with Mental Illness among Portuguese Nursing Students. *J. Pers. Med.* **2022**, *12*, 326. [CrossRef]
18. Sousa, L.; Gemito, L.; Ferreira, R.; Pinho, L.; Fonseca, C.; Lopes, M. Programs Addressed to Family Caregivers/Informal Caregivers Needs: Systematic Review Protocol. *J. Pers. Med.* **2022**, *12*, 145. [CrossRef]
19. Rocha, P.; Baixinho, C.L.; Marques, A.; Henriques, A. Safety-Promoting Interventions for the Older Person with Hip Fracture on Returning Home: A Protocol for a Systematic Review. *J. Pers. Med.* **2022**, *12*, 654. [CrossRef]
20. Tilinca, M.C.; Tiuca, R.A.; Tilea, I.; Varga, A. The SGLT-2 Inhibitors in Personalized Therapy of Diabetes Mellitus Patients. *J. Pers. Med.* **2021**, *11*, 1249. [CrossRef]
21. Cortés-Pérez, I.; Zagalaz-Anula, N.; Ibancos-Losada, M.d.R.; Nieto-Escámez, F.A.; Obrero-Gaitán, E.; Osuna-Pérez, M.C. Virtual Reality-Based Therapy Reduces the Disabling Impact of Fibromyalgia Syndrome in Women: Systematic Review with Meta-Analysis of Randomized Controlled Trials. *J. Pers. Med.* **2021**, *11*, 1167. [CrossRef]
22. Loureiro, F.; Ferreira, M.; Sarreira-de-Oliveira, P.; Antunes, V. Interventions to Promote a Healthy Sexuality among School Adolescents: A Scoping Review. *J. Pers. Med.* **2021**, *11*, 1155. [CrossRef]
23. Zaharia, A.-C.; Dumitrescu, O.-M.; Radu, M.; Rogoz, R.-E. Adherence to Therapy in Glaucoma Treatment—A Review. *J. Pers. Med.* **2022**, *12*, 514. [CrossRef] [PubMed]

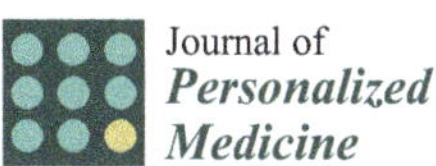

Journal of
*Personalized
Medicine*

Article

A Novel Boot Camp Program to Help Guide Personalized Exercise in People with Parkinson Disease

Josefa Domingos [1,2,3], John Dean [2], Travis M. Cruickshank [4,5], Katarzyna Śmiłowska [6], Júlio Belo Fernandes [3] and Catarina Godinho [3,*]

1 Department of Neurology, Center of Expertise for Parkinson & Movement Disorders, Donders Institute for Brain, Cognition and Behaviour, Radboud University Medical Center, 6500HB Nijmegen, The Netherlands; domingosjosefa@gmail.com
2 Triad Solutions, Aurora, CO 80012, USA; john@johnmdean.com
3 Grupo de Patologia Médica, Nutrição e Exercício Clínico (PaMNEC)—Centro de Investigação Interdisciplinar Egas Moniz (CiiEM), Escola Superior de Saúde Egas Moniz, Caparica, 2829-511 Almada, Portugal; juliobelo01@gmail.com
4 Centre for Precision Health, Edith Cowan University, Joondalup, WA 6027, Australia; t.cruickshank@ecu.edu.au
5 Perron Institute for Neurological and Translational Science, Nedlands, WA 6009, Australia
6 Department of Neurology, Silesian Center of Neurology, 40-055 Katowice, Poland; kasia.smilowska@gmail.com
* Correspondence: cgcgodinho@gmail.com; Tel.: +351-91-007-7492

Abstract: Given the variety of exercise programs available for people with Parkinson's disease (PD), such individuals may struggle to make decisions about what exercise to perform. The objective of this study was to assess the usefulness, satisfaction, and preferences regarding participation in a PD-personalized educational and exercise boot camp program. Attendees participated in a four-day program consisting of exercise sessions, workshops, and social activities. We collected demographic and clinical information. We assessed satisfaction and preferences immediately after. At one-month follow-up, participants assessed usefulness and changes in exercise habits. Eight individuals diagnosed with PD, with a mean age of 59.5 ± 6.8 years, participated. All participants felt "very satisfied" and likely to attend future events. The two favorite sessions were: cognitive stepping and dance-based movements. At one-month follow-up, participants considered the program "very useful" and reported changes in their exercise routine. Our results suggest that the boot camp program was considered useful and capable of influencing participants' exercise habits.

Keywords: Parkinson disease; personalized medicine; clinical exercise; exercise prescription; boot camp; physiotherapy

Citation: Domingos, J.; Dean, J.; Cruickshank, T.M.; Śmiłowska, K.; Fernandes, J.B.; Godinho, C. A Novel Boot Camp Program to Help Guide Personalized Exercise in People with Parkinson Disease. *J. Pers. Med.* **2021**, *11*, 938. https://doi.org/10.3390/jpm11090938

Academic Editor: Edward J. Modestino

Received: 26 July 2021
Accepted: 18 September 2021
Published: 20 September 2021

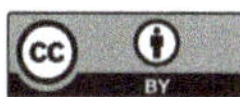

1. Introduction

Parkinson's disease (PD) is a neurodegenerative disease that results in a gradual reduction in activities of daily living and quality of life [1]. Increasing evidence suggests that individuals with PD benefit from continuous ongoing exercise to improve and maintain physical functioning and help them better manage the disease [2,3].

As such, people with PD are currently encouraged to play an active role in self-management and acquire the exercise tools in their community to manage their disease [4]. Yet, there is a variety of rehabilitation, exercise, and physical activity programs that are now available for individuals with PD. Some of the more common approaches highlighted in recent literature include amplitude-based movements [5–8], dance [9–11], Tai Chi [12,13], Qigong [14,15], Nordic walking [16,17], boxing [18–20], and aquatic exercise [21,22].

Translation of therapies into practice in the community setting has, however, proven difficult. Engaging in a regular rehabilitation and clinical exercise interventions and guaranteeing ongoing adherence requires finding the proper program that really fits the patients' needs and preferences, as well as bypasses common perceived barriers to exercise in PD [23,24].

Just telling people about the benefits of these exercises and expecting them to make decisions is debatable. Making the choice about which type of exercise programs to perform, understanding the evidence, safety issues, and the adaptations needed for each program [25] may be difficult. Considering the benefits of such programs, there is a need to overcome these translation issues.

Several lines of evidence have suggested that boot camps represent an effective and useful means of teaching [26,27]. Despite knowledge of this success, few studies have investigated the usefulness of delivering exercise education via boot camps for individuals with PD.

No study has attempted to encompass the range of these different approaches all in one intervention or program in PD. Providing access to a boot camp program that provides participants the opportunity to familiarize themselves with types of exercise programs while guiding them as to what works best and potentially guiding their exercise choices may be of critical importance. Here, we present a PD-personalized educational and physical activity boot camp program that provides participants the opportunity to familiarize themselves with common evidenced exercise programs.

Our primary objective was to assess the patients' perceived usefulness (or helpfulness) and utilization (or how much they changed their exercise routines and made use of the knowledge) of the program to facilitate exercise choice and lifestyle behavior over time. Secondary objectives included the assessment of satisfaction, preferences, and adverse events.

2. Methods

2.1. Design

We used a single group pre-test and post-test design.

2.2. Sampling and Recruitment

The sampling method selection was non-probabilistic by convenience. Following European Parkinson guidelines regarding the recommended number of individuals per group [3], we included eight individuals with PD, invited via email from a Parkinson's patient association. All participants had to be able to ambulate independently, able to tolerate a minimum 1 h of exercise, and able to attend all 4 days of the boot camp. Care partners were also invited to attend.

2.3. Participants

Eight individuals with PD (5 women) participated in the program with a mean age of 59.5 ± 6.8 years. All participants were participating for the first time in a boot camp. The participants' demographics and clinical characteristics can be found on Table 1.

Table 1. Participants' general and clinical characteristics.

Participant	Gender	Age	Time since Diagnose	Main Problems	Perceived Health (Now and Compared to Last Year)	Fall History
1	F	66	10 years PD	My inability to help my husband in a casual spontaneous way The lack of reliability and independence Fear of loss of mind, dignity, feeling powerlessness Fear of falling Dyskinesia and appearing to be drunk	Poor, the same as last year	1 fall outdoors, 2 months ago Near falls occasionally
2	F	61	2.8 years PD	Slowness Balance and walking Speech & swallowing Apathy	Very good and about the same	1 fall outdoors 6 months ago, couldn't get up. Near falls occasionally
3	M	59	8 years PD	Stiff neck and bad posture Walking	Good, about the same	No falls Near falls occasionally
4	M	60	8 years PD	Walking indoors Walking outdoors Time management & relaxing	Good, somewhat worse than one year ago	Frequent falls. Weekly, don't pick my feet up. Daily near falls A little fear of falling
5	F	57	4 years PD	Walking Walking and talking	Good, somewhat worse than one year ago	No Falls No Near falls
6	F	70	6.5 years PD	Imbalance Walking coordination Anxiety, frustration, self-confidence Driving, being able to see in the dark	Fair, much less now than a year ago	2 Falls last 6 months Near falls once per week
7	F	60	1.8 years PD	Night (early morning) and morning stiffness (pre-medication) OFF phases Lower back and sometimes neck pain Memory / Concentration—recalling names or a particular word Being able to stay focused on one thing	Fair, much less now than a year ago	No Falls No near falls Some fear of falling
8	M	45	9 years PD	Lack of sleep, Restlessness Freezing/walking Unfit/overweight Stiffness	Good, about the same	No Falls Near falls occasionally

2.4. Ethics and Procedures

This study follows the principles of the Declaration of Helsinki. The study was approved by the Egas Moniz Research Ethics Board. Participants completed an informed consent form before starting the program and received an information sheet explaining how their data would be used.

2.5. Program

The boot camp program consisted of four days of training featuring sessions that were 30–60 min each for a total average of 4 h per day. The boot camp began with an overview of general group goals based on a pre-assessment questionnaire. After, it focused on alternating between exercise, educational sessions, and social patient–family interactions. See Table 2 for topics presented on each day. To provide an engaging educational experience, therapists used various formats to teach, including multimedia presentations, hands-on activities during lectures, exercise sessions, and interactive discussions (question-and-answer periods that allowed participants to learn from the therapists but also from each other). The tips and tricks sessions, for example, included trying the cueing strategies taught and exploring solutions for better management of issues associated with PD reported on a pre camp questionnaires. Presenters' slides and tangible information to easily reference later were shared with all participants.

Table 2. Description of the boot camp educational and exercise sessions' topics.

Days	Educational and Exercise Sessions	Format
Day 1	One-on-one brief assessments and introductions	Education
	Exercise in Parkinson Disease: why, what and how.	Education
	Introduction to variety of exercises.	Practice
	New exercise ingredient in PD: cognitive-motor training.	Education
	Cognitive Stepping with amplitude-based movements.	Practice
Day 2	Review of Day 1, goals for the day	Education
	Changes in voice, communication and swallowing in PD	Education
	Voice, Breathing & Movement session	Practice
	Educational session: Walking/freezing/talking difficulties	Education
	Walk & Talk dual task program	Practice
	Nordic walking with integrated voice training session	Both
Day 3	Review of Day 2, goals for the day	Education
	Hydrotherapy: impact on mobility	Education
	Exercise Session: Using boxing for mobility and voice training in PD	Practice
	Tips & Tricks for transfers in daily life and exercise	Both
	Exercises for transfers: rhythm, amplitude & speed	Practice
Day 4	Review of the Camp, future goals & community resources	Education
	Tips & Tricks for bypassing barriers to exercise.	Education
	Goodbye Drum-based dancing activity	Practice
	Adapted Tai Chi	Practice
	'Take home messages' test activity	Education

The exercise sessions included practicing examples of amplitude-based interventions [5–8], Nordic walking [16,17], multitask cognitive and motor exercise challenges [2,28–30], hydrotherapy [21,22,31] and tai-chi [12,13], dance-based movements [9–11], as well as a boxing session [18–20].

All sessions were delivered in a group format. To guarantee safety, two volunteers were available to provide support to people if needed. The intensity of the physical activity sessions was delivered according to patient's tolerance and started ranging from a low to moderate intensity of aerobic exercise (40–60% HRR (or VO2R). Due to the group format, patients were taught to self-assess and monitor their effort throughout each session. The volumes of the aerobic based sessions were $\geq$30/40 min of continuous or intermittent exercise per session based on the exercise recommendations in European guideline for physiotherapy for Parkinson's disease [3]. The program was led by a physiotherapist and a speech therapist with specialized training and experience in PD (Josefa Domingos and John Dean). A local physiotherapist was invited to the program to be able to carry on exercise classes if requested by participants.

Social activities (e.g., mealtimes, resting breaks) promoted interaction with peers and contributed to peoples' feeling more acquainted with each other, adding to a positive group dynamic.

2.6. Data Collection

Participants completed an online pre-assessment structured questionnaire before the program, a post-assessment immediately after, and a one-month follow-up.

The pre-assessment collected general information on demographics, top 5 clinical problems, past medical conditions, disease management strategies used, current exercise, preferred exercise modalities, and perceived barriers/facilitators to performing exercise. The pre-assessments also inquired about the participant's goals and expectations for attending the boot camp.

Immediately after the program, we assessed satisfaction, preferences, and any adverse events via online anonymous questionnaire. Patients were asked to rate on 4-point scales how satisfied they were with boot camp (1 = not satisfied, 2 = neither, 3 = satisfied, and 4 = very satisfied), whether they would recommend the program to a friend (1 = Yes, 2 = No, 3 = Maybe), and how likely are they to return to a similar program (1 = very likely, 2 = likely, 3 = neither, and 4 = unlikely). They were also asked which sessions they preferred (1 = Educational sessions; 2 = Dance-based amplitude movements; 3 = Voice & Breathing; 4 = Boxing session; 5 = Walk & Talk dual task training; 6 = Cognitive stepping program; 7 = Hydrotherapy activity; 8 = Nordic walking; 9 = On the floor activities; 10 = Drum-based dance activity) and if there was any type of problem encountered during the program.

A follow-up anonymous questionnaire emailed to each participant one month after the boot camp asked the participants to assess the perceived usefulness of the program in the management of the current participant's exercise habits, as well as to assess the utilization (or how much they changed their exercise routines and made use of the knowledge and experience of the bootcamp). Usefulness was assessed based upon the patients' perceived (self-reported) usefulness of the program. Patients were asked to rate on 4-point scales how useful the boot camp was in helping them manage their current exercise habits (1 = not useful, 2 = neither useful, nor useless, 3 = useful, and 4 = very useful). Utilization was based upon changes in exercise habits that were made after the program.

2.7. Data Analysis

Data were extracted to a spreadsheet. Using the IBM Statistic Package for the Social Sciences software, version 26.0 descriptive statistics were adopted to analyze data.

3. Results

Participants most frequently reported their expectation for the boot camp was to learn more about specialized exercise. See patients' exercise habits and expectations for the boot camp in Table 3.

Table 3. Participants' current exercise habits, perceived exercise barrier's, facilitators and expectations for the boot camp.

Participant	Current Exercise Habits	Perceived Barriers to Exercise	Perceived Factors That Would Facilitate Exercising	Expectations for the Exercise Camp Program
1	Current: yes Which: stretching Frequency: daily Average time: 15 min	Fluctuations in health	Caregiver/partner are supportive, accessing instructors with PD expertise	"To try to find a way back, relearn how to exercise, get a shared goal. Learn from others. Reduce need to take pills"
2	Current: yes Which: walking, ball activities. Frequency: every other day Average time: 20 min	Poor coordination Fear of looking silly Accessing instructors with PD expertise is difficult	Perceived benefit and visible improvement after exercising, able to work out during working hours	"Improve my coordination and health without the use of drugs"
3	Current: yes Which: cycling, walking Frequency: cycling twice a week, walking every day. Average time: 60 min	Fluctuations in health Not easy to access specialized exercises	Perceiving benefit and visible improvement after exercising, accessing instructors with PD expertise	"To understand what exercises would be best for me, also being with fellow sufferers of similar abilities"
4	Current: yes Which: Cycling Frequency: 1 per week Average time: 45 min	Fluctuations in health Lack of time to exercise Always something to do for Parkinson society	Perceiving the benefit after exercising	"To access the "feel good factor" & challenge myself more, see what I should do for exercise"
5	Current: yes Which: walking the dog Frequency: Daily Average time: 30 min	Fluctuations in health Lack of time to exercise Job restrictions	Accessing instructors with PD expertise	"I would like to gain knowledge and further my skills in managing the disease through exercise"
6	Current: yes Which: golf, walking Frequency: 2 times a week Average time: 60 min	Fluctuations in health Lack of confidence exercising outside of rehab setting Weather conditions Living in a rural area without access to specialized care	Perceiving benefit and improvement after exercising, easy access to the gym or exercise facility, accessing instructors with PD expertise, fun things in group with people fitness same as me	"To boost confidence and fitness levels, in fun environment"
7	Current: yes Which: Parkinson Choir, Conductive Education Frequency: choir 1 per week; education 1 per month Average time: 75 min	Fluctuations in health Fear of falling, effect of weather conditions	Caregiver/partner being supportive, easy access to the gym or specific exercise facility, accessing instructors with PD expertise	"To identify a daily/weekly exercise regime with ones that will be more beneficial to me"
8	Current: yes Which: Jiu-jitsu Frequency: once a week Average time: 60 min	Fluctuations in health Lack of time to exercise Lack of interest Job restrictions	Easy accessing to the gym or exercise facility, accessing instructors with PD expertise, able to workout during working hours	"Get tips for getting fitter and do more specific exercises"

3.1. Percieved Usefulness and Utilization

Participants considered the boot camp very useful (seven in eight; 87.5 %) and useful (one in eight; 12.5%) in managing their current exercise habits. At one-month follow-up, seven participants reported making changes in their exercise routine after the boot camp, and one participant said, "Not really changed anything; I need more time in my day". The participants that made changes mentioned specifically: "I do exercise more frequently now"; "Introduced the "power" breathing that I learnt in the program", "Taking daily commitment to exercise seriously", "Joined a gym to do more exercise", "I do more walking periods and cognitive games", "I started Nordic walking" and, "started sessions with the physiotherapist involved in the program".

3.2. Satisfaction

After the program, all participants had favorable feedback, with all (100%) feeling very satisfied, likely to attend future events, and "would recommend to another person with PD".

3.3. Preferences

About six in eight (75 %) participants felt that many of the exercises and activities were new to them. The two training sessions that participants enjoyed the most were: dual task cognitive stepping (six in eight; 75 %) and dance-like movements (six in eight; 75 %). The two sessions that participants enjoyed less were: Nordic walking (two in eight) and boxing training (two in eight).

3.4. Safety

No falls, major injuries, or adverse events occurred during the program. One patient could not attend boxing sessions due to a superficial finger injury.

4. Discussion

Our study aimed to assess the usefulness, utilization, satisfaction, and preferences regarding participation in a PD-personalized educational and clinical exercise boot camp program. Based on our results, the boot camp was perceived to be useful by all eight participants with mild and moderate PD. Overall, seven out of eight participants referred they had made changes in their exercise routines one month after. The patients reported high satisfaction levels and there were no severe adverse events. Given the benefits of ongoing exercise in PD and the number of current options, the importance of offering guidance for safe, PD-specific, exercise programs for this population cannot be underestimated [18,25]. Importantly, this paper could help pave the way forward to delivering personalized exercise education through online boot camps during the COVID-19 pandemic crisis.

After the program, the patients were highly satisfied. Several positive aspects may have contributed to the high patient satisfaction reported. First, the information from the questionnaire prior to the program allowed for better tailoring of the program to all the participants' needs. Besides clinical information on health status, the questionnaires also provided with logistical information based on questions such as "What would be a good time for you to start the activities?", "If you are bringing someone, please tell us who and what would you like them to learn from the boot camp?", and "What topics and activities would you like to be addressed in the boot camp?". Personalized exercise programs that are appropriately designed and delivered increase patient satisfaction with care options [32]. Shared goal setting should always be considered during the initiation and implementation of exercise interventions. Second, intrinsic motivation, via experiencing the actual benefit of each exercise, and enjoying participation are important factors for long-term training adherence [33,34].

The ability to try out the exercises can make a significant difference in one's ability to judge the preference, usefulness, and long-term utilization of the varied exercise options. It ultimately determines the degree to which individuals can judge information effectively and use it to make smart exercise selections. Third, delivering the program in a group format allowed participants to experience the beneficial effects of social support and motivation from fellow patients [35]. Fourth, most of the participants (six in eight; 75 %) felt that many of the exercises and activities were new to them, even though all participants were already doing some sort of exercise on a weekly basis. They reported initially having clear expectations for the boot camp to gain more knowledge on specific PD exercises. Accessing specialized care was considered initially as one of the most common factors that would facilitate exercising (six in eight participants).

Implementing such a program was not without some limitations. First, some patients might not have future access to personalized exercise programs presented. As such, we invited a local physiotherapist to the program to help ensure that participants would have an opportunity to access specialized care if needed. This was an innovated solution to facilitate access to personalized care. Interestingly, most participants preferred to include changes in their daily routine activities with only one preferring to book sessions with the physiotherapist after completing the program. However, measuring the knowledge of participants immediately after the program would have brought better insights concerning reasons for change or no change (utilization) one month after. Second, even though participants were told to invite their families and caregivers, only one participant decided to bring a caregiver. Nevertheless, all participants were confident that they could contact the physiotherapist any time they needed additional information or insight. The influence of the caregiver should be a key factor to be better explored in future programs. Third, the group format imposed some safety concerns. We limited registrations to eight people with PD to assure a safe and efficient setting according to current recommendations [3]. Fourth, the nature of the study, with a small sample size and single center design, imposes restrictions on the generalizability of the findings. We included a heterogeneous group of people with PD with different backgrounds and did not specifically include participants with more advanced stages of PD. Further research is needed to measure its effectiveness on other subtypes and profiles of people and against other educational programs.

5. Conclusions

Our findings demonstrate that trying out different exercises can support judgments and decisions and thus may be a viable tool for more effective exercise prescription programs for the PD community. It is easily replicable, improves patients' knowledge about exercise, and based on the reported interest of participants in attending another similar program as well as the benefits they perceived of the usefulness of the program, is likely to be well-received by health care professionals world-wide.

Author Contributions: J.D. (Josefa Domingo): Conceptualization; Data curation; Formal analysis; Investigation; Methodology; Writing and Project administration. J.D. (John Dean): Conceptualization; Methodology and Writing and Reviewing. T.M.C.: Writing and Reviewing. K.Ś.: Conceptualization; Writing and Reviewing. J.B.F.: Formal analysis; Methodology; Writing and Reviewing. C.G.: Conceptualization; Data curation; Formal analysis; Investigation; Methodology; Writing; Reviewing and Editing. All authors have read and agreed to the published version of the manuscript.

Funding: This research did not receive any specific grant from funding agencies in the public, commercial, or not-for-profit sectors.

Institutional Review Board Statement: The study was conducted according to the guidelines of the Declaration of Helsinki, and approved by the Institutional Review Board of Egas Moniz Higher School of Health Board of Directors (ID 70; 17/02/2021).

Informed Consent Statement: Informed consent was obtained from all subjects involved in the study.

Data Availability Statement: The data presented in this study are available on request from the first author.

Acknowledgments: This publication is financed by national funds through the FCT—Foundation for Science and Technology, I.P., under the project UIDB/04585/2020. The researchers would like to

J. Pers. Med. **2021**, 11, 938

thank the Centro de Investigação Interdisciplinar Egas Moniz (CiiEM) for the support provided for the publication of this article.

Conflicts of Interest: The authors declare that they have no conflict of interests.

Ethical Approval: Before conducting the study, a research protocol was analysed and approved by the Institutional Ethics Committee of Egas Moniz Higher School of Health (ID 948; Date: 25/03/2021).

References

1. Fereshtehnejad, S.M.; Postuma, R.B. Subtypes of Parkinson's Disease: What Do They Tell Us About Disease Progression? *Curr. Neurol. Neurosci. Rep.* **2017**, 17, 34. [CrossRef]
2. Conradsson, D.; Löfgren, N.; Nero, H.; Hagströmer, M.; Ståhle, A.; Lökk, J.; Franzén, E. The Effects of Highly Challenging Balance Training in Elderly With Parkinson's Disease: A Randomized Controlled Trial. *Neurorehabilit. Neural Repair* **2015**, 29, 827–836. [CrossRef]
3. Keus, S.; Munneke, M.; Graziano, M.; Paltamaa, J.; Pelosin, E.; Domingos, J.; Brühlmann, S.; Ramaswamy, B.; Prins, J.; Struiksma, C.; et al. *European Physiotherapy Guideline for Parkinson's Disease*; KNGF/ParkinsonNet: Nemegen, The Netherlands, 2014.
4. Dineen-Griffin, S.; Garcia-Cardenas, V.; Williams, K.; Benrimoj, S.I. Helping patients help themselves: A systematic review of self-management support strategies in primary health care practice. *PLoS ONE* **2019**, 14, e0220116. [CrossRef]
5. Fox, C.; Ebersbach, G.; Ramig, L.; Sapir, S. LSVT LOUD and LSVT BIG: Behavioral Treatment Programs for Speech and Body Movement in Parkinson Disease. *Parkinson's Dis.* **2012**, 2012, 391946. [CrossRef] [PubMed]
6. Millage, B.; Vesey, E.; Finkelstein, M.; Anheluk, M. Effect on Gait Speed, Balance, Motor Symptom Rating, and Quality of Life in Those with Stage I Parkinson's Disease Utilizing LSVT BIG(R). *Rehabil. Res. Pract.* **2017**, 2017, 9871070. [CrossRef]
7. Isaacson, S.; O'Brien, A.; Lazaro, J.D.; Ray, A.; Fluet, G. The JFK BIG study: The impact of LSVT BIG®® on dual task walking and mobility in persons with Parkinson's disease. *J. Phys. Ther. Sci.* **2018**, 30, 636–641. [CrossRef]
8. Ramig, L.; Halpern, A.; Spielman, J.; Fox, C.; Freeman, K. Speech treatment in Parkinson's disease: Randomized controlled trial (RCT). *Mov. Disord.* **2018**, 33, 1777–1791. [CrossRef] [PubMed]
9. Carapellotti, A.M.; Stevenson, R.; Doumas, M. The efficacy of dance for improving motor impairments, non-motor symptoms, and quality of life in Parkinson's disease: A systematic review and meta-analysis. *PLoS ONE* **2020**, 15, e0236820. [CrossRef]
10. Aguiar, L.; Priscila, R.; Morris, M. Therapeutic Dancing for Parkinson's Disease. *Int. J. Gerontol.* **2016**, 10, 64–70. [CrossRef]
11. Kalyani, H.; Sullivan, K.A.; Moyle, G.; Brauer, S.; Jeffrey, E.R.; Kerr, G.K. Impacts of dance on cognition, psychological symptoms and quality of life in Parkinson's disease. *NeuroRehabilitation* **2019**, 45, 273–283. [CrossRef]
12. Liu, H.H.; Yeh, N.C.; Wu, Y.F.; Yang, Y.R.; Wang, R.Y.; Cheng, F.Y. Effects of Tai Chi Exercise on Reducing Falls and Improving Balance Performance in Parkinson's Disease: A Meta-Analysis. *Parkinson's Dis.* **2019**, 2019, 9626934. [CrossRef]
13. Choi, H.J. Effects of therapeutic Tai chi on functional fitness and activities of daily living in patients with Parkinson disease. *J. Exerc. Rehabil.* **2016**, 12, 499–503. [CrossRef]
14. Liu, X.L.; Chen, S.; Wang, Y. Effects of Health Qigong Exercises on Relieving Symptoms of Parkinson's Disease. *Evid.-Based Complement. Altern. Med.* **2016**, 2016, 5935782. [CrossRef]
15. Chen, S.; Zhang, Y.; Wang, Y.T.; Liu, X.; Song, W.; Du, X. The effect of Qigong-based therapy on patients with Parkinson's disease: A systematic review and meta-analysis. *Clin. Rehabil.* **2020**, 34, 1436–1448. [CrossRef]
16. Wróblewska, A.; Gajos, A.; Smyczyńska, U.; Bogucki, A. The Therapeutic Effect of Nordic Walking on Freezing of Gait in Parkinson's Disease: A Pilot Study. *Parkinson's Dis.* **2019**, 2019, 3846279. [CrossRef]
17. Monteiro, E.P.; Franzoni, L.T.; Cubillos, D.M.; de Oliveira Fagundes, A.; Carvalho, A.R.; Oliveira, H.B.; Pantoja, P.D.; Schuch, F.B.; Rieder, C.R.; Martinez, F.G.; et al. Effects of Nordic walking training on functional parameters in Parkinson's disease: A randomized controlled clinical trial. *Scand. J. Med. Sci. Sports* **2017**, 27, 351–358. [CrossRef]
18. Morris, M.E.; Ellis, T.D.; Jazayeri, D.; Heng, H.; Thomson, A.; Balasundaram, A.P.; Slade, S.C. Boxing for Parkinson's Disease: Has Implementation Accelerated Beyond Current Evidence? *Front. Neurol.* **2019**, 10, 1222. [CrossRef]
19. Combs, S.A.; Diehl, M.D.; Chrzastowski, C.; Didrick, N.; McCoin, B.; Mox, N.; Staples, W.H.; Wayman, J. Community-based group exercise for persons with Parkinson disease: A randomized controlled trial. *NeuroRehabilitation* **2013**, 32, 117–124. [CrossRef]
20. Domingos, J.; Radder, D.; Riggare, S.; Godinho, C.; Dean, J.; Graziano, M.; de Vries, N.M.; Ferreira, J.; Bloem, B.R. Implementation of a Community-Based Exercise Program for Parkinson Patients: Using Boxing as an Example. *J. Parkinson's Dis.* **2019**, 9, 615–623. [CrossRef]
21. Perez-de la Cruz, S.; Garcia Luengo, A.V.; Lambeck, J. Effects of an Ai Chi fall prevention programme for patients with Parkinson's disease. *Neurologia* **2016**, 31, 176–182. [CrossRef]
22. Kurt, E.E.; Buyukturan, B.; Buyukturan, O.; Erdem, H.R.; Tuncay, F. Effects of Ai Chi on balance, quality of life, functional mobility, and motor impairment in patients with Parkinson's disease. *Disabil. Rehabil.* **2018**, 40, 791–797. [CrossRef] [PubMed]
23. Afshari, M.; Yang, A.; Bega, D. Motivators and Barriers to Exercise in Parkinson's Disease. *J. Parkinson's Dis.* **2017**, 7, 703–711. [CrossRef]
24. Prakash, P.; Scott, T.F.; Baser, S.M.; Leichliter, T.; Schramke, C.J. Self-Reported Barriers to Exercise and Factors Impacting Participation in Exercise in Patients with Parkinson's Disease. *Mov. Disord. Clin. Pract.* **2021**, 8, 631–633. [CrossRef]

25. Domingos, J.; Dean, J.; Godinho, C.; Melo, F. Proliferation of community exercise programs with limited evidence and expertise: Safety implications. *Mov. Disord.* **2018**, *33*, 1365–1366. [CrossRef]

26. Lamba, S.; Wilson, B.; Natal, B.; Nagurka, R.; Anana, M.; Sule, H. A suggested emergency medicine boot camp curriculum for medical students based on the mapping of Core Entrustable Professional Activities to Emergency Medicine Level 1 milestones. *Adv. Med. Educ. Pract.* **2016**, *7*, 115–124.

27. Heimroth, J.; Jones, V.M.; Howard, J.D.; Sutton, E.R.H. Utilizing Surgical Bootcamps to Teach Core Entrustable Professional Activities to Senior Medical Students. *Am. Surg.* **2018**, *84*, 783–788. [CrossRef]

28. Altmann, L.J.; Stegemöller, E.; Hazamy, A.A.; Wilson, J.P.; Okun, M.S.; McFarland, N.R.; Wagle Shukla, A.; Hass, C.J. Unexpected dual task benefits on cycling in Parkinson disease and healthy adults: A neuro-behavioral model. *PLoS ONE* **2015**, *10*, e0125470. [CrossRef] [PubMed]

29. Fernandes, A.; Rocha, N.; Santos, R.; Tavares, J.M. Effects of dual-task training on balance and executive functions in Parkinson's disease: A pilot study. *Somatosens. Mot. Res.* **2015**, *32*, 122–127. [CrossRef]

30. Strouwen, C.; Molenaar, E.; Münks, L.; Keus, S.; Zijlmans, J.; Vandenberghe, W.; Bloem, B.R.; Nieuwboer, A. Training dual tasks together or apart in Parkinson's disease: Results from the DUALITY trial. *Mov. Disord.* **2017**, *32*, 1201–1210. [CrossRef]

31. Carroll, L.M.; Volpe, D.; Morris, M.E.; Saunders, J.; Clifford, A.M. Aquatic Exercise Therapy for People With Parkinson Disease: A Randomized Controlled Trial. *Arch. Phys. Med. Rehabil.* **2017**, *98*, 631–638. [CrossRef]

32. Fernandes, J.B.; Fernandes, S.B.; Almeida, A.S.; Vareta, D.A.; Miller, C.A. Older Adults' Perceived Barriers to Participation in a Falls Prevention Strategy. *J. Pers. Med.* **2021**, *11*, 450. [CrossRef]

33. Collado-Mateo, D.; Lavín-Pérez, A.M.; Peñacoba, C.; Del Coso, J.; Leyton-Román, M.; Luque-Casado, A.; Gasque, P.; Fernández-Del-Olmo, M.Á.; Amado-Alonso, D. Key Factors Associated with Adherence to Physical Exercise in Patients with Chronic Diseases and Older Adults: An Umbrella Review. *Int. J. Environ. Res. Public Health* **2021**, *18*, 2023. [CrossRef] [PubMed]

34. Teixeira, P.J.; Carraca, E.V.; Markland, D.; Silva, M.N.; Ryan, R.M. Exercise, physical activity, and self-determination theory: A systematic review. *Int. J. Behav. Nutr. Phys. Act.* **2012**, *9*, 78. [CrossRef]

35. King, L.A.; Wilhelm, J.; Chen, Y.; Blehm, R.; Nutt, J.; Chen, Z.; Serdar, A.; Horak, F.B. Effects of Group, Individual, and Home Exercise in Persons With Parkinson Disease: A Randomized Clinical Trial. *J. Neurol. Phys. Ther.* **2015**, *39*, 204–212. [CrossRef] [PubMed]

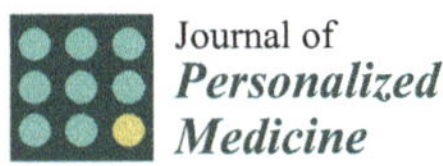
Journal of
*Personalized
Medicine*

MDPI

Article

The Role of Pain Catastrophizing and Pain Acceptance in Performance-Based and Self-Reported Physical Functioning in Individuals with Fibromyalgia and Obesity

Giorgia Varallo [1,2], Federica Scarpina [3,4], Emanuele Maria Giusti [1,2,*], Carlos Suso-Ribera [5], Roberto Cattivelli [1,2], Anna Guerrini Usubini [1,2], Paolo Capodaglio [6,7] and Gianluca Castelnuovo [1,2]

1   Psychology Research Laboratory, Istituto Auxologico Italiano IRCCS, San Giuseppe Hospital, 28824 Verbania, Italy; g.varallo@auxologico.it (G.V.); r.cattivelli@auxologico.it (R.C.); anna.guerriniusubini@unicatt.it (A.G.U.); gianluca.castelnuovo@auxologico.it (G.C.)
2   Department of Psychology, Catholic University of Milan, 20123 Milan, Italy
3   "Rita Levi Montalcini" Department of Neurosciences, University of Turin, 10124 Turin, Italy; f.scarpina@auxologico.it
4   Unit of Neurology and Neurorehabilitation, Istituto Auxologico Italiano IRCCS, San Giuseppe Hospital, 28824 Verbania, Italy
5   Department of Basic and Clinical Psychology and Psychobiology, Jaume I University, 12071 Castellon de la Plana, Spain; susor@uji.es
6   Orthopaedic Rehabilitation Unit and Research Laboratory in Biomechanics and Rehabilitation, Istituto Auxologico Italiano IRCCS, San Giuseppe Hospital, 28824 Verbania, Italy; p.capodaglio@auxologico.it
7   Department of Surgical Sciences, Physical and Rehabilitation Medicine, University of Turin, 10121 Turin, Italy
*   Correspondence: e.giusti@auxologico.it; Tel.: +39-0323-4338

Citation: Varallo, G.; Scarpina, F.; Giusti, E.M.; Suso-Ribera, C.; Cattivelli, R.; Guerrini Usubini, A.; Capodaglio, P.; Castelnuovo, G. The Role of Pain Catastrophizing and Pain Acceptance in Performance-Based and Self-Reported Physical Functioning in Individuals with Fibromyalgia and Obesity. *J. Pers. Med.* **2021**, *11*, 810. https://doi.org/10.3390/jpm11080810

Academic Editors: Fábio G. Teixeira, Catarina Godinho and Júlio Belo Fernandes

Received: 26 July 2021
Accepted: 17 August 2021
Published: 19 August 2021

Publisher's Note: MDPI stays neutral with regard to jurisdictional claims in published maps and institutional affiliations.

Abstract: Impaired physical functioning is one of the most critical consequences associated with fibromyalgia, especially when there is comorbid obesity. Psychological factors are known to contribute to perceived (i.e., subjective) physical functioning. However, physical function is a multidimensional concept encompassing both subjective and objective functioning. The contribution of psychological factors to performance-based (i.e., objective) functioning is unclear. This study aims to investigate the contribution of pain catastrophizing and pain acceptance to both self-reported and performance-based physical functioning. In this cross-sectional study, 160 participants completed self-report measures of pain catastrophizing, pain acceptance, and pain severity. A self-report measure and a performance-based test were used to assess physical functioning. Higher pain catastrophizing and lower pain acceptance were associated with poorer physical functioning at both self-reported and performance-based levels. Our results are consistent with previous evidence on the association between pain catastrophizing and pain acceptance with self-reported physical functioning. This study contributes to the current literature by providing novel insights into the role of psychological factors in performance-based physical functioning. Multidisciplinary interventions that address pain catastrophizing and pain acceptance are recommended and might be effective to improve both perceived and performance-based functioning in women with FM and obesity.

Keywords: fibromyalgia; physical functioning; obesity; pain catastrophizing; pain acceptance; chronic pain; rehabilitation; clinical psychology; performance-based test

1. Introduction

Fibromyalgia (FM) is a complex chronic pain condition that predominantly affects women [1,2]. It is characterized by widespread pain, fatigue, cognitive impairment, and a decline in physical functioning. Although the aetiology of FM is still unclear, central sensitization might play a crucial role [3,4]. However, an interplay between genetic/biological and psychosocial factors appears to be necessary to explain the development and maintenance of this disease [5,6].

Impaired physical functioning is one of the most critical consequences associated with FM [1,7,8]. Reduced physical functional capacity is a significant obstacle to daily activities [9–11] and has a negative effect on the individual's quality of life [3,12]. For example, women with FM have difficulties performing activities crucial to remaining physically independent, which increases their need for assistance from others [9].

The physical decline associated with FM is further exacerbated when individuals have comorbid obesity [13–15]. Obesity is an important condition to consider in FM owing to its high prevalence in this population, which can be partly attributed to the decreased activity levels in individuals with FM [7,13,16]. Obesity contributes to the disability burden associated with FM [13]. In particular, obesity is associated with increased pain severity and decreased physical functioning in FM [13,14,16–18]. Individuals with FM and obesity experience severe functional limitations owing to the combination of two issues: persistent pain related to FM and restricted movement imposed by obesity [13,19–21]. Thus, both conditions can interact with and exacerbate each other. Specifically, the chronic pain and fatigue associated with FM can lead to sedentary behavior, physical inactivity, and weight gain, which can negatively impact physical health and pain status, creating a vicious cycle [22].

In recent years, there has been a growing consensus on the importance of improving physical functioning rather than just reducing pain severity in people with chronic pain [23–25]. Consistent with this idea, efforts are being made to shift the focus of pain management from reducing pain to improving the quality of life [25–27]. As a consequence, modifiable psychological factors like pain-related cognitions and beliefs about experience of pain that partly explain individual differences in the adaptation to chronic pain, such as pain catastrophizing and pain acceptance, have gained ground in pain research in the past decades [28–32].

Pain catastrophizing is defined as a set of exaggerated and negative cognitive-emotional responses to actual or anticipated painful sensations [33]. According to the fear-avoidance model, which is a theoretical model developed to outline how pain-related cognitions influence pain experience [34–36], pain catastrophizing is a key cognitive factor associated with poor functioning in individuals with chronic pain. Indeed, the tendency to exaggerate and ruminate on pain experiences, combined with the tendency to feel helpless during pain episodes (i.e., pain catastrophizing), are known to lead to fear of movement and activity aversion [36]. As a result, individuals with chronic pain who tend to catastrophize engage in a variety of safety behaviors (i.e., movement avoidance, guarded movement) to prevent the worsening of pain symptoms [37]. Eventually, these behaviors lead to a cycle of avoidance; deconditioning; and, as a result, increased disability [7,38,39].

Pain catastrophizing has been observed in individuals with FM [40] and has been robustly associated with physical impairment in FM and other pain conditions [41–44]. However, the role of pain catastrophizing in individuals with chronic pain conditions and comorbid obesity remains less clear. Somers et al. reported higher levels of pain catastrophizing in individuals with severe obesity and osteoarthritis compared with individuals with less severe degrees of obesity and overweight [45]. Shelby and colleagues observed that higher levels of pain catastrophizing were associated with higher levels of disability in older adults with overweight, obesity, and osteoarthritis [46]. On the contrary, we recently observed no significant association between pain catastrophizing and physical disability in a sample of individuals with obesity and chronic low back pain [32]. These contradictory and heterogeneous findings could be attributed to the characteristics of participants in terms of age, clinical condition, and level of obesity, among other factors. However, the scarcity of evidence about the role of pain catastrophizing in individuals with FM and comorbid obesity justifies the need for more research.

Pain acceptance is another psychological factor that has received increasing attention in chronic pain research [47]. It refers to the willingness to experience painful sensations without attempting to avoid them, as well as the willingness to continue significant activities despite the presence of pain [48]. While the fear-avoidance model considers pain catastrophizing as a major contributor to pain-related disability, the psychological flexibility model of pain identifies pain acceptance as a key factor underlying individual differences in the pain adaptation [49]. The psychological flexibility model emphasizes the importance of an individual's ability to flexibly change or persist with a behavior considering personal goals and values in a setting of competing psychological influences (such as acceptance of pain) and situational conditions [49]. Persisting in value-oriented behaviors despite uncomfortable experiences, such as pain, is essential to living a full and meaningful life according to this framework [50]. Indeed, pain acceptance appears to facilitate participation in valued activities and the pursuit of personal goals [51], which results in reduced pain interference with daily activities and less perceived disability [47,51,52].

The combination of both pain catastrophizing and pain acceptance might be important to consider in pain research. Previous studies have generally focused on the identification of psychological factors that have a negative impact on physical functioning in individuals with chronic pain [31,40,53–56]. However, in recent years, resilience factors have also gained ground in pain research [57]. Pain acceptance has emerged as a crucial component in the adaptation to chronic pain. Pain acceptance is, in fact, increasingly targeted in rehabilitative interventions that emphasize the promotion of resources rather than the restoration or modification of only negative and dysfunctional behaviors [58]. In summary, while pain catastrophizing may act as a barrier to a favorable adaptation to chronic pain (i.e., risk or vulnerability factor), pain acceptance might be a facilitator (i.e., resilience factor) [59].

To date, research into physical functioning in individuals with chronic pain and FM has mostly relied on self-report measures [25,41,60–69]. Performance-based measures, which focus on actual rather than perceived functional ability, have generally been neglected. Importantly, however, self-report and performance-based measures provide different, but complementary information about physical functioning [70]. Physical function is a multidimensional construct that should encompass both subjective (i.e., self-reported functional capacity) and objective (i.e., impaired movement) aspects [25,71–73]. While self-report measures assess what individuals "believe they can do", performance-based tests evaluate what they "can actually do" [70]. The contribution of psychological factors tends to be greater for subjective aspects that involve a cognitive evaluation (such as perceived functioning) rather than actual performance in daily activities [74]. Therefore, past research might have revealed strong associations between psychological factors and self-report measures of physical functioning because they assessed subjective perceptions. Importantly, performance-based and self-reported physical functions are not significantly correlated in individuals with heterogeneous musculoskeletal chronic pain [71]. In addition, a study highlighted that individuals with FM report worse subjective physical functioning compared with objective performance [75]. Therefore, research that evaluates and compares the contribution of psychological factors to perceived and performance-based functioning outcomes is necessary to advance interdisciplinary interventions for chronic pain.

In summary, the goal of the present study is to investigate the contribution of pain catastrophizing (vulnerability factor) and pain acceptance (resilience factor) to the physical functioning of individuals with FM and comorbid obesity. We hypothesized that pain catastrophizing [41–43,52,56] would be associated with reduced physical functioning, while pain acceptance would be associated with better physical functioning [47,60,62,76]. We also hypothesized that the contribution of psychological variables will be greater for perceived versus performance-based functioning [74].

2. Materials and Methods

2.1. Procedure and Participants

A cross-sectional study was conducted. An a priori power analysis was performed using G. Power (version 3.1.9.4) [77] to calculate the required sample size to detect statistical significance. Setting a conservative small-to-medium effect size of the predictors (0.10), an alpha of 0.05, and a power of 0.90, a minimum sample size of $n = 130$ was required to detect the hypothesized effects.

From January 2019 to September 2019, 160 women were consecutively recruited at the start of a one-month-long hospitalization program for weight loss and physical therapy at the Orthopaedic Rehabilitation Unit of the IRCCS Istituto Auxologico Italiano (Piancavallo, Italy). Data collection was conducted during the first week of the diagnostic assessment, before starting a physical therapy and nutritional rehabilitative program for weight loss.

Participants were included in this study if they (a) had a FM diagnosis provided by a rheumatologist according to Wolfe et al. criteria [1]; (b) met the American College of Rheumatology (ACR) Research Criteria for fibromyalgia [78,79], as measured by the Fibromyalgia Survey Questionnaire in its Italian version [53]; (c) were over 18 years; and (d) were able to sign an informed consent form and could complete the questionnaires.

Patients were excluded if they (a) had psychiatric disorders with psychotic symptoms or severe personality disorders; (b) had previously or were currently receiving psychological treatment for FM; and (c) had comorbid acute pain conditions or comorbid chronic pain conditions different from FM.

2.2. Measures

Sociodemographic and clinical data. Participants completed a self-report protocol that included age, weight (in kilograms), and height (in centimeters), job status (i.e., employed, unemployed, or disability pension), current opioid use, and pain duration (in years).

Fibromyalgia symptomatology. The Italian version of the fibromyalgia survey questionnaire (FSQ) [53] was used to assess the ACR fibromyalgia research criteria [78,79]. This measure, which is recommended in [78,80], was administered to evaluate the level of symptomatology required to confirm the diagnosis of FM. Individuals must meet the following research criteria: (1) widespread pain index ≥ 7 and symptom severity scale score ≥ 5 OR widespread pain index of 4–6 and symptom severity scale score ≥ 9; (2) symptoms have generally been present for at least 3 months.

Pain severity. The numeric pain rating scale (NPRS) [81] was used to assess pain severity levels. It consists of an 11-point scale (anchors 0 = "no pain"; 10 = "worst possible pain"). The Numeric Pain Rating Scale is a well-validated and widely used measure of pain severity in chronic pain conditions [82].

Pain catastrophizing. The pain catastrophizing scale (PCS) [83] is a self-report measure of pain-related catastrophic thinking. It consists of 13 items on a five-point Likert scale (from 0 = "not at all" to 4 = "all the time"). The total score ranges from 0 to 52, with higher scores indicating higher levels of pain catastrophizing [84]. The Italian version [84] has psychometric properties comparable with the original version. In the current study, internal consistency was excellent (Cronbach's $\alpha = 0.89$).

Pain acceptance. The chronic pain acceptance questionnaire (CPAQ) is a measure of pain acceptance [85–87] that consists of 20 items scored on a 7-point Likert scale (0 = "never true" to 6 = "always true"). The maximum total score is 120, with higher scores indicating greater acceptance. The Italian version of the questionnaire was used [88], which, in line with the original version, has obtained good psychometric properties. In the present study, the internal consistency of this measure was excellent (Cronbach's $\alpha = 0.90$).

Self-report physical functioning limitations. Self-reported physical functioning limitations were assessed using the physical functioning subscale of the fibromyalgia impact questionnaire—revised (PF-FIQR). The FIQR is a 21-item measure. The items use an 11-point numeric rating scale ranging from 0 to 10, with 10 representing "worst" functioning scores. All questions are related to the functioning of the last 7 days. Higher total scores indicate a higher impact of the disease and worse functioning. The FIQR assesses three domains: (a) 'physical function', (b) 'overall impact', and (c) 'symptoms'. The total score, which assesses the impact of FM on overall functioning, can also be computed. Considering the aim of the present study, the physical function subscale was used. Specifically, the physical functioning subscale of the FIQR includes nine items developed to evaluate the level of physical impairment. This scale has been used in previous research [38,75,89,90]. Scores on the physical functioning subscale of the FIQR range from 0 to 30, with higher scores indicating worse physical functioning. The FIQR and its subscales have good psychometric properties and good discriminant ability [38]. In the current study, internal consistency was good (Cronbach's α = 0.82).

Performance-based physical functioning. The 6-min walking test (6MWT) is a performance-based test used to evaluate the ability to walk and is a simple and inexpensive measure of physical functioning. The 6MWT has been used in research with persons with FM [38,90,91] with good applicability and reliability findings [38,92]. In this test, the participant is required to walk for six minutes along a rectangular course of 45.7 m. Walking distance in meters is measured with higher scores, indicating better physical performance. The distance walked during the 6MWT has been found to be shorter in females with FM compared with healthy women (i.e., discriminant validity) [9]. Furthermore, the 6MWT has good reproducibility and is recommended for the assessment of walking ability in individuals with obesity [93]. Women with obesity have also been found to walk significantly shorter distances during the 6MWT compared with their normal-weight counterparts [94,95].

2.3. Statistical Analysis

Counts and percentages were used to describe categorical variables, whereas means and standard deviations were used to describe continuous variables. Height in meters and weight in kilograms were used to compute body mass index (i.e., BMI, as the weight in kilograms divided by the square of height in meters (kg/m^2) [96]), which is considered as an indicator of obesity (BMI $\geq$ 30) [96].

Pearson bivariate analyses were performed to evaluate the associations between the numeric pain rating scale (i.e., pain severity), the pain catastrophizing scale (i.e., pain catastrophizing), the chronic pain acceptance questionnaire (i.e., pain acceptance), the physical functioning scale of the fibromyalgia impact questionnaire (i.e., self-reported physical functioning), and the 6-min walking test (i.e., performance-based physical functioning).

To answer our research question, we used multivariate hierarchical regression analyses, as done in previous studies [28,29,33,34]. Before the multivariate regression, we checked the assumptions of normality, linearity, homoscedasticity, and multicollinearity of the data. To evaluate the contribution of pain catastrophizing and pain acceptance, self-reported physical functioning limitations and performance-based physical functioning were independently introduced as dependent factors in two separate regressions. In both models, age [97,98], opioid use [98,99], and pain duration [100,101] were entered into the first step as covariates to control for their relationship with the outcome measures. Pain severity was entered in the second step, because of its association with physical functioning [38,102]. Pain catastrophizing and pain acceptance were entered simultaneously in the third and last step. The change in explained variance (ΔR^2) was used to evaluate the additional variance of the dependent variables accounted for by the variables included in each block. The significance was evaluated using a criterion of $p < 0.05$. Data were analyzed using the Jamovi software [103].

3. Results

The participant's characteristics are reported in Table 1.

Table 1. Means and standard deviations of sociodemographic characteristics and clinical measures. The theoretical range and actual range are reported. $n = 160$.

Sociodemographic Characteristics			$n = 160$
Age in years (mean $\pm$ SD)			43.6 ± 7.25
Body mass index (mean $\pm$ SD)			44.3 ± 7.15
Pain duration in years (mean $\pm$ SD)			7.08 ± 2.70
Current opioid use (%)			13.1%
Employed (%)			71.9%
Full-time			22.5%
Part-time			49.4%
Clinical measures	Theoretical range	Sample's range	Mean $\pm$ SD
Widespread pain index	0–19	7–18	13.8 ± 2.70
Symptoms' severity	0–12	5–11	8.13 ± 1.85
Numeric pain rating scale	0–10	3–9	5.67 ± 1.58
Pain catastrophizing scale	0–52	0–44	27.3 ± 10.3
Chronic pain acceptance questionnaire	0–120	21–74	51.7 ± 11.2
Physical functioning subscale	0–30	9–29	17.7 ± 4.77
6-Min walking test in meters	NA *	201–402	306 ± 59.4

Note. * NA: Not applicable.

3.1. Correlations

Pearson's correlations between measures are reported in Table 2. Pain catastrophizing and pain acceptance were significantly and negatively correlated ($r = -0.49$, $p < 0.001$). Pain catastrophizing was significantly and positively associated with pain severity ($r = 0.42$, $p < 0.001$), perceived limitations in physical functioning ($r = 0.43$, $p < 0.001$), and performance-based physical functioning ($r = -0.57$, $p < 0.001$). On the contrary, pain acceptance was significantly and negatively related to pain severity ($r = -0.39$, $p < 0.001$) and limitations in physical functioning ($r = -0.47$, $p < 0.001$), and linked to improved performance-based physical functioning ($r = 0.52$, $p < 0.001$). Perceived physical limitations and performance-based physical functioning were correlated in the negative direction ($r = -0.53$, $p < 0.001$), because higher scores on the self-report physical functioning limitations measure correspond to greater disability, while higher scores on the performance-based test reflect better physical functioning.

Table 2. Pearson correlation coefficients between study variables. $n = 160$.

	1	2	3	4
1. Pain severity (NPRS)	-			
2. Pain catastrophizing (PCS)	0.42 *	-		
3. Pain acceptance (CPAQ)	−0.39 *	−0.49 *	-	
4. Self-reported physical functioning limitations (PF-FIQR)	0.36 *	0.43 *	−0.47 *	-
5. Performance-based physical functioning (6MWT)	−0.38 *	−0.57 *	0.52 *	−0.53 *

Note. NPRS: numeric pain rating scale; PCS: pain catastrophizing scale; CPAQ: chronic pain acceptance questionnaire; PF-FIQR: physical functioning subscale of the firbomyalgia impact questionnaire; 6MWT: 6-minute walking test. * $p < 0.001$.

3.2. Hierarchical Regression Relative to Self-Reported Physical Functioning Limitations

The first multivariate hierarchical regression was conducted using self-report physical functioning limitations as the dependent variable (Table 3). The demographic characteristics (i.e., pain duration, age, current opioid use, and body mass index) included in the first step explained a nonsignificant 4% ($R^2 = 0.04$) variance in self-report physical functioning limitations in the first step ($F_{(4, 155)} = 1.78$; $p = 0.14$). Pain severity, which was included in the second step, significantly contributed an additional 12% of the explained variance ($\Delta F_{(1, 154)} = 22.60$; $p < 0.001$; $\Delta R^2 = 0.12$) of self-report physical functioning limitations. The third step, which included pain catastrophizing and pain acceptance, significantly explained an additional 17% of the variance of self-reported physical functioning limitations ($\Delta F_{(2, 152)} = 20.10$; $p < 0.001$; $\Delta R^2 = 0.17$).

Table 3. Multivariate hierarchical regression predicting self-report physical functioning limitations.

	Step 1		Step 2		Step 3	
Factors	B (SE)	p	B (SE)	p	B (SE)	p
Pain duration	−0.04 (0.14)	0.792	0.02 (0.13)	856	−0.07 (0.12)	0.566
Age	−0.01 (0.05)	0.826	0.02 (0.05)	0.707	−0.01 (0.04)	0.929
Current opioid use	2.86 (1.13)	0.012	2.70 (1.06)	0.110	2.66 (0.95)	0.006
Body mass index	0.01 (0.05)	0.897	−0.04 (0.05)	0.400	−0.09 (0.23)	0.054
Pain severity			1.09 (0.23)	<0.001	0.44 (0.23)	0.060
Pain catastrophizing					0.12 (0.04)	0.003
Pain acceptance					−0.13 (0.03)	<0.001

In the final model, opioid use (B = 2.66, p = 0.006), pain acceptance (B = −0.13, $p < 0.001$), and pain catastrophizing (B = 0.12, $p \leq 0.001$) contributed unique variance to the prediction of self-reported physical functioning limitations. Pain severity, which was significantly associated with self-report physical functioning limitations in the second step, became nonsignificant when accounting for the contribution of pain catastrophizing and pain acceptance.

3.3. Hierarchical Regression Relative to Performance-Based Physical Functioning

A second multivariate hierarchical regression was conducted using performance-based physical functioning as the dependent variable (Table 4). The first step, which included demographic variables (i.e., pain duration, age, current opioid use, body mass index), explained a significant 12% (R^2 = 0.12) variance in performance-based physical functioning (F (4155) = 5.23, $p \leq 0.001$). In the second step, pain severity contributed an additional 14% variance in performance-based physical functioning (ΔF (1154) = 28.9; $p < 0.001$; ΔR^2 = 0.139). Next, pain catastrophizing and pain acceptance included in the third step significantly explained an additional 23% variance of performance-based physical functioning (ΔF (2152) = 33.3; $p < 0.001$; ΔR^2 = 0.226).

Table 4. Multivariate hierarchical regression predicting performance-based physical functioning.

	Step 1		Step 2		Step 3	
Factors	B (SE)	p	B (SE)	p	B (SE)	p
Pain duration	−3.85 (1.66)	0.022	−4.65 (1.54)	0.003	−3.37 (1.30)	0.010
Age	−1.07 (0.62)	0.089	−1.16 (0.58)	0.045	−0.81 (0.49)	0.099
Current opioid use	−37.79 (13.47)	0.006	−35.68 (0.59)	0.005	−35.99 (10.43)	<0.001
Body mass index	−1.02 (0.63)	0.109	−0.36 (0.59)	0.544	0.29 (0.51)	0.574
Pain severity			−14.46 (2.69)	<0.001	−5.05 (2.54)	0.048
Pain catastrophizing					−2.21 (0.43)	<0.001
Pain acceptance					1.45 (0.37)	<0.001

Pain duration, current opioid use, and pain severity were significantly associated with performance-based physical functioning in the final model. Additionally, both pain catastrophizing (B = −0.364; $p < 0.001$) and pain acceptance (B = 0.272; $p \leq 0.001$) uniquely and significantly contributed to performance-based physical functioning.

4. Discussion

In this study, we aimed to explore the association between pain catastrophizing and pain acceptance with self-reported and performance-based physical functioning in individuals with FM and obesity. We confirmed our hypothesis that higher pain catastrophizing and lower pain acceptance would be significantly associated with poorer physical functioning when assessed with a self-reported and a performance-based measure. Specifically, both pain catastrophizing and pain acceptance were significant predictors of self-reported and performance-based physical functioning, even after controlling for body mass index, pain duration, current opioid use, and pain severity. Contrary to our hypotheses, however, the contribution of psychological variables was stronger for performance-based compared with self-reported physical functioning.

Research has repeatedly shown that pain catastrophizing and pain acceptance are important predictors of self-reported physical functioning in samples with acute [104,105] and chronic pain [105,106], including FM [41,107–110]. Our findings are consistent with the previous evidence. Previous research, however, has primarily focused on subjective measures of functional capacity. Our work contributes to the literature by combining a self-reported measure with a performance-based test that provides a more objective evaluation of physical functioning. The present study revealed that psychological factors contribute not only to perceived physical functioning, but also to actual functioning. Importantly, both pain catastrophizing and pain acceptance uniquely contributed to the prediction of self-reported and performance-based functioning, implying that the two factors are likely to influence physical functioning via distinct pathways. Ultimately, the fact that the two psychological factors contributed significantly to physical functioning when included in the same multivariate analysis supports the idea that they should both be independently targeted in multidisciplinary interventions. In addition, this contributes to the validity of different psychological models to understand the pain experience, such as the fear-avoidance model and the psychological flexibility model.

Individuals who catastrophize tend to appraise pain as a catastrophic and harmful experience and frequently ruminate and feel hopeless about it [43,111]. Based on the present results, the tendency to catastrophize about pain might negatively affect both the individual's perception of what they are capable of accomplishing in terms of physical performance (i.e., what I think I can do) as well as their actual physical performance (i.e., what I can do). We propose a mechanism to explain why this might occur. Pain catastrophizing might increase the level of attention and awareness of painful sensations [112], thus increasing protective behaviors. Individuals with chronic pain who catastrophize engage in a variety of safety behaviors (e.g., activity avoidance, movement restriction, and guarded movement) to prevent the worsening of pain symptoms [37]. Obesity, in turn, might increase avoidance in chronic musculoskeletal pain conditions [113]. In particular, the belief that excessive weight causes additional damage or increases pain might play an additional role in restricting activity, which, combined with skin friction, discomfort, and respiratory difficulties [114], might result in the avoidance of movements and, in turn, impediment to weight loss [113].

On the other hand, the willingness to persist with important activities without attempting to avoid pain (i.e., acceptance) might have a positive influence on both subjective and actual physical functioning [47,51,52]. Individuals who accept pain as an unpleasant experience that they are willing to undergo in order to achieve their goals might be more likely to move and engage in valued activities despite the pain. In addition, acceptance might facilitate the adaptation to chronic pain by focusing on one's personal goals rather than on pain control, thereby preventing the implementation of pain-avoidance behaviors [47,51,52]. Taking all the previous points into account, reducing pain catastrophizing and enhancing pain acceptance by implementing psychological interventions might help individuals with chronic pain to reduce the adoption of unnecessary and detrimental protective behaviors that perpetuate a cycle of avoidance, deconditioning, and increased disability [7,38,39].

Interestingly, we observed that the self-reported measure of physical function and the performance-based test were significantly and moderately related. Our results are consistent with those of Mannerkorpi and colleagues [38], but not with the findings of Greenberg and colleagues, who found no significant relationship between subjective and objective measures of physical functioning in individuals with heterogeneous chronic pain [71]. These discrepancies could be owing to differences in sample characteristics or measurements used across studies, or they might suggest that the relationship between subjective and objective components of physical functioning might be modulated differently in clinical conditions. While acknowledging this, owing to the scarcity of existing studies, more research is still needed to determine the extent to which self-report and objective measures of functioning are associated in different populations. Such studies are important because they investigate whether a subjective assessment of physical functioning can be used as a reliable alternative measure in objective tests of physical functioning, which are generally more time-consuming.

An interesting and unexpected finding was that the contribution of psychological factors was greater for performance-based physical functioning as opposed to self-reported physical functioning, while psychological aspects have a greater impact on factors that require cognitive evaluation [74]. One possible explanation for the findings is that the performance-based test might be interpreted as both pain-provoking and/or actually painful to perform. Thus, attention directed at a potential or actual pain-inducing movement might activate the repertoire of pain-related cognitive/coping strategies in a more prominent and influential way to motivate different behaviors. For example, individuals who tend to catastrophize about pain might be encouraged to restrict movement when they experience pain in real-world contexts, while those who accept pain might be prompted to persist in movement in this same scenario. More studies are needed to confirm this hypothesis, which could lead to an interesting line of future research.

Body mass index was not significantly related to self-reported and performance-based physical functioning. This result contradicted previous evidence [13,115,116]. It should be noted, however, that the variability in body mass index was limited in our sample because only individuals with obesity were included. In addition, recent studies have argued that body mass index may be an inadequate and oversimplified measure that does not properly capture the complexity of obesity [117,118]. Different indices of obesity could be used in future studies, such as the level of adiposity and the distribution of adipose tissue [119,120].

Among other control factors, current opioid use was found to be significantly associated with both self-reported and performance-based physical functioning. Individuals who are currently on opioid therapy might rely on this medication because of their low level of both subjective and objective physical functioning. Instead, pain duration and pain severity were only significantly related to performance-based physical functioning. The biological function of pain is to alter behavior by prioritizing protection and avoidance [121], and it seems likely that pain has a more pronounced effect on physical performance than on its perception [122]. Relative to pain duration, it is possible that individuals with a longer history of chronic pain have implemented dysfunctional coping strategies over the years (such as avoidance of movement and activities due to pain persistence despite treatment) that lead to the development of deconditioning and disuse, thus worsening the actual ability to move [35,123].

The findings of this study could have several clinical implications. According to our results, measures of pain catastrophizing and pain acceptance should be included in the assessment of biopsychosocial aspects of pain in FM and obesity to provide a more complete picture of the factors that significantly affect physical functioning. Furthermore, our findings suggest that pain catastrophizing and pain acceptance should be treatment targets in psychological evidence-based intervention to improve physical functioning in individuals with FM, and obesity should include pain catastrophizing and pain acceptance as treatment targets. In support of this hypothesis, Baranoff and colleagues [47] highlighted how changes in pain catastrophizing and pain acceptance accounted for changes in self-reported and performance-based disability in individuals with chronic pain, primarily located in the lower back. Importantly, because both pain catastrophizing and pain acceptance are significant predictors of both perceived and actual physical functioning, multidisciplinary interventions targeting both factors are likely to improve both aspects of functional capacity. More research is required to test this hypothesis in individuals with FM, especially when it is associated with obesity.

Finally, it is important to note that the willingness to move and engage in physical activity is critical in the management of both FM and obesity. Physical activity improves physical functioning in individuals with FM [124–129] as well as in those with obesity [130–132]. Consequently, current and previous research supports the idea that it might be beneficial to reduce pain catastrophizing and enhance pain acceptance in order to promote adherence to physical activity and a healthy, active lifestyle in individuals with FM and obesity. More research is needed to determine what other factors might be important in promoting physical activity compliance.

This study has some limitations. We did not include a control group (for example, individuals who are only affected by FM or obesity). In addition, we focused only on two psychological factors. While both are important factors according to the pain literature, other psychological factors, such as kinesiophobia [31] or pain self-efficacy [133], might also play a role in physical functioning. Furthermore, while the self-report questionnaire used referred to a period in the past (e.g., the previous week), the performance-based measure was based on the present moment. While most available measures refer to this timeframe, the development of self-reported measures that refer to the current time of assessment could be used to mitigate this mismatch. In addition, the pain severity measure used in this study assesses the intensity of perceived pain at the time of completion. As there can be variability in the levels of perceived pain in fibromyalgia even within a single day [134–136], measures that assess medial pain intensity over a week could be implemented to address this limitation. Finally, because we focused on individuals with FM and obesity as a comorbid condition, the findings might not be generalizable to other populations.

5. Conclusions

Our findings suggest that pain catastrophizing and pain acceptance should be addressed to improve performance-based and self-reported physical functioning in individuals with FM and obesity. If these components are ignored, rehabilitative interventions may neglect critical factors associated with the maintenance of poor physical functioning and physical health.

Author Contributions: G.V. conceived and designed the study protocol and performed the data collections with R.C. and A.G.U.; G.V. carried out literature searches; G.V. designed and carried out the statistical analysis; G.V. drafted the manuscript; G.V., F.S., E.M.G. and C.S.-R. interpreted the data; F.S., E.M.G. and C.S.-R. collaborated in drafting the manuscript; P.C. supervised the enrollment of participants; E.M.G. and G.C. supervised the psychological data collection. All authors critically reviewed and contribute to the final version of the paper. All authors have read and agreed to the published version of the manuscript.

Funding: This research received no external funding.

Institutional Review Board Statement: The study was conducted according to the guidelines of the Declaration of Helsinki of 1975, as revised in 1983, and approved by the Ethics Committee of Instituto Auxologico Italiano (code V.0.4 30-05-2017).

Informed Consent Statement: Informed consent was obtained from all subjects involved in the study.

Data Availability Statement: The data presented in this study are available on request from the corresponding author. The data are not publicly available because they contain information that could compromise the privacy of research participants.

Conflicts of Interest: The authors declare no conflict of interest.

References

1. Wolfe, F.; Clauw, D.J.; Fitzcharles, M.-A.; Goldenberg, D.L.; Häuser, W.; Katz, R.L.; Mease, P.J.; Russell, A.S.; Russell, I.J.; Walitt, B. 2016 Revisions to the 2010/2011 fibromyalgia diagnostic criteria. *Semin. Arthritis Rheum.* **2016**, *46*, 319–329. [CrossRef]
2. Marques, A.P.; Santo, A.D.S.D.E.; Berssaneti, A.A.; Matsutani, L.A.; Yuan, S.L.K. Prevalence of fibromyalgia: Literature review update. *Rev. Bras. Reum.* **2017**, *57*, 356–363. [CrossRef]
3. Clauw, D.J. Fibromyalgia. *JAMA* **2014**, *311*, 1547–1555. [CrossRef] [PubMed]

4. Siracusa, R.; Paola, R.; Cuzzocrea, S.; Impellizzeri, D. Fibromyalgia: Pathogenesis, Mechanisms, Diagnosis and Treatment Options Update. *Int. J. Mol. Sci.* **2021**, *22*, 3891. [CrossRef] [PubMed]
5. Stisi, S.; Cazzola, M.; Buskila, D.; Spath, M.; Giamberardino, M.; Sarzi-Puttini, P.; Arioli, G.; Alciati, A.; Leardini, G.; Gorla, R.; et al. Etiopathogenetic mechanisms of fibromyalgia syndrome. *Reumatismo* **2011**, *60*, 25–35. [CrossRef]
6. Ghiggia, A.; Torta, R.; Tesio, V.; Di Tella, M.; Romeo, A.; Colonna, F.; Geminiani, G.C.; Fusaro, E.; Batticciotto, A.; Castelli, L. Psychosomatic syndromes in fibromyalgia. *Clin. Exp. Rheumatol.* **2017**, *35*, 106–111. [PubMed]
7. Bennett, R.M.; Jones, J.; Turk, D.C.; Russell, I.J.; Matallana, L. An internet survey of 2596 people with fibromyalgia. *BMC Musculoskelet. Disord.* **2007**, *8*, 27. [CrossRef] [PubMed]
8. Turk, D.C.; Dworkin, R.H.; Revicki, D.; Harding, G.; Burke, L.B.; Cella, D.; Cleeland, C.S.; Cowan, P.; Farrar, J.T.; Hertz, S.; et al. Identifying important outcome domains for chronic pain clinical trials: An IMMPACT survey of people with pain. *Pain* **2008**, *137*, 276–285. [CrossRef] [PubMed]
9. Jones, J.; Rutledge, D.N.; Jones, K.D.; Matallana, L.; Rooks, D.S. Self-Assessed Physical Function Levels of Women with Fibromyalgia: A National Survey. *Women's Health Issues* **2008**, *18*, 406–412. [CrossRef]
10. Kingsley, J.D.; Panton, L.B.; Toole, T.; Sirithienthad, P.; Mathis, R.; McMillan, V. The Effects of a 12-Week Strength-Training Program on Strength and Functionality in Women with Fibromyalgia. *Arch. Phys. Med. Rehabil.* **2005**, *86*, 1713–1721. [CrossRef]
11. Verbunt, J.A.; Pernot, D.H.; Smeets, R.J. Disability and quality of life in patients with fibromyalgia. *Health Qual. Life Outcomes* **2008**, *6*, 8. [CrossRef]
12. Costa, I.D.S.; Gamundí, A.; Miranda, J.G.V.; França, L.G.S.; De Santana, C.N.; Montoya, P. Altered Functional Performance in Patients with Fibromyalgia. *Front. Hum. Neurosci.* **2017**, *11*, 14. [CrossRef]
13. Okifuji, A.; Donaldson, G.W.; Barck, L.; Fine, P.G. Relationship Between Fibromyalgia and Obesity in Pain, Function, Mood, and Sleep. *J. Pain* **2010**, *11*, 1329–1337. [CrossRef]
14. Aparicio, V.A.; Ortega, F.B.; Carbonell-Baeza, A.; Camiletti, D.; Ruiz, J.R.; Delgado-Fernández, M. Relationship of Weight Status with Mental and Physical Health in Female Fibromyalgia Patients. *Obes. Facts* **2011**, *4*, 443–448. [CrossRef]
15. Kim, C.-H.; Luedtke, C.A.; Vincent, A.; Thompson, J.M.; Oh, T.H. Association of body mass index with symptom severity and quality of life in patients with fibromyalgia. *Arthritis Care Res.* **2012**, *64*, 222–228. [CrossRef] [PubMed]
16. Vincent, A.; Clauw, D.; Oh, T.H.; Whipple, M.O.; Toussaint, L.L. Decreased Physical Activity Attributable to Higher Body Mass Index Influences Fibromyalgia Symptoms. *PM&R* **2014**, *6*, 802–807. [CrossRef]
17. Kim, C.-H.; Luedtke, C.A.; Vincent, A.; Thompson, J.M.; Oh, T.H. Association Between Body Mass Index and Response to a Brief Interdisciplinary Treatment Program in Fibromyalgia. *Am. J. Phys. Med. Rehabil.* **2012**, *91*, 574–583. [CrossRef] [PubMed]
18. Arranz, L.; Canela, M.; Rafecas, M.; Rafecas, M. Relationship between body mass index, fat mass and lean mass with SF-36 quality of life scores in a group of fibromyalgia patients. *Rheumatol. Int.* **2011**, *32*, 3605–3611. [CrossRef] [PubMed]
19. D'Onghia, M.; Ciaffi, J.; Lisi, L.; Mancarella, L.; Ricci, S.; Stefanelli, N.; Meliconi, R.; Ursini, F. Fibromyalgia and obesity: A comprehensive systematic review and meta-analysis. *Semin. Arthritis Rheum.* **2021**, *51*, 409–424. [CrossRef] [PubMed]
20. Wearing, S.C.; Hennig, E.; Byrne, N.; Steele, J.; Hills, A.P. The biomechanics of restricted movement in adult obesity. *Obes. Rev.* **2006**, *7*, 13–24. [CrossRef]
21. Larsson, U.E.; Mattsson, E. Functional limitations linked to high body mass index, age and current pain in obese women. *Int. J. Obes.* **2001**, *25*, 893–899. [CrossRef]
22. Okifuji, A.; Hare, B. The association between chronic pain and obesity. *J. Pain Res.* **2015**, *8*, 399–408. [CrossRef]
23. Turk, D.C.; Dworkin, R.H.; Allen, R.R.; Bellamy, N.; Brandenburg, N.; Carr, D.B.; Cleeland, C.; Dionne, R.; Farrar, J.T.; Galer, B.S.; et al. Core outcome domains for chronic pain clinical trials: IMMPACT recommendations. *Pain* **2003**, *106*, 337–345. [CrossRef] [PubMed]
24. Turk, D.C.; Dworkin, R.H. What should be the core outcomes in chronic pain clinical trials? *Arthritis Res. Ther.* **2004**, *6*, 151–154. [CrossRef] [PubMed]
25. Jackson, W.; Zale, E.L.; Berman, S.J.; Malacarne, A.; Lapidow, A.; Schatman, M.E.; Kulich, R.; Vranceanu, A.-M. Physical functioning and mindfulness skills training in chronic pain: A systematic review. *J. Pain Res.* **2019**, *12*, 179–189. [CrossRef] [PubMed]
26. Severeijns, R.; Vlaeyen, J.; Hout, M.A.V.D.; Weber, W.E. Pain Catastrophizing Predicts Pain Intensity, Disability, and Psychological Distress Independent of the Level of Physical Impairment. *Clin. J. Pain* **2001**, *17*, 165–172. [CrossRef] [PubMed]
27. Pincus, T.; Burton, A.K.; Vogel, S.; Field, A. A Systematic Review of Psychological Factors as Predictors of Chronicity/Disability in Prospective Cohorts of Low Back Pain. *Spine* **2002**, *27*, E109–E120. [CrossRef]
28. Gatchel, R.J.; Peng, Y.B.; Peters, M.; Fuchs, P.; Turk, D.C. The biopsychosocial approach to chronic pain: Scientific advances and future directions. *Psychol. Bull.* **2007**, *133*, 581–624. [CrossRef]
29. Segura-Jiménez, V.; Borges-Cosic, M.; Soriano-Maldonado, A.; Estévez-López, F.; Alvarez-Gallardo, I.C.; Herrador-Colmenero, M.; Delgado-Fernández, M.; Ruiz, J.R. Association of sedentary time and physical activity with pain, fatigue, and impact of fibromyalgia: The al-Ándalus study. *Scand. J. Med. Sci. Sports* **2015**, *27*, 83–92. [CrossRef] [PubMed]
30. Crombez, G.; Vlaeyen, J.; Heuts, P.H.; Lysens, R. Pain-related fear is more disabling than pain itself: Evidence on the role of pain-related fear in chronic back pain disability. *Pain* **1999**, *80*, 329–339. [CrossRef]

31. Varallo, G.; Scarpina, F.; Giusti, E.M.; Cattivelli, R.; Usubini, A.G.; Capodaglio, P.; Castelnuovo, G. Does Kinesiophobia Mediate the Relationship between Pain Intensity and Disability in Individuals with Chronic Low-Back Pain and Obesity? *Brain Sci.* **2021**, *11*, 684. [CrossRef] [PubMed]

32. Varallo, G.; Giusti, E.M.; Scarpina, F.; Cattivelli, R.; Capodaglio, P.; Castelnuovo, G. The Association of Kinesiophobia and Pain Catastrophizing with Pain-Related Disability and Pain Intensity in Obesity and Chronic Lower-Back Pain. *Brain Sci.* **2020**, *11*, 11. [CrossRef]

33. Quartana, P.J.; Campbell, C.M.; Edwards, R.R. Pain catastrophizing: A critical review. *Expert Rev. Neurother.* **2009**, *9*, 745–758. [CrossRef] [PubMed]

34. Keefe, F.J.; Rumble, M.E.; Scipio, C.D.; Giordano, L.A.; Perri, L.M. Psychological aspects of persistent pain: Current state of the science. *J. Pain* **2004**, *5*, 195–211. [CrossRef]

35. Leeuw, M.; Goossens, M.; Linton, S.J.; Crombez, G.; Boersma, K.; Vlaeyen, J. The Fear-Avoidance Model of Musculoskeletal Pain: Current State of Scientific Evidence. *J. Behav. Med.* **2006**, *30*, 77–94. [CrossRef]

36. Crombez, G.; Eccleston, C.; Van Damme, S.; Vlaeyen, J.; Karoly, P. Fear-Avoidance Model of Chronic Pain. *Clin. J. Pain* **2012**, *28*, 475–483. [CrossRef]

37. Vlaeyen, J.W.; Linton, S.J. Fear-avoidance and its consequences in chronic musculoskeletal pain: A state of the art. *Pain* **2000**, *85*, 317–332. [CrossRef]

38. Mannerkorpi, K.; Svantesson, U.; Broberg, C. Relationships Between Performance-Based Tests and Patients' Ratings of Activity Limitations, Self-Efficacy, and Pain in Fibromyalgia. *Arch. Phys. Med. Rehabil.* **2006**, *87*, 259–264. [CrossRef]

39. Gaudreault, N.; Boulay, P. Cardiorespiratory fitness among adults with fibromyalgia. *Breathe* **2018**, *14*, e25–e33. [CrossRef]

40. Edwards, R.R.; Cahalan, C.; Mensing, G.; Smith, M.T.; Haythornthwaite, J.A. Pain, catastrophizing, and depression in the rheumatic diseases. *Nat. Rev. Rheumatol.* **2011**, *7*, 216–224. [CrossRef] [PubMed]

41. Paschali, M.; Lazaridou, A.; Paschalis, T.; Napadow, V.; Edwards, R. Modifiable Psychological Factors Affecting Functioning in Fibromyalgia. *J. Clin. Med.* **2021**, *10*, 803. [CrossRef]

42. Suso-Ribera, C.; García-Palacios, A.; Botella, C.; Ribera-Canudas, M.V. Pain Catastrophizing and Its Relationship with Health Outcomes: Does Pain Intensity Matter? *Pain Res. Manag.* **2017**, *2017*, 9762864. [CrossRef]

43. Edwards, R.R.; Bingham, C.O.; Bathon, J.; Haythornthwaite, J.A. Catastrophizing and pain in arthritis, fibromyalgia, and other rheumatic diseases. *Arthritis Care Res.* **2006**, *55*, 325–332. [CrossRef] [PubMed]

44. Larice, S.; Ghiggia, A.; Di Tella, M.; Romeo, A.; Gasparetto, E.; Fusaro, E.; Castelli, L.; Tesio, V. Pain appraisal and quality of life in 108 outpatients with rheumatoid arthritis. *Scand. J. Psychol.* **2019**, *61*, 271–280. [CrossRef] [PubMed]

45. Somers, T.J.; Keefe, F.J.; Carson, J.W.; Pells, J.J.; Lacaille, L. Pain catastrophizing in borderline morbidly obese and morbidly obese individuals with osteoarthritic knee pain. *Pain Res. Manag.* **2008**, *13*, 401–406. [CrossRef]

46. Shelby, R.A.; Somers, T.J.; Keefe, F.J.; Pells, J.J.; Dixon, K.E.; Blumenthal, J.A. Domain Specific Self-Efficacy Mediates the Impact of Pain Catastrophizing on Pain and Disability in Overweight and Obese Osteoarthritis Patients. *J. Pain* **2008**, *9*, 912–919. [CrossRef] [PubMed]

47. Baranoff, J.; Hanrahan, S.; Kapur, D.; Connor, J. Acceptance as a process variable in relation to catastrophizing in multidisciplinary pain treatment. *Eur. J. Pain* **2012**, *17*, 101–110. [CrossRef]

48. Thompson, M.; McCracken, L.M. Acceptance and Related Processes in Adjustment to Chronic Pain. *Curr. Pain Headache Rep.* **2011**, *15*, 144–151. [CrossRef]

49. Vowles, K.; McCracken, L.; Sowden, G.; Ashworth, J. Psychological Flexibility in Coping with Chronic Pain: Further examination of the brief pain coping inventory-2. *Clin. J. Pain* **2014**, *30*, 324–330. [CrossRef]

50. McCracken, L.M.; Morley, S. The Psychological Flexibility Model: A Basis for Integration and Progress in Psychological Approaches to Chronic Pain Management. *J. Pain* **2014**, *15*, 221–234. [CrossRef]

51. McCracken, L.M. Learning to live with the pain: Acceptance of pain predicts adjustment in persons with chronic pain. *Pain* **1998**, *74*, 21–27. [CrossRef]

52. Vowles, K.E.; McCracken, L.M.; Eccleston, C. Patient functioning and catastrophizing in chronic pain: The mediating effects of acceptance. *Health Psychol.* **2008**, *27*, S136–S143. [CrossRef]

53. Varallo, G.; Ghiggia, A.; Arreghini, M.; Capodaglio, P.; Manzoni, G.M.; Giusti, E.M.; Castelli, L.; Castelnuovo, G. The Reliability and Agreement of the Fibromyalgia Survey Questionnaire in an Italian Sample of Obese Patients. *Front. Psychol.* **2020**, *12*, 187. [CrossRef]

54. Marshall, P.W.M.; Schabrun, S.; Knox, M.F. Physical activity and the mediating effect of fear, depression, anxiety, and catastrophizing on pain related disability in people with chronic low back pain. *PLoS ONE* **2017**, *12*, e0180788. [CrossRef] [PubMed]

55. Giusti, E.M.; Manna, C.; Varallo, G.; Cattivelli, R.; Manzoni, G.M.; Gabrielli, S.; D'Amario, F.; Lacerenza, M.; Castelnuovo, G. The Predictive Role of Executive Functions and Psychological Factors on Chronic Pain after Orthopaedic Surgery: A Longitudinal Cohort Study. *Brain Sci.* **2020**, *10*, 685. [CrossRef]

56. Keefe, F.J.; Brown, G.K.; Wallston, K.A.; Caldwell, D.S. Coping with rheumatoid arthritis pain: Catastrophizing as a maladaptive strategy. *Pain* **1989**, *37*, 51–56. [CrossRef]

57. Ramírez-Maestre, C.; de la Vega, R.; Sturgeon, J.A.; Peters, M. Editorial: Resilience Resources in Chronic Pain Patients: The Path to Adaptation. *Front. Psychol.* **2019**, *10*, 2848. [CrossRef]

58. Sturgeon, J.A.; Zautra, A.J. Resilience: A New Paradigm for Adaptation to Chronic Pain. *Curr. Pain Headache Rep.* **2010**, *14*, 105–112. [CrossRef]
59. Sturgeon, J.A.; Zautra, A.J. Psychological Resilience, Pain Catastrophizing, and Positive Emotions: Perspectives on Comprehensive Modeling of Individual Pain Adaptation. *Curr. Pain Headache Rep.* **2013**, *17*, 1–9. [CrossRef]
60. Kanzler, K.E.; Pugh, J.A.; McGeary, D.D.; Hale, W.J.; Mathias, C.W.; Kilpela, L.S.; Karns-Wright, T.E.; Robinson, P.J.; Dixon, S.A.; Bryan, C.J.; et al. Mitigating the Effect of Pain Severity on Activity and Disability in Patients with Chronic Pain: The Crucial Context of Acceptance. *Pain Med.* **2019**, *20*, 1509–1518. [CrossRef]
61. DiBenedetto, D.; Wawrzyniak, K.M.; Finkelman, M.; Kulich, R.J.; Chen, L.; Schatman, M.E.; Stone, M.T.; Mao, J. Relationships between Opioid Dosing, Pain Severity, and Disability in a Community-Based Chronic Pain Population: An Exploratory Retrospective Analysis. *Pain Med.* **2019**, *20*, 2155–2165. [CrossRef]
62. Craner, J.R.; Sperry, J.A.; Koball, A.M.; Morrison, E.J.; Gilliam, W.P. Unique Contributions of Acceptance and Catastrophizing on Chronic Pain Adaptation. *Int. J. Behav. Med.* **2017**, *24*, 542–551. [CrossRef] [PubMed]
63. Yu, L.; Kioskli, K.; McCracken, L.M. The Psychological Functioning in the COVID-19 Pandemic and Its Association with Psychological Flexibility and Broader Functioning in People With Chronic Pain. *J. Pain* **2021**, *22*, 926–939. [CrossRef] [PubMed]
64. Suso-Ribera, C.; Camacho-Guerrero, L.; Osma, J.; Suso-Vergara, S.; Gallardo-Pujol, D. A Reduction in Pain Intensity Is More Strongly Associated with Improved Physical Functioning in Frustration Tolerant Individuals: A Longitudinal Moderation Study in Chronic Pain Patients. *Front. Psychol.* **2019**, *10*, 907. [CrossRef]
65. Ferreira-Valente, M.A.; Pais-Ribeiro, J.; Jensen, M.P. Associations Between Psychosocial Factors and Pain Intensity, Physical Functioning, and Psychological Functioning in Patients with Chronic Pain. *Clin. J. Pain* **2014**, *30*, 713–723. [CrossRef] [PubMed]
66. Goesling, J.; Henry, M.J.; Moser, S.E.; Rastogi, M.; Hassett, A.L.; Clauw, D.J.; Brummett, C. Symptoms of Depression Are Associated with Opioid Use Regardless of Pain Severity and Physical Functioning among Treatment-Seeking Patients with Chronic Pain. *J. Pain* **2015**, *16*, 844–851. [CrossRef]
67. Matos, M.; Bernardes, S.; Goubert, L. The relationship between perceived promotion of autonomy/dependence and pain-related disability in older adults with chronic pain: The mediating role of self-reported physical functioning. *J. Behav. Med.* **2016**, *39*, 704–715. [CrossRef] [PubMed]
68. Jensen, M.P.; Nielson, W.R.; Turner, J.A.; Romano, J.M.; Hill, M.L. Readiness to self-manage pain is associated with coping and with psychological and physical functioning among patients with chronic pain. *Pain* **2003**, *104*, 529–537. [CrossRef]
69. Karasawa, Y.; Yamada, K.; Iseki, M.; Yamaguchi, M.; Murakami, Y.; Tamagawa, T.; Kadowaki, F.; Hamaoka, S.; Ishii, T.; Kawai, A.; et al. Association between change in self-efficacy and reduction in disability among patients with chronic pain. *PLoS ONE* **2019**, *14*, e0215404. [CrossRef]
70. Terwee, C.B.; van der Slikke, R.; van Lummel, R.C.; Benink, R.J.; Meijers, W.G.; de Vet, H.C. Self-reported physical functioning was more influenced by pain than performance-based physical functioning in knee-osteoarthritis patients. *J. Clin. Epidemiol.* **2006**, *59*, 724–731. [CrossRef]
71. Greenberg, J.; Mace, R.A.; Popok, P.J.; Kulich, R.J.; Patel, K.V.; Burns, J.W.; Somers, T.J.; Keefe, F.J.; Schatman, M.E.; Vrancenanu, A.-M. Psychosocial Correlates of Objective, Performance-Based, and Patient-Reported Physical Function Among Patients with Heterogeneous Chronic Pain. *J. Pain Res.* **2020**, *13*, 2255–2265. [CrossRef]
72. World Health Organization. *World Report on Disability*; World Health Organization: Geneva, Switzerland, 2011.
73. Taylor, A.M.; Phillips, K.; Patel, K.V.; Turk, D.C.; Dworkin, R.H.; Beaton, D.; Clauw, D.J.; Gignac, M.A.M.; Markman, J.D.; Williams, D.A.; et al. Assessment of physical function and participation in chronic pain clinical trials: IMMPACT/OMERACT recommendations. *Pain* **2016**, *157*, 1836. [CrossRef]
74. Suso-Ribera, C.; Borba, V.M.; Martín-Brufau, R.; Suso-Vergara, S.; García-Palacios, A. Individual differences and health in chronic pain: Are sex-differences relevant? *Health Qual. Life Outcomes* **2019**, *17*, 128. [CrossRef] [PubMed]
75. Estévez-López, F.; Álvarez-Gallardo, I.C.; Segura-Jiménez, V.; Soriano-Maldonado, A.; Borges-Cosic, M.; Pulido-Martos, M.; Aparicio, V.A.; Carbonell-Baeza, A.; Delgado-Fernández, M.; Geenen, R. The discordance between subjectively and objectively measured physical function in women with fibromyalgia: Association with catastrophizing and self-efficacy cognitions. The al-Ándalus project. *Disabil. Rehabil.* **2018**, *40*, 329–337. [CrossRef] [PubMed]
76. Ramírez-Maestre, C.; Esteve, R.; López-Martínez, A.E. Fear-Avoidance, Pain Acceptance and Adjustment to Chronic Pain: A Cross-Sectional Study on a Sample of 686 Patients with Chronic Spinal Pain. *Ann. Behav. Med.* **2014**, *48*, 402–410. [CrossRef] [PubMed]
77. Faul, F.; Erdfelder, E.; Buchner, A.; Lang, A.-G. Statistical power analyses using G*Power 3.1: Tests for correlation and regression analyses. *Behav. Res. Methods* **2009**, *41*, 1149–1160. [CrossRef]
78. Wolfe, F.; Clauw, D.J.; Fitzcharles, M.-A.; Goldenberg, D.L.; Häuser, W.; Katz, R.S.; Mease, P.; Russell, A.S.; Russell, I.J.; Winfield, J.B. Fibromyalgia Criteria and Severity Scales for Clinical and Epidemiological Studies: A Modification of the ACR Preliminary Diagnostic Criteria for Fibromyalgia. *J. Rheumatol.* **2011**, *38*, 1113–1122. [CrossRef]
79. Wolfe, F. Fibromyalgia Research Criteria. *J. Rheumatol.* **2014**, *41*, 187. [CrossRef]
80. Carrillo-De-La-Peña, M.T.; Triñanes, Y.; González-Villar, A.J.; Romero-Yuste, S.; Gomez-Perretta, C.; Arias, M.; Wolfe, F. Convergence between the 1990 and 2010 ACR diagnostic criteria and validation of the Spanish version of the Fibromyalgia Survey Questionnaire (FSQ). *Rheumatol. Int.* **2014**, *35*, 141–151. [CrossRef]

81. Ritter, P.L.; González, V.M.; Laurent, D.D.; Lorig, K.R. Measurement of pain using the visual numeric scale. *J. Rheumatol.* **2006**, *33*, 574–580.
82. Breivik, H.; Borchgrevink, P.C.; Allen, S.M.; Rosseland, L.A.; Romundstad, L.; Hals, E.K.B.; Kvarstein, G.; Stubhaug, A. Assessment of pain. *Br. J. Anaesth.* **2008**, *101*, 17–24. [CrossRef]
83. Sullivan, M.J.L.; Bishop, S.R.; Pivik, J. The Pain Catastrophizing Scale: Development and validation. *Psychol. Assess.* **1995**, *7*, 524–532. [CrossRef]
84. Monticone, M.; Baiardi, P.; Ferrari, S.; Foti, C.; Mugnai, R.; Pillastrini, P.; Rocca, B.; Vanti, C. Development of the Italian version of the Pain Catastrophising Scale (PCS-I): Cross-cultural adaptation, factor analysis, reliability, validity and sensitivity to change. *Spine* **2012**, *35*, 1241–1246. [CrossRef] [PubMed]
85. Vowles, K.E.; McCracken, L.M. Acceptance and values-based action in chronic pain: A study of treatment effectiveness and process. *J. Consult. Clin. Psychol.* **2008**, *76*, 397–407. [CrossRef]
86. McCracken, L.M.; Yang, S.-Y. The role of values in a contextual cognitive-behavioral approach to chronic pain. *Pain* **2006**, *123*, 137–145. [CrossRef]
87. McCracken, L.M.; Vowles, K.; Eccleston, C. Acceptance of chronic pain: Component analysis and a revised assessment method. *Pain* **2004**, *107*, 159–166. [CrossRef] [PubMed]
88. Bernini, O.; Pennato, T.; Cosci, F.; Berrocal, C. The Psychometric Properties of the Chronic Pain Acceptance Questionnaire in Italian Patients with Chronic Pain. *J. Health Psychol.* **2010**, *15*, 1236–1245. [CrossRef]
89. Ayán, C.; Martín, V.; Alonso-Cortés, B.; Álvarez, M.; Valencia, M.; Barrientos, M. Relationship between aerobic fitness and quality of life in female fibromyalgia patients. *Clin. Rehabil.* **2007**, *21*, 1109–1113. [CrossRef] [PubMed]
90. Carbonell-Baeza, A.; Ruiz, J.; Aparicio, V.A.; Ortega, F.B.; Delgado-Fernández, M. The 6-Minute Walk Test in Female Fibromyalgia Patients: Relationship with Tenderness, Symptomatology, Quality of Life, and Coping Strategies. *Pain Manag. Nurs.* **2013**, *14*, 193–199. [CrossRef] [PubMed]
91. Carbonell-Baeza, A.; Aparicio, V.A.; Ortega, F.B.; Cuevas, A.M.; Alvarez, I.C.; Ruiz, J.R.; Delgado-Fernandez, M. Does a 3-month multidisciplinary intervention improve pain, body composition and physical fitness in women with fibromyalgia? *Br. J. Sports Med.* **2011**, *45*, 1189–1195. [CrossRef]
92. Pankoff, B.; Overend, T.; Lucy, D.; White, K. Validity and responsiveness of the 6-minute walk test for people with fibromyalgia. *J. Rheumatol.* **2000**, *27*, 2666–2670.
93. Larsson, U.E.; Reynisdottir, S. The six-minute walk test in outpatients with obesity: Reproducibility and known group validity. *Physiother. Res. Int.* **2008**, *13*, 84–93. [CrossRef] [PubMed]
94. Mattsson, E.; Larsson, U.E.; Rössner, S. Is walking for exercise too exhausting for obese women? *Int. J. Obes.* **1997**, *21*, 380–386. [CrossRef] [PubMed]
95. De Souza, S.A.F.; Faintuch, J.; Fabris, S.M.; Nampo, F.K.; Luz, C.; Fabio, T.L.; Sitta, I.S.; Fonseca, I.C.D.B. Six-minute walk test: Functional capacity of severely obese before and after bariatric surgery. *Surg. Obes. Relat. Dis.* **2009**, *5*, 540–543. [CrossRef] [PubMed]
96. WHO. *World Health Organization Technical Report Series Obesity: Preventing and Managing the Global Epidemic*; Report of a WHO Consultation on Obesity; WHO: Geneva, Switzerland, 2000; ISBN 9241208945.
97. Hunter, J. Demographic Variables and Chronic Pain. *Clin. J. Pain* **2001**, *17*, S14–S19. [CrossRef]
98. Ferrari, S.; Vanti, C.; Pellizzer, M.; Dozza, L.; Monticone, M.; Pillastrini, P. Is there a relationship between self-efficacy, disability, pain and sociodemographic characteristics in chronic low back pain? A multicenter retrospective analysis. *Arch. Physiother.* **2019**, *9*, 1–9. [CrossRef]
99. Fillingim, R.B.; Doleys, D.M.; Edwards, R.R.; Lowery, D. Clinical Characteristics of Chronic Back Pain as a Function of Gender and Oral Opioid Use. *Spine* **2003**, *28*, 143–150. [CrossRef] [PubMed]
100. Rijken, M.; Spreeuwenberg, P.; Schippers, J.; Groenewegen, P.P. The importance of illness duration, age at diagnosis and the year of diagnosis for labour participation chances of people with chronic illness: Results of a nationwide panel-study in the Netherlands. *BMC Public Health* **2013**, *13*, 803. [CrossRef]
101. Chaney, J.M.; Uretsky, D.L.; Mullins, L.L.; Doppler, M.J.; Palmer, W.R.; Wees, S.J.; Klein, H.S.; Doud, D.K.; Reiss, M.L. Differential effects of age and illness duration on pain-depression and disability-depression relationships in rheumatoid arthritis. *Int. J. Rehabil. Health* **1996**, *2*, 101–112. [CrossRef]
102. Carbonell-Baeza, A.; Aparicio, V.A.; Sjöström, M.; Ruiz, J.R.; Delgado-Fernandez, M. Pain and functional capacity in female fibromyalgia patients. *Pain Med.* **2011**, *12*, 1667–1675. [CrossRef] [PubMed]
103. Jamovi (Version 1.2) The Jamovi Project 2020. Available online: https://www.jamovi.org/about.html (accessed on 16 August 2021).
104. Ramírez-Maestre, C.; Esteve, R.; Ruiz-Párraga, G.; Gómez-Pérez, L.; López-Martínez, A.E. The Key Role of Pain Catastrophizing in the Disability of Patients with Acute Back Pain. *Int. J. Behav. Med.* **2017**, *24*, 239–248. [CrossRef]
105. Wertli, M.M.; Eugster, R.; Held, U.; Steurer, J.; Kofmehl, R.; Weiser, S. Catastrophizing—A prognostic factor for outcome in patients with low back pain: A systematic review. *Spine J.* **2014**, *14*, 2639–2657. [CrossRef]
106. Ferreira-Valente, A.; Solé, E.; Sánchez-Rodríguez, E.; Sharma, S.; Pathak, A.; Jensen, M.P.; Miró, J.; de la Vega, R. Does Pain Acceptance Buffer the Negative Effects of Catastrophizing on Function in Individuals with Chronic Pain? *Clin. J. Pain* **2021**, *37*, 339–348. [CrossRef] [PubMed]

107. Catala, P.; Suso-Ribera, C.; Gutierrez, L.; Perez, S.; Lopez-Roig, S.; Peñacoba, C. Is thought management a resource for functioning in women with fibromyalgia irrespective of pain levels? *Pain Med.* **2021**, *22*, 1827–1836. [CrossRef]
108. Tangen, S.F.; Helvik, A.-S.; Eide, H.; Fors, E.A. Pain acceptance and its impact on function and symptoms in fibromyalgia. *Scand. J. Pain* **2020**, *20*, 727–736. [CrossRef]
109. Rodero, B.; Casanueva, B.; Luciano, J.V.; Gili, M.; Serrano-Blanco, A.; García-Campayo, J. Relationship between behavioural coping strategies and acceptance in patients with fibromyalgia syndrome: Elucidating targets of interventions. *BMC Musculoskelet. Disord.* **2011**, *12*, 143. [CrossRef]
110. Trainor, H.; Baranoff, J.; Henke, M.; Winefield, H. Functioning with fibromyalgia: The role of psychological flexibility and general psychological acceptance. *Aust. Psychol.* **2019**, *54*, 214–224. [CrossRef]
111. Gracely, R.H.; Geisser, M.E.; Giesecke, T.; Grant, M.A.B.; Petzke, F.; Williams, D.A.; Clauw, D.J. Pain catastrophizing and neural responses to pain among persons with fibromyalgia. *Brain* **2004**, *127*, 835–843. [CrossRef]
112. Roelofs, J.; Peters, M.L.; McCracken, L.; Vlaeyen, J. The pain vigilance and awareness questionnaire (PVAQ): Further psychometric evaluation in fibromyalgia and other chronic pain syndromes. *Pain* **2003**, *101*, 299–306. [CrossRef]
113. Cooper, L.; Ells, L.; Ryan, C.; Martin, D. Perceptions of adults with overweight/obesity and chronic musculoskeletal pain: An interpretative phenomenological analysis. *J. Clin. Nurs.* **2018**, *27*, e776–e786. [CrossRef] [PubMed]
114. Hulens, M.; Vansant, G.; Claessens, A.L.; Lysens, R.; Muls, E. Predictors of 6-minute walk test results in lean, obese and morbidly obese women. *Scand. J. Med. Sci. Sports* **2003**, *13*, 98–105. [CrossRef] [PubMed]
115. Neumann, L.; Lerner, E.; Glazer, Y.; Bolotin, A.; Shefer, A.; Buskila, D. A cross-sectional study of the relationship between body mass index and clinical characteristics, tenderness measures, quality of life, and physical functioning in fibromyalgia patients. *Clin. Rheumatol.* **2008**, *27*, 1543–1547. [CrossRef] [PubMed]
116. Yunus, M.B.; Arslan, S.; Aldag, J.C. Relationship between body mass index and fibromyalgia features. *Scand. J. Rheumatol.* **2002**, *31*, 27–31. [CrossRef] [PubMed]
117. Urquhart, D.M.; Berry, P.; Wluka, A.; Strauss, B.J.; Wang, Y.; Proietto, J.; Jones, G.; Dixon, J.B.; Cicuttini, F.M. Increased Fat Mass Is Associated with High Levels of Low Back Pain Intensity and Disability. *Spine* **2011**, *36*, 1320–1325. [CrossRef]
118. Han, T.; Schouten, J.S.; Lean, M.; Seidell, J. The prevalence of low back pain and associations with body fatness, fat distribution and height. *Int. J. Obes.* **1997**, *21*, 600–607. [CrossRef]
119. Donnelly, J.E.; Smith, B.; Jacobsen, D.J.; Kirk, E.; DuBose, K.; Hyder, M.; Bailey, B.; Washburn, R. The role of exercise for weight loss and maintenance. *Best Pract. Res. Clin. Gastroenterol.* **2004**, *18*, 1009–1029. [CrossRef]
120. Egger, G.; Dixon, J. Non-nutrient causes of low-grade, systemic inflammation: Support for a 'canary in the mineshaft' view of obesity in chronic disease. *Obes. Rev.* **2010**, *12*, 339–345. [CrossRef]
121. Attridge, N.; Noonan, D.; Eccleston, C.; Keogh, E. The disruptive effects of pain on n-back task performance in a large general population sample. *Pain* **2015**, *156*, 1885–1891. [CrossRef]
122. Hodges, P.; Smeets, R. Interaction Between Pain, Movement, and Physical Activity: Short-term benefits, long-term consequences, and targets for treatment. *Clin. J. Pain* **2015**, *31*, 97–107. [CrossRef]
123. Celletti, C.; Castori, M.; La Torre, G.; Camerota, F. Evaluation of Kinesiophobia and Its Correlations with Pain and Fatigue in Joint Hypermobility Syndrome/Ehlers-Danlos Syndrome Hypermobility Type. *BioMed Res. Int.* **2013**, *2013*, 1–7. [CrossRef]
124. Busch, A.J.; Barber, K.A.; Overend, T.J.; Peloso, P.M.J.; Schachter, C.L. Exercise for treating fibromyalgia syndrome. *Cochrane Database Syst. Rev.* **2007**, *17*, CD003786. [CrossRef] [PubMed]
125. Fontaine, K.R.; Conn, L.; Clauw, D.J. Effects of lifestyle physical activity on perceived symptoms and physical function in adults with fibromyalgia: Results of a randomized trial. *Arthritis Res. Ther.* **2010**, *12*, R55. [CrossRef]
126. Macfarlane, G.J.; Kronisch, C.; Dean, L.; Atzeni, F.; Häuser, W.; Flüß, E.; Choy, E.; Kosek, E.; Amris, K.; Branco, J.; et al. EULAR revised recommendations for the management of fibromyalgia. *Ann. Rheum. Dis.* **2016**, *76*, 318–328. [CrossRef] [PubMed]
127. Da Costa, D.; Abrahamowicz, M.; Lowensteyn, I.; Bernatsky, S.; Dritsa, M.; Fitzcharles, M.-A.; Dobkin, P.L. A randomized clinical trial of an individualized home-based exercise programme for women with fibromyalgia. *Rheumatology* **2005**, *44*, 1422–1427. [CrossRef] [PubMed]
128. Meiworm, L.; Jakob, E.; Walker, U.A.; Peter, H.H.; Keul, J. Patients with fibromyalgia benefit from aerobic endurance exercise. *Clin. Rheumatol.* **2000**, *19*, 253–257. [CrossRef]
129. Rooks, D.S.; Silverman, C.B.; Kantrowitz, F.G. The effects of progressive strength training and aerobic exercise on muscle strength and cardiovascular fitness in women with fibromyalgia: A pilot study. *Arthritis Care Res.* **2002**, *47*, 22–28. [CrossRef] [PubMed]
130. Petridou, A.; Siopi, A.; Mougios, V. Exercise in the management of obesity. *Metabolism* **2018**, *92*, 163–169. [CrossRef]
131. Oppert, J.-M.; Bellicha, A.; Ciangura, C. Physical activity in management of persons with obesity. *Eur. J. Intern. Med.* **2021**, *20*, S0953–S6205. [CrossRef]
132. Johns, D.J.; Hartmann-Boyce, J.; Jebb, S.A.; Aveyard, P. Diet or Exercise Interventions vs Combined Behavioral Weight Management Programs: A Systematic Review and Meta-Analysis of Direct Comparisons. *J. Acad. Nutr. Diet.* **2014**, *114*, 1557–1568. [CrossRef]
133. Alamam, D.M.; Leaver, A.; Alsobayel, H.I.; Moloney, N.; Lin, J.; Mackey, M.G. Low Back Pain–Related Disability Is Associated with Pain-Related Beliefs Across Divergent Non–English-Speaking Populations: Systematic Review and Meta-Analysis. *Pain Med.* **2021**. [CrossRef]

134. Williams, D.A.; Gendreau, M.; Hufford, M.R.; Groner, K.; Gracely, R.H.; Clauw, D.J. Pain Assessment in Patients with Fibromyalgia Syndrome: A consideration of methods for clinical trials. *Clin. J. Pain* **2004**, *20*, 348–356. [CrossRef] [PubMed]
135. Clauw, D.J.; Crofford, L.J. Chronic widespread pain and fibromyalgia: What we know, and what we need to know. *Best Pract. Res. Clin. Rheumatol.* **2003**, *17*, 685–701. [CrossRef]
136. Harris, R.E.; Williams, D.A.; McLean, S.; Sen, A.; Hufford, M.; Gendreau, R.M.; Gracely, R.H.; Clauw, D.J. Characterization and consequences of pain variability in individuals with fibromyalgia. *Arthritis Rheum.* **2005**, *52*, 3670–3674. [CrossRef] [PubMed]

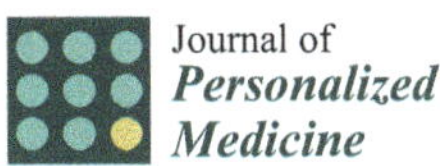

Journal of
Personalized Medicine

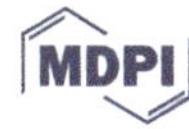

Personalised Approach to Diagnosing and Managing Ischemic Stroke with a Plasma-Soluble Urokinase-Type Plasminogen Activator Receptor

Katarzyna Śmiłowska [1,2,*], Marek Śmiłowski [3], Robert Partyka [1], Danuta Kokocińska [1] and Przemysław Jałowiecki [1]

1   Department of Emergency Medicine, Faculty of Medical Sciences, Medical University of Silesia, 40-055 Katowice, Poland; robertpartyka@op.pl (R.P.); dkokocinska@op.pl (D.K.); olaf@pro.onet.pl (P.J.)
2   Department of Neurology, 5th Regional Hospital in Sosnowiec, Plac Medyków 1, 41-200 Sosnowiec, Poland
3   Department of Hematology and Bone Marrow Transplantation, Medical University of Silesia, 40-055 Katowice, Poland; marek.smilowski2@gmail.com
*   Correspondence: kasia.smilowska@gmail.com

Citation: Śmiłowska, K.; Śmiłowski, M.; Partyka, R.; Kokocińska, D.; Jałowiecki, P. Personalised Approach to Diagnosing and Managing Ischemic Stroke with a Plasma-Soluble Urokinase-Type Plasminogen Activator Receptor. *J. Pers. Med.* **2022**, *12*, 457. https://doi.org/10.3390/jpm12030457

Academic Editors: Fábio G. Teixeira, Catarina Godinho and Júlio Belo Fernandes

Received: 15 February 2022
Accepted: 10 March 2022
Published: 14 March 2022

Publisher's Note: MDPI stays neutral with regard to jurisdictional claims in published maps and institutional affiliations.

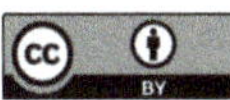

Abstract: Background: The increasing incidence of ischemic stroke has led to the search for a novel biomarker to predict the course of disease and the risk of mortality. Recently, the role of the soluble urokinase plasminogen activator receptor (suPAR) as a biomarker and indicator of immune system activation has been widely examined. Therefore, the aim of the current study was to assess the dynamics of changes in serum levels of suPAR in ischemic stroke and to evaluate the prognostic value of suPAR in determining mortality risk. Methods: Eighty patients from the Department of Neurology, diagnosed with ischemic stroke, were enrolled in the study. Residual blood was obtained from all the patients on the first, third and seventh days after their ischemic stroke and the concentrations of suPAR and C-reactive protein (CRP), as well as the number of leukocytes and National Institute of Health's Stroke Scale (NIHSS) scores, were evaluated. Results: On the first day of ischemic stroke, the average suPAR concentration was 6.55 ng/mL; on the third day, it was 8.29 ng/mL; on the seventh day, it was 9.16 ng/mL. The average CRP concentration on the first day of ischemic stroke was 4.96 mg/L; on the third day, it was 11.76 mg/L; on the seventh day, it was 17.17 mg/L. The number of leukocytes on the first day of ischemic stroke was $7.32 \times 10^3/\text{mm}^3$; on the third day, it was $9.27 \times 10^3/\text{mm}^3$; on the seventh day, it was $10.41 \times 10^3/\text{mm}^3$. Neurological condition, which was assessed via the NIHSS, on the first day of ischemic stroke, was scored at 10.71 points; on the third day, it was scored at 12.34 points; on the seventh day, it was scored at 13.75 points. An increase in the values of all the evaluated parameters on the first, third and seventh days of hospitalisation was observed. The patients with hypertension, ischemic heart disease and type 2 diabetes showed higher suPAR and CRP concentrations at the baseline as well as on subsequent days of hospitalisation. The greatest sensitivity and specificity were characterised by suPAR-3, where a value above 10.5 ng/mL resulted in a significant increase in mortality risk. Moreover, an NIHSS-1 score above 12 points and a CRP-3 concentration above 15.6 mg/L significantly increased the risk of death in the course of the disease. Conclusions: The plasma suPAR concentration after ischemic stroke is strongly related to the patient's clinical status, with a higher concentration on the first and third days of stroke resulting in a poorer prognosis at a later stage of treatment. Therefore, assessing the concentration of this parameter has important prognostic value.

Keywords: stroke; ischemia; biomarkers; mortality risk

1. Introduction

Clinically, stroke is defined as a focal or global cerebral dysfunction, of a vascular origin, that occurs suddenly and lasts at least 24 h [1]. Over 12 to 15 million people worldwide are afflicted by this disease annually [2,3]. Approximately 15% of patients die within one month after having a stroke, and only 10% present a complete withdrawal of neurological deficits. The risk of recurrent ischemic stroke is 5 to 25% annually and is higher in the first weeks following the stroke [4–6]. In general, 25% of the patients present mild neurological symptoms, while 40% experience permanent disability, both motor and cognitive, at a moderate or severe level; another 10% of the patients require continuous nursing care due to neurological disability [7]. This leads to a reduction in daily activities due to varying degrees of neurological deficits [8]. Therefore, the increasing incidence of stroke has prompted researchers to search for new diagnostic biomarkers to enable early disease detection, quick, tailored treatment and, ideally, prognostic value.

Functional impairment from ischemic stroke is the result of not only structural brain damage but also accompanying immune dysregulation [9]. Therefore, the role of inflammatory biomarkers, such as plasma-soluble urokinase-type plasminogen activator receptor (suPAR), C-reactive protein (CRP), procalcitonin (PCT) and white blood cells (WBC), has been strongly argued to predict the course of ischemic stroke and to determine its mortality risk [10]. Increased concentrations of inflammatory markers in the blood occur independent of the infection, and, thus, monitoring these parameters is useful in predicting the course of ischaemic stroke [11].

Urokinase plasminogen activator (uPA) and its receptor (uPAR) play an important role in the pathogenesis of vascular diseases [12]. As a result of the activation of the immune system accompanying a stroke, the concentration of suPAR in body fluids increases with the severity of the immune response [13,14]. So far, evidence is limited regarding whether the increase in suPAR concentration is merely a consequence of the activation of the immune system or also has the potential to enhance immune response [15]. The latter hypothesis is supported by the fact that uPA and its receptor are involved in the conversion of plasminogen to plasmin. Proper blood clotting, conditioned by the dissolution of fibrin at the site of vascular injury, depends on plasminogen activation by a tissue plasminogen activator (t-PA). The uPA–uPAR complex increases plasminogen activity on the cell surface by initiating a proteolysis reaction, which enables cell migration [16]. Moreover, the uPA–uPAR complex has an effect on leukocytes independent of plasminogen activation. The uPA fragments may act as a chemotactin for neutrophils and a mitogen for lymphocytes. Urokinase from the uPA–uPAR complex determines the effective process of adhesion, increasing the interaction with integrins and vitronectin [17]. The interaction of uPAR with β2-integrin increases the migration of inflammatory cells as well as the mobilisation and activation of leukocytes. Moreover, uPAR facilitates migration through plasmin generation on the cell surface (after binding its ligand-uPA) with the subsequent dissolution of the extracellular matrix and plays a role in the mobilisation and activation of leukocytes via interaction with β2-integrins.

Atherosclerotic plaque in the carotid arteries causes an increased concentration of macrophages and leads to the release of uPAR from their surface [18]. Moreover, uPAR plays a role in the pathogenesis of vascular diseases, which is usually accompanied by inflammation [19,20]. Atherosclerotic plaque lesions induce an inflammatory process, which is initiated by low density lipoprotein (LDL) molecules in the subendothelial area of arteries [21]. These molecules induce endothelial cell activation and inflammatory cell recruitment through chemokines and adhesion molecules [22]. The accumulation of inflammatory cells leads to the degeneration of components that stabilise the vascular wall, leading to the weakening of the plaque and increasing the risk of rupture [23]. The degeneration of the extracellular matrix also involves the fibrinolytic system through the activation of plasminogen, which is converted from an inactive proenzyme to plasmin by two activators: tissue plasminogen activator (t-PA) and urokinase plasminogen activator (u-PA). This, in turn, is connected to the cellular uPA receptor. Moreover, the conversion of plasminogen to plasmin leads to fibrin degeneration [24]. A soluble form of defragmented uPAR becomes detectable in body fluids [25]. The plasma concentration of suPAR increases, reflecting the activation of the immune system caused by bacterial and viral infections, sepsis or cancer [26,27].

Ischemic stroke has a two-phase effect on the peripheral immune system. In the initial phase, a generalised inflammatory process results in the massive production of classical inflammatory markers, such as cytokines and chemokines [28]. As a result, the blood–brain barrier enables the infiltration of lymphocytes [29–31]. This process leads to secondary brain injury but also plays a protective role as it contributes to the regeneration of nervous tissue.

Damage to the blood–brain barrier results in a local inflammatory reaction that occurs as early as 30 min after the ischemic episode. Neutrophils begin to accumulate in the region of infarction, with the highest concentration occurring between one and three days after ischemia [29]. Neutrophils participate in the inflammatory process by releasing pro-inflammatory mediators [32]. In addition, monocytes are involved in the process, transforming into macrophages in the nervous tissue. They release interleukin-6 (IL-6), which is responsible for immune response within both the central and peripheral nervous systems [33]. Activated T lymphocytes are also involved in the local inflammatory response. Their highest concentration can be observed on the seventh day after the stroke [34]. These lymphocytes—specifically $CD4^+$ and $CD8^+$ lymphocytes—exert adverse effects by producing interferon-γ and interleukin-17 (IL-17). T-regulatory lymphocytes, in turn, produce interleukin 10 (IL-10), a modulating anti-inflammatory response [35]. Pro-inflammatory cytokines activate local microglial cells and induce the migration of immune cells to the site of ischemia [36].

Stroke-induced immunosuppression (SIIS) occurs after the early inflammatory response [37]. SIIS limits the regeneration of the nervous tissue, worsening the prognosis of and leading to severe complications from the stroke—specifically infections, which occur in up to 65% of patients [38]. The most common infections involve the urinary and respiratory tracts [39]. The increased risk of infection is a result of decreased activation of T lymphocytes and a significant decrease in the number of T and B cells [31]. The activation of the immune system also increases the concentration of inflammatory biomarkers (e.g., CRP, erythrocyte sedimentation rate, white blood cells (WBC), peripheral neutrophils), indicating worse prognosis [40–43].

We hypothesised that ischemic stroke, which activates the immune system, leads to changes in the concentration of plasma suPAR. Therefore, we sought to accomplish the following objectives: (1) assess the dynamics of changes in plasma suPAR concentrations on the first, third and seventh days after ischemic stroke; (2) conduct a comparative analysis of changes in suPAR concentrations in relation to the neurological status of patients, assessed using the National Institute of Health's Stroke Scale (NIHSS); (3) assess the correlation between the concentration of suPAR, the concentration of CRP and leukocyte count; (4) assess the prognostic value of suPAR in determining the risk of death among patients with ischemic stroke in comparison with the prognostic value of CRP, the NIHSS and WBC.

2. Material and Methods

Eighty patients with ischemic stroke were included in the study in the Department of Neurology of the Regional Hospital in Pszczyna, Poland. The diagnosis was made based on clinical symptoms and neuroimaging studies. Ethical approval for this study was obtained from the Medical University of Silesia in Katowice (no: KNW/0022/KB/85/13). The study was conducted between 2013 and 2017.

The inclusion criteria were as follows: (1) symptoms of stroke up to 24 h prior to admission; (2) >18 years old for both males and females; (3) no other causes of neurological deficits after brain imaging; (4) clinical diagnosis of ischemic stroke. Patients were excluded from participation if they had (1) clinical or laboratory features of infection upon admission to hospital; (2) stroke not ischemic in nature (e.g., haemorrhagic stroke, subarachnoid haemorrhage); (3) other causes of neurological deficits (epileptic seizure with Todd paresis); (4) symptoms of transient ischemic attack (TIA); (5) electrolyte disturbances; (6) cancer diagnosis; (7) stroke located in the posterior cranial fossa.

SuPARnostic kits (ViroGates, Lyngby, Denmark) were used to determine the suPAR concentration. Blood was collected on the first, third and seventh days after ischemic stroke. The material was centrifuged at a rate of 3000 rpm for 10 min. The obtained plasma was frozen at $-20\ ^{\circ}$C. The plasma was then quantitatively analysed using the SuPARnostic ELISA assay (ViroGates, Lyngby, Denmark) to determine the suPAR concentration.

Statistical Methods

The type of distribution of the examined parameters was evaluated using the Shapiro–Wilk test. A Student's *t*-test for both related and unrelated variables was used to evaluate mean values whose distribution was close to normal. The statistical analysis assumed a level of significance of $p < 0.05$.

If the distribution differed from the normal distribution, the following procedures were applied accordingly: a Wilcoxon test and a Mann–Whitney U-test. The correspondence of the distribution with the normal distribution was assessed using a chi-square test. For the analysis of non-parametric variables (prevalence), either the non-parametric chi-square independence test or the Fischer precision test was used. Correlations were investigated using the chi-square test. In order to assess the correlation between the examined variables, a significance level of $p < 0.05$ was adopted. To determine the relationship between suPAR, NIHSS, CRP and WBC and the mortality rate, a logistic regression analysis was used, taking into account the risk factors of stroke. The cut-off points for each parameter were determined using area under the curve (AUC) receiver operating characteristic (ROC) analysis, on the basis of which predictive values were obtained for each parameter and a quotient of the likelihood of the occurrence of a given event was determined. In the case of AUC ROC analysis, a significance range of 0.8 to 0.95 was used.

3. Results

3.1. Study Population

The final analysis included data obtained from 80 patients (37 women and 43 men) who met the inclusion criteria. The demographic characteristics of the study group are presented in Table 1.

Table 1. Demographic characteristics.

Risk Factor	Value
Age	70.4 ± 7.9
Gender (F/M)	37/43
Arterial hypertension (%)	56%
Ischemic heart disease (%)	35%
Atrial fibrillation (%)	44%
Type 2 diabetes mellitus (%)	51%
Smoking (%)	23%
Hypercholesterolemia (%)	38%

3.2. Values of the Tested Parameters

The average values of the tested parameters (suPAR, NIHSS, CRP and WBC) are presented in Table 2. On the first day following ischemic stroke, the suPAR (suPAR-1) concentration was 6.55 ng/mL and exceeded the reference values for healthy subjects (4.5 ng/mL). The CRP concentration on the first day following ischemic stroke (CRP-1) was in the upper limit of the normal range (4.96 mg/L; N < 5mg/L), while the number of WBC was 7.32 thousand/mm^3 and was, therefore, in the normal range (n 9.8 thd/mm^3).

Table 2. suPAR, NIHSS, CRP and WBC values on the first, third and seventh day after ischemic stroke.

Parameter	First Day	Third Day	Seventh Day
suPAR [ng/mL]	6.55 ± 1.66	8.29 ± 3.49	9.16 ± 3.84
NIHSS [pts]	10.71 ± 5.52	12.34 ± 6.42	13.75 ± 8.61
CRP [mg/L]	4.96 ± 2.34	11.76 ± 13.34	17.17 ± 20.13
WBC [thd/mm^3]	7.32 ± 1.7	9.27 ± 3.57	10.41 ± 3.53

3.3. Assessment of the Change in suPAR, NIHSS, CRP and WBC

Comparing the average suPAR-1 values with those of suPAR-3 and suPAR-7, we observed a statistically significant increase in the suPAR concentration on the third day of hospitalisation (suPAR-3) in comparison with the first day (suPAR-1) ($p < 0.05$) and on the seventh day of hospitalisation (suPAR-7) in comparison with the first and third days ($p < 0.05$).

Based on the analyses, a statistically significant difference was observed in the NIHSS score on the third day of hospitalisation (NIHSS-3) in comparison with the first day of hospitalisation (NIHSS-1) ($p < 0.05$) and on the seventh day of hospitalisation (NIHSS-7) in comparison with the first and third days ($p < 0.05$). A significant increase in the CRP concentration was observed on the third day of hospitalisation (CRP-3) compared to the first day (CRP-1) ($p < 0.05$) and on the seventh day (CRP-7) compared to the first and third days ($p < 0.05$).

The increase in the number of WBC on the third day of hospitalisation (WBC-3) compared to the first day (WBC-1) was also statistically significant ($p < 0.05$), as was the increase in the number of WBC on the seventh day of hospitalisation (WBC-7) compared to the first and third days ($p < 0.05$).

3.4. Analysis of suPAR in Correlation to NIHSS

3.4.1. Day I

Statistical analysis revealed a correlation between the suPAR concentration on the first day of hospitalisation (suPAR-1) and neurological status assessed based on the NIHSS (NIHSS-1) ($r = 0.48$; $p < 0.05$), as well as an average positive correlation between the suPAR-1 concentration and NIHSS-3 ($r = 0.47$; $p < 0.05$) and NIHSS-7 ($r = 0.41$; $p < 0.05$).

3.4.2. Day III

On the third day of hospitalisation, a weak positive correlation between the suPAR-3 concentration and NIHSS-3 ($r = 0.28$; $p < 0.05$) was found.

3.4.3. Day VII

On the seventh day of hospitalisation, a weak positive correlation between the suPAR-7 concentration and NIHSS-7 ($r = 0.27$; $p < 0.05$) and an average positive correlation between the suPAR-7 concentration and the neurological status of the patient at the same time (NIHSS-7) ($r = 0.41$; $p < 0.05$) was observed.

3.5. The Correlation between Concentrations of suPAR, CRP and WBC

An average positive correlation between the concentration of suPAR-1 and the concentration of CRP-1 ($r = 0.43$; $p < 0.05$) and a weak positive correlation between the concentrations of suPAR-1 and WBC-7 ($r = 0.23$; $p < 0.05$) were identified. There was also a weak positive correlation between the concentrations of suPAR-3 and WBC-7 ($r = 0.26$; $p < 0.05$) as well as between the concentrations of suPAR-7 and WBC-7 ($r = 0.38$; $p < 0.05$).

There was an average positive correlation between CRP-1 and NIHSS-1 ($r = 0.48$; $p < 0.05$), between CRP-1 and NIHSS-3 ($r = 0.39$; $p < 0.05$) and between CRP-1 and NIHSS-7 ($r = 0.36$; $p < 0.05$).

3.6. Impact of Risk Factors on the Assessed Parameters

We analysed the relation between individual risk factors of ischemic stroke, such as hypertension, ischemic heart disease, atrial fibrillation, type 2 diabetes mellitus, smoking and hypercholesterolemia, and their influence on the evaluated parameters.

The patients with arterial hypertension exhibited higher concentrations of suPAR-1, suPAR-3 and suPAR-7, as well as CRP-1, CRP-3 and CRP-7, than the patients without arterial hypertension. Other parameters (NIHSS and WBC) did not differ significantly in the groups of patients with and without hypertension.

In the patients with ischemic heart disease, significant differences were found in both suPAR (suPAR-1, suPAR-3 and suPAR-7) and CRP (CRP-1, CRP-3 and CRP-7) concentrations. There was no correlation between the NIHSS values and the number of WBC in this group of patients.

No differences were found in the parameters after taking into consideration patients with atrial fibrillation.

The patients with type 2 diabetes mellitus showed increased suPAR values in all the time periods (suPAR-1, suPAR-3 and suPAR-7) and in CRP-3 and CRP-7 values in comparison with the patients without diabetes. The remaining parameters did not differ significantly.

Smokers showed higher concentrations of suPAR-3 and suPAR-7, NIHSS-3 and NIHSS-7, as well as CRP-7, compared to non-smokers.

The patients with hypercholesterolemia did not show any differences in the values of the evaluated parameters in comparison with the patients without hypercholesterolemia, except for CRP-7.

3.7. Prognostic Value of Assessed Parameters and Mortality Rate

During hospitalisation, 11 patients died (14%). Death occurred on average 17 days after the ischemic episode. All the deaths were related either directly (e.g., brain oedema) or indirectly (e.g., infectious complications) to the stroke. As shown in Table 3, the patients with comorbidities, such as arterial hypertension, ischemic heart disease, type 2 diabetes mellitus and smoking, had a higher mortality risk. Similarly, higher concentrations of suPAR-1, suPAR-3, suPAR-7, CRP-3 and CRP-7, as well as the neurological status of the patient (NIHSS-1, NIHSS-3 and NIHSS-7), were also associated with a higher mortality risk (Table 4).

Table 3. Risk factors for ischemic stroke and post-stroke mortality.

Death	Yes ($n = 11$)	No ($n = 69$)	p
Age	69.5 ± 4.9	70.6 ± 8.3	-
Sex (F/M)	4/7	33/36	-
Arterial hypertension (%)	100	49	$p < 0.05$
Ischemic heart disease (%)	78	59	$p < 0.05$
Atrial fibrillation (%)	45	43	-
Type 2 diabetes mellitus (%)	73	48	$p < 0.05$
Smoking (%)	73	14	$p < 0.05$
Hypercholesterolemia (%)	58	45	-

Table 4. Comparison assessed parameters (suPAR, NIHSS, CRP, WBC) and post-stroke mortality.

Death	Yes (*n* = 11)	No (*n* = 69)	*p*
suPAR on day I	8.48	6.24	$p < 0.05$
suPAR on day III	10.74	7.90	$p < 0.05$
suPAR on day VII	12.52	8.62	$p < 0.05$
NIHSS on day I	14.45	10.12	$p < 0.05$
NIHSS on day III	16.00	11.75	$p < 0.05$
NIHSS on day VII	17.36	13.17	$p < 0.05$
CRP on day I	5.91	4.81	-
CRP on day III	9.27	12.16	$p < 0.05$
CRP on day VII	12.68	17.88	$p < 0.05$
WBC on day I	7.40	7.31	-
WBC on day III	8.84	9.34	-
WBC on day VII	10.62	10.38	-

In contrast, atrial fibrillation and hypercholesterolemia were not associated with mortality risk.

3.8. AUC ROC Analysis of the Prognostic Value of suPAR

To determine the risk factors influencing the concentrations of the assessed parameters, a multifactor analysis was conducted to assess their prognostic value in the study group with regard to gender, age, presence of ischemic heart disease, presence of arterial hypertension, presence of type 2 diabetes mellitus and smoking status. The selected group of patients was statistically analysed in order to determine the prognostic value of these parameters in predicting the risk of post-stroke mortality.

Moreover, suPAR-3 had the highest sensitivity and specificity, with a cut-off point of 12.7 ng/mL, indicating an increased risk of post-stroke mortality. A concentration of suPAR-1 exceeding 8.4 ng/mL was associated with a higher risk of death. NIHSS-1 ($\geq$14 points) and CRP-3 (concentration above 14.6 mg/L) were correlated with a significant increase in mortality risk (Table 5).

Table 5. Comparison of prognostic value of individual parameters.

Parameter	Sensitivity	Specificity	95% CI	Cut-Off Point	Chance Quotient	AUC (0.8–0.95)
suPAR-1 [ng/mL]	90.9	61.8	0.7–0.9	7.64	2.82	0.80
suPAR-3 [ng/mL]	81.8	81.2	0.8–0.9	10.5	8.06	0.89
NIHSS-1 [pkt]	81.8	75.4	0.7–0.9	12.0	2.99	0.83
CRP-3 [mg/L]	81.8	81.5	0.7–0.9	15.6	4.83	0.81
WBC-7 [thd/mm^3]	72.7	82.4	0.7–0.9	13.7	2.04	0.80

4. Discussion

To our knowledge, this was the first study to examine the prognostic value of suPAR concerning ischemic stroke. The majority of the previous studies have focused on suPAR concentrations with regard to ischemic heart disease, cancer, infections or type 2 diabetes mellitus.

The suPAR concentration increased on the first day following ischemic stroke, with further increases in the subsequent days. The increases in CRP and WBC were observed later, starting on the third and seventh days after the stroke, respectively. Folyovich et al. made a similar observation, reporting that the suPAR concentrations increased immediately after the stroke and continued to increase for the next seven days, while CRP and WBC increased only on the seventh day after the stroke [31].

Based on our results, a suPAR-1 concentration above 7.64 ng/mL increases the mortality risk almost threefold, while a suPAR-3 concentration above 10.49 ng/mL increases the mortality risk by up to eightfold. We also found that an NIHSS score of >12 on the first day after a stroke increases the mortality risk threefold. At the same time, a CRP-3 concentration >15.6 mg/L was associated with a fivefold increase in the mortality risk. The prognostic value of WBC was found to be significant only on the seventh day following the stroke, doubling the mortality risk. The AUC in the ROC analysis for suPAR-3 was the largest, amounting to 0.89, and this parameter had the highest prognostic value on the third day after the stroke.

The concentration of suPAR, similar to that of CRP, plays an important role in predicting the course of disease and the risk of mortality among patients with life-threatening conditions. This argument applies not only to stroke but also to cancer and infectious diseases. The relationship between suPAR levels and mortality risk has been observed in malaria, tuberculosis, HIV infections, urinary tract infections and bacterial meningitis, as well as in neoplastic diseases, such as colorectal cancer, ovarian cancer and multiple myeloma [44–50]. Increased suPAR concentrations indicated a poor prognosis in bacteraemia [51,52], and its prognostic role was also demonstrated in patients with acute respiratory distress syndrome (ARDS)—i.e., the suPAR concentration correlated with the severity of ARDS [53]. In HIV infections, a higher concentration of suPAR was observed in patients with a lower number of $CD4^+$ lymphocytes, a higher viral load and greater AIDS-related mortality. Patients diagnosed with fatal sepsis also had significantly higher suPAR concentrations than those with non-fatal sepsis. As a single biomarker, suPAR had a higher prognostic value than CRP and PCT, increasing even further when analysed in combination with the above biomarkers. Increased concentrations of suPAR were associated with an increased likelihood of being transferred to the intensive care unit [54,55]. Moreover, in this case, the suPAR concentrations correlated with the assessment scales typically used in intensive care units, such as APACHE-II, SAPS-II or SOFA. Donadello et al. demonstrated that, in sepsis, a suPAR concentration of >5.5 ng/mL has a high prognostic value, exceeding that of both CRP and PCT [56]. Donadello et al. pointed out that sepsis generates many reactions from both inflammatory and anti-inflammatory mediators, activating cellular and also humoral responses. Likewise, in a study by Kofoed et al., the prognostic value of suPAR was compared with that of CRP and PCT in patients with sepsis [55,56]. The prognostic value of suPAR was higher than that of other markers and was comparable to the SOFA or SAPS II score; further, combining suPAR with age generated a better prognostic result than the SAPS II score alone.

4.1. Markers of Inflammation in Stroke

Emsley et al. reported that the CRP concentrations may already be elevated on the day of the stroke, with the highest concentrations occurring 5 to 7 days thereafter and remaining stable for the subsequent three months [57]. These results are similar to those reported in our study, although the time points were slightly different. Additionally, the dynamics of changes in leukocyte counts reported by Emsley et al. were slightly different than those we reported. On the first day of measurement, the number of WBC did not exceed the reference values (9.8 thousand/mm^3), although they did significantly differ from those in the control group (6.2 thousand/mm^3). Emsley et al. also observed an increase in the number of WBC above the normal count between five and seven days following stroke and, as in the case of CRP, these values were maintained for three months thereafter. These observations were made after the exclusion of the infectious factor on admission to the hospital. According to the authors, two mechanisms may be the cause of the increase in CRP and WBC. On the one hand, strokes cause the rapid activation of the immune system, which persists in the first days following the stroke; on the other hand, it is possible that increased levels of inflammatory parameters may result from a "low-activity" inflammatory process preceding the stroke, one that develops asymptomatically in the body, contributing to the vascular incident.

The above hypothesis could be confirmed by observations made by Rost et al., which also indicated the contribution of a "low-activity" inflammatory process to the aetiology of stroke and transient cerebral ischemia [58]. During 12 to 14 years of observation, the authors found that CRP concentrations in the upper range of normal values increased the risk of ischemic brain incidents threefold in women and twofold in men, including after considering the co-occurrence of risk factors such as smoking, cholesterol, systolic blood pressure or type 2 diabetes mellitus. The authors stated that the relationship between CRP concentrations and risk of stroke was linear and that the high values of this relationship can be treated as an independent risk factor for stroke. A similar relationship has also been demonstrated for both stroke and ischemic heart disease [41,59–63]. This was confirmed by observations of patients for whom the use of rosuvastatin resulted in a decrease in CRP concentrations with a simultaneous decrease in the risk of myocardial infarction [64,65].

Studies on unstable atherosclerotic plaque in the carotid arteries have shown that their inflammatory activity increases shortly after the ischemic incident and decreases as the atherosclerotic plaque stabilises [66]. Symptomatic atherosclerotic plaque within the carotid arteries may differ in composition, and, thus, in symptomatology, and the nature of plaque damage, e.g., in amaurosis fugax, differs from that observed in transient cerebral ischemia or stroke [67,68]. Therefore, suPAR concentrations may be a potential marker of inflammatory process activity in atherosclerotic plaque and serve as a measure of its stability. Olson et al. reported elevated suPAR levels immediately after the vascular incident in patients with both ischemic stroke and transient cerebral ischemia [69]. By measuring the suPAR concentrations in blood flowing through carotid arteries containing unstable atherosclerotic plaque and comparing them with suPAR concentrations in blood flowing through the radial artery and the antecubital fossa vein, the authors demonstrated that suPAR can be released through the plaque. However, statistical analysis did not determine whether the assessment of suPAR concentrations could provide knowledge about the inflammatory process activity in the plaque or whether such knowledge was restricted to assessing the risk of ischemia development in the course of atherosclerosis. A correlation between suPAR concentrations and age and the coexistence of diabetes was found. In a paper by Elkind et al., the results of studies of patients who underwent internal carotid endarterectomy were analysed [70]. Blood samples collected a day before the procedure showed significantly higher suPAR concentrations in patients with symptomatic plaques than in patients with asymptomatic plaques, but there was no correlation between suPAR concentrations in plaques and plasma levels in the same patient. The suPAR concentration positively correlated with the concentrations of other biomarkers of inflammation, such as high-sensitive CRP (hsCRP) and creatinine, as well as tumour necrosis factor-α (TNF-α), interleukin-1b (IL-1b) or interleukin-6 (IL-6). The suPAR concentration in both atherosclerotic plaque and plasma correlated positively with risk factors such as age, presence of diabetes and female sex. Atherosclerotic plaque damage results in a series of cellular and molecular damage, including lipoproteins, morphotic elements, mechanical vascular damage and inflammatory factors [71]. CRP and suPAR, as acute-phase proteins, are an indicator of the ongoing inflammatory process and highlight the advancement of atherosclerotic plaque [72]. Although they are not stroke-specific markers, such as interleukin 1 (Il-1), interleukin 6 (Il-6) or tumour necrosis factor-α (TNF-α), they suggest the existence of immunological activation in the course of the inflammatory process and tissue damage [58].

Thus, patients with stroke with a thrombotic aetiology, underlying the atherosclerotic plaque process even before the stroke, may show higher concentrations of suPAR and CRP compared to patients with stroke with a cardiovascular aetiology [27]. However, the growth of these markers often takes place within the accepted normal ranges [13]. The gold standard for the evaluation of this process in clinical practice is the determination of high-sensitivity CRP, but the role of suPAR as a more stable molecule, and thus having a greater practical application, is also increasingly indicated [66,73].

Idicula et al. observed that the median CRP concentration on hospital admission was 3 mg/L—but, in some patients, the stroke symptoms increased despite the absence of infection, which was positively correlated with the neurological condition assessed on the NIHSS on admission [74]. High levels of CRP on admission were positively correlated with worse functional status on discharge (measured using the Rankin and Barthel scales) and high mortality rates estimated 2.5 years after stroke. The research also confirmed the positive correlation between suPAR and CRP concentrations and the functional status of patients. Idicula et al. also stated that, in cardiovascular stroke, the CRP concentration after the stroke was higher than that in thrombotic stroke, likely due to higher severity, which leads to higher activation of the immune system [74].

4.2. The Role of Lymphocytes

Many authors, in addition to evaluating the usefulness of commonly used markers of inflammation, such as suPAR, CRP and WBC, have highlighted the role of T lymphocytes in immune processes in the course of a stroke. In the analysis by Folyovich et al., it was noted that, in the first hours after a stroke, the number of CD64$^+$ lymphocytes suddenly increased and then dropped to lower values than in the control group after seven days [31]. Observing this correlation, the authors suggested that there were two-phase changes in the immune system: the initial activation of the immune system is followed by its suppression, which may result in the development of a secondary infection. The authors assumed that, on the basis of observation of the dynamics of CD64$^+$ lymphocyte count changes, it is possible to obtain reliable information about the risk of infection development in the days following stroke. Vogelgesang et al., on the other hand, found that stroke causes an immediate and significant decrease in the number of peripheral CD4$^+$ and CD8$^+$ lymphocytes [75]. This decrease is most visible in the first 12 h after the stroke, while, in the following days, it gradually returns to normal values. They also showed that normalisation is delayed in patients with follow-up infection. They assumed that the fluctuations in CD4$^+$ and CD8$^+$ lymphocytes were due to the fact that stroke leads not only to a local inflammatory nervous tissue response reflected in a generalised inflammatory response but also to significant immunosuppression associated with a decrease in peripheral T lymphocytes. This number, determined one day after a stroke, may also be a prognostic factor in the onset of post-stroke infection. In this study, an inverse correlation between the number of T lymphocytes and the NIHSS results was also found. This means that the degree of immunosuppression is reflected in an increasing neurological deficit. The increase in the number of WBC in the work of Vogelgesang et al. was observed at the time of admission, and, in consecutive days of hospitalisation (2nd, 7th and 14th), increased values were observed [75]. In our own observations, an increase in the number of WBC occurred only on the seventh day after stroke, constituting an active parameter but one that is not very useful in the first days after the vascular incident.

Yan et al. observed a significant increase in the number of CD4$^+$ lymphocytes immediately after stroke [29]. This lymphocytic line includes regulatory T lymphocytes, which play a role in suppressing the immune response, maintaining immune homeostasis and preventing autoimmunity. It was found that activated T lymphocytes, penetrating through the blood–brain barrier, contribute to secondary damage to nerve tissue in the ischemic zone. It is possible, however, that they also play a protective or regenerative and repairing role within the damaged tissue. This may be due to the presence of cytokines and growth factors supplied by lymphocytes to the lesion site as well as the modulation of microglia activation [76,77].

4.3. suPAR and Stroke Risk Factors

In our study, we observed that the coexistence of diseases such as ischemic heart disease, hypertension and type 2 diabetes resulted in higher concentrations of suPAR and CRP in patients in comparison to those not affected by these diseases. In the group of patients with hypercholesterolemia, no differences in suPAR concentration were observed, and higher CRP concentrations were observed only in the patients on the seventh day after stroke. In the patients with atrial fibrillation, no significant differences in the parameters were found. Cigarette smokers differed only in the range of suPAR-3, suPAR-7 and CRP-7. Similar observations were made by many researchers. Haupt et al. found that suPAR levels were elevated in patients with hypertension, diabetes, smoking, alcohol consumption and an unhealthy diet [78]. Higher suPAR concentrations were also found in patients with previous myocardial infarction. On the other hand, the suPAR concentrations among those who quit smoking were comparable to those of patients who never smoked. Concentrations of suPAR were also closely related to biochemical parameters, such as total cholesterol and TG. It was also observed that risk factors such as hypertension, ischemic heart disease, type 2 diabetes and cigarette smoking increase the mortality risk in patients with stroke. These data are consistent with the observations made by Rallidis et al., who observed a significantly higher mortality rate in patients with hypertension and diabetes [79]. However, they did not observe these correlations in patients with ischemic heart disease, hypercholesterolemia, smoking and obesity. The above-mentioned authors also observed that the CRP concentrations were significantly elevated at the time of hospital admission among patients who later died. This parameter was an independent prognostic factor of early mortality-related complications. An increase in CRP concentrations by one unit caused an increase in the risk of early death by 14%.

On the other hand, Persson et al. noted that elevated suPAR concentrations occur in patients with ischemic heart disease and smokers [65]. In their analysis of smokers and non-smokers, they demonstrated that the risk of cardiovascular disease was related to the concentrations of suPAR in both groups. The authors also found a correlation between the concentration of Lp-PLA2 protein and the risk of cardiovascular disease. Concentrations of suPAR were only poorly associated with other markers of inflammation, such as hsCRP and WBC, which is consistent with other publications [52,80].

5. Conclusions

To conclude, suPAR can serve as a biomarker of mortality risk in patients with ischemic stroke. The plasma concentration of suPAR increases on the first day following the ischemic stroke and corresponds with the severity of the disease.

Author Contributions: Conceptualization, K.Ś., D.K., R.P. and P.J. Methodology, K.Ś., M.Ś., R.P. and P.J. Formal Analysis, K.Ś. and M.Ś. Investigation, K.Ś., M.Ś. and R.P. Writing—Original Draft Preparation K.Ś. and M.Ś. Writing—Review & Editing, R.P., D.K. and P.J. Supervision D.K. and P.J. Funding Acquisition K.Ś. All authors have read and agreed to the published version of the manuscript.

Funding: K.S. received a grant from Medical University of Silesia for Ph.D. students (grant number: KNW-2-023/D/4/N).

Institutional Review Board Statement: The study was conducted according to the guidelines of the Declaration of Helsinki and approved by the Institutional Review Board (or Ethics Committee) of Bioethics Committee of Medical University of Silesia in Katowice (KNW/0022/KB/85/13).

Informed Consent Statement: Patient consent was waived based on Bioethics Committee agreement due to the use of the residual blood.

Data Availability Statement: The data presented in this study are available on request from the corresponding author. The data are not publicly available due to privacy issues.

Conflicts of Interest: Authors declare no conflict of interest.

References

1. Sacco, R.L.; Adams, R.; Albers, G.; Alberts, M.J.; Benavente, O.; Furie, K.; Goldstein, L.B.; Gorelick, P.; Halperin, J.; Harbaugh, R.; et al. Guidelines for prevention of stroke in patients with ischemic stroke or transient ischemic attack: A statement for healthcare professionals from the American Heart Association/American Stroke Association Council on Stroke: Co-sponsored by the Council on Cardiovascular Radiology and Intervention: The American Academy of Neurology affirms the value of this guideline. *Stroke* **2006**, *37*, 577–617. [PubMed]
2. Katan, M.; Luft, A. Global Burden of Stroke. *Skull Base* **2018**, *38*, 208–211. [CrossRef] [PubMed]
3. Global, regional, and national burden of stroke and its risk factors, 1990-2019: A systematic analysis for the Global Burden of Disease Study 2019. *Lancet Neurol.* **2021**, *20*, 795–820. [CrossRef]
4. Meschia, J.F.; Bushnell, C.; Boden-Albala, B.; Braun, L.T.; Bravata, D.M.; Chaturvedi, S.; Creager, M.A.; Eckel, R.H.; Elkind, M.S.V.; Fornage, M.; et al. Guidelines for the primary prevention of stroke: A statement for healthcare professionals from the American Heart Association/American Stroke Association. *Stroke* **2014**, *45*, 3754–3832. [CrossRef]
5. Donkor, E.S. Stroke in the21stCentury: A Snapshot of the Burden, Epidemiology, and Quality of Life. *Stroke Res. Treat.* **2018**, *2018*, 3238165. [CrossRef]
6. Brønnum-Hansen, H.; Davidsen, M.; Thorvaldsen, P. Long-Term Survival and Causes of Death After Stroke. *Stroke* **2001**, *32*, 2131–2136. [CrossRef]
7. Donnan, G.A.; Fisher, M.; Macleod, M.; Davis, S.M. Stroke. *Lancet* **2008**, *371*, 1612–1623. [CrossRef]
8. Flynn, R.; MacWalter, R.; Doney, A. The cost of cerebral ischaemia. *Neuropharmacology* **2008**, *55*, 250–256. [CrossRef]
9. Javidi, E.; Magnus, T. Autoimmunity After Ischemic Stroke and Brain Injury. *Front. Immunol.* **2019**, *10*, 686. [CrossRef]
10. Kofoed, K.; Andersen, O.; Kronborg, G.; Tvede, M.; Petersen, J.; Eugen-Olsen, J.; Larsen, K. Use of plasma C-reactive protein, procalcitonin, neutrophils, macrophage migration inhibitory factor, soluble urokinase-type plasminogen activator receptor, and soluble triggering receptor expressed on myeloid cells-1 in combination to diagnose infections: A prospective study. *Crit. Care* **2007**, *11*, R38. [CrossRef]
11. Sproston, N.R.; Ashworth, J.J. Role of C-Reactive Protein at Sites of Inflammation and Infection. *Front. Immunol.* **2018**, *9*, 754. [CrossRef]
12. Li, P.; Gao, Y.; Ji, Z.; Zhang, X.; Xu, Q.; Li, G.; Guo, Z.; Zheng, B.; Guo, X. Role of urokinase plasminogen activator and its receptor in metastasis and invasion of neuroblastoma. *J. Pediatr. Surg.* **2004**, *39*, 1512–1519. [CrossRef]
13. Persson, M.; Östling, G.; Smith, G.; Hamrefors, V.; Melander, O.; Hedblad, B.; Engström, G. Soluble urokinase plasminogen activator receptor: A risk factor for carotid plaque, stroke, and coronary artery disease. *Stroke* **2014**, *45*, 18–23. [CrossRef] [PubMed]
14. Riisbro, R.; Christensen, I.; Høgdall, C.; Brünner, N. Soluble Urokinase Plasminogen Activator Receptor Measurements: Influence of Sample Handling. *Int. J. Biol. Markers* **2001**, *16*, 233–239. [CrossRef] [PubMed]
15. Thunø, M.; Macho, B.; Eugen-Olsen, J. suPAR: The molecular crystal ball. *Dis. Markers* **2009**, *27*, 157–172. [CrossRef] [PubMed]
16. Mahmood, N.; Mihalcioiu, C.; Rabbani, S.A. Multifaceted Role of the Urokinase-Type Plasminogen Activator (uPA) and Its Receptor (uPAR): Diagnostic, Prognostic, and Therapeutic Applications. *Front. Oncol.* **2018**, *8*, 24. [CrossRef]
17. De Lorenzi, V.; Sarra Ferraris, G.M.; Madsen, J.B.; Lupia, M.; Andreasen, P.A.; Sidenius, N. Urokinase links plasminogen activation and cell adhesion by cleavage of the RGD motif in vitronectin. *EMBO Rep.* **2016**, *17*, 982–998. [CrossRef] [PubMed]
18. Shah, P.K. Mechanisms of plaque vulnerability and rupture. *J. Am. Coll. Cardiol.* **2003**, *41*, S15–S22. [CrossRef]
19. Nicholl, S.M.; Roztocil, E.; Davies, M.G. Plasminogen Activator System and Vascular Disease. *Curr. Vasc. Pharm.* **2006**, *4*, 101–116. [CrossRef]
20. Fuhrman, B. The urokinase system in the pathogenesis of atherosclerosis. *Atherosclerosis* **2012**, *222*, 8–14. [CrossRef] [PubMed]
21. Skålén, K.; Gustafsson, M.; Rydberg, E.K.; Hultén, L.M.; Wiklund, O.; Innerarity, T.L.; Borén, J. Subendothelial retention of atherogenic lipoproteins in early atherosclerosis. *Nature* **2002**, *417*, 750–754. [CrossRef] [PubMed]
22. Hansson, G.K. Inflammation, Atherosclerosis, and Coronary Artery Disease. *N. Engl. J. Med.* **2005**, *352*, 1685–1695. [CrossRef] [PubMed]
23. Newby, A.C. Metalloproteinases and Vulnerable Atherosclerotic Plaques. *Trends Cardiovasc. Med.* **2007**, *17*, 253–258. [CrossRef]
24. Collen, D. The plasminogen (fibrinolytic) system. *Thromb. Haemost.* **1999**, *82*, 259–270. [CrossRef]
25. Beaufort, N.; LeDuc, D.; Rousselle, J.-C.; Magdolen, V.; Luther, T.; Namane, A.; Chignard, M.; Pidard, D. Proteolytic Regulation of the Urokinase Receptor/CD87 on Monocytic Cells by Neutrophil Elastase and Cathepsin G. *J. Immunol.* **2003**, *172*, 540–549. [CrossRef]
26. Svensson, P.A.; Olson, F.J.; Hägg, D.A.; Ryndel, M.; Wiklund, O.; Karlström, L.; Hulthe, J.; Carlsson, L.M.S.; Fagerberg, B. Urokinase-type plasminogen activator receptor is associated with macrophages and plaque rupture in symptomatic carotid atherosclerosis. *Int. J. Mol. Med.* **2008**, *22*, 459–464. [PubMed]
27. Persson, M.; Engström, G.; Björkbacka, H.; Hedblad, B. Soluble urokinase plasminogen activator receptor in plasma is associated with incidence of CVD. Results from the Malmö Diet and Cancer Study. *Atherosclerosis* **2012**, *220*, 502–505. [CrossRef] [PubMed]
28. Offner, H.; Subramanian, S.; Parker, S.M.; E Afentoulis, M.; A Vandenbark, A.; Hurn, P.D. Experimental Stroke Induces Massive, Rapid Activation of the Peripheral Immune System. *J. Cereb. Blood Flow Metab.* **2005**, *26*, 654–665. [CrossRef]

29. Yan, J.; Greer, J.; Etherington, K.; Cadigan, G.P.; Cavanagh, H.; Henderson, R.D.; O'Sullivan, J.; Pandian, J.D.; Read, S.; McCombe, P.A. Immune activation in the peripheral blood of patients with acute ischemic stroke. *J. Neuroimmunol.* **2009**, *206*, 112–117. [CrossRef]

30. Arumugam, T.; Granger, D.N.; Mattson, M.P. Stroke and T-Cells. *Neuromolecular Med.* **2005**, *7*, 229–242. [CrossRef]

31. Folyovich, A.; Biro, E.M.; Orbán, C.; Bajnok, A.; Varga, V.; Béres-Molnár, K.A.; Vásárhelyi, B.; Toldi, G. Relevance of novel inflammatory markers in stroke-induced immunosuppression. *Bmc Neurol.* **2014**, *14*, 41. [CrossRef] [PubMed]

32. Yilmaz, G.; Arumugam, T.V.; Stokes, K.Y.; Granger, D.N. Role of T lymphocytes and interferon-gamma in ischemic stroke. *Circulation* **2006**, *113*, 2105–2112. [CrossRef] [PubMed]

33. Loddick, S.A.; Turnbull, A.V.; Rothwell, N.J. Cerebral Interleukin-6 is Neuroprotective during Permanent Focal Cerebral Ischemia in the Rat. *J. Cereb. Blood Flow Metab.* **1998**, *18*, 176–179. [CrossRef] [PubMed]

34. Schroeter, M.; Jander, S.; Witte, O.W.; Stoll, G. Local immune responses in the rat cerebral cortex after middle cerebral artery occlusion. *J. Neuroimmunol.* **1994**, *55*, 195–203. [CrossRef]

35. Chatila, T.A. Role of regulatory T cells in human diseases. *J. Allergy Clin. Immunol.* **2005**, *116*, 949–959. [CrossRef]

36. Neumann, S.; Shields, N.J.; Balle, T.; Chebib, M.; Clarkson, A.N. Innate Immunity and Inflammation Post-Stroke: An α7-Nicotinic Agonist Perspective. *Int. J. Mol. Sci.* **2015**, *16*, 29029–29046. [CrossRef]

37. Faura, J.; Bustamante, A.; Miró-Mur, F.; Montaner, J. Stroke-induced immunosuppression: Implications for the prevention and prediction of post-stroke infections. *J. Neuroinflammation* **2021**, *18*, 127. [CrossRef]

38. Vargas, M.; Horcajada, J.P.; Obach, V.; Revilla, M.; Cervera, A.; Torres, F.; Planas, A.M.; Mensa, J.; Chamorro, Á. Clinical consequences of infection in patients with acute stroke: Is it prime time for further antibiotic trials? *Stroke* **2006**, *37*, 461–465. [CrossRef]

39. Weimar, C.; Roth, M.P.; Zillessen, G.; Glahn, J.; Wimmer, M.L.; Busse, O.; Haberl, R.L.; Diener, H.-C. German Stroke Data Bank Collaborators. Complications following Acute Ischemic Stroke. *Eur. Neurol.* **2002**, *48*, 133–140. [CrossRef]

40. Syrjänen, J.; Teppo, A.M.; Valtonen, V.V.; Iivanainen, M.; Maury, C.P. Acute phase response in cerebral infarction. *J. Clin. Pathol.* **1989**, *42*, 63–68. [CrossRef]

41. Muir, K.W.; Weir, C.; Alwan, W.; Squire, I.B.; Lees, K.R. C-Reactive Protein and Outcome After Ischemic Stroke. *Stroke* **1999**, *30*, 981–985. [CrossRef] [PubMed]

42. Vila, N.; Filella, X.; Deulofeu, R.; Ascaso, C.; Abellana, R.; Chamorro, A. Cytokine-induced inflammation and long-term stroke functional outcome. *J. Neurol. Sci.* **1999**, *162*, 185–188. [CrossRef]

43. Boysen, G.; Christensen, H. Stroke severity determines body temperature in acute stroke. *Stroke* **2001**, *32*, 413–417. [CrossRef] [PubMed]

44. Eugen-Olsen, J.; Gustafson, P.; Sidenius, N.; Fischer, T.K.; Parner, J.; Aaby, P.; Gomes, V.F.; Lisse, I. The serum level of soluble urokinase receptor is elevated in tuberculosis patients and predicts mortality during treatment: A community study from Guinea-Bissau. *Int. J. Tuberc. Lung Dis.* **2002**, *6*, 686–692. [PubMed]

45. Ostrowski, S.R.; Ullum, H.; Goka, B.Q.; Høyer-Hansen, G.; Obeng-Adjei, G.; Pedersen, B.K.; Akanmori, B.D.; Kurtzhals, J.A.L. Plasma concentrations of soluble urokinase-type plasminogen activator receptor are increased in patients with malaria and are associated with a poor clinical or a fatal outcome. *J. Infect. Dis.* **2005**, *191*, 1331–1341. [CrossRef]

46. Rabna, P.; Andersen, A.; Wejse, C.; Oliveira, I.; Gomes, V.F.; Haaland, M.B.; Aaby, P.; Eugen-Olsen, J. High mortality risk among individuals assumed to be TB-negative can be predicted using a simple test. *Trop. Med. Int. Heal.* **2009**, *14*, 986–994. [CrossRef]

47. Ostrowski, S.R.; Piironen, T.; Høyer-Hansen, G.; Gerstoft, J.; Pedersen, B.K.; Ullum, H. High plasma levels of intact and cleaved soluble urokinase receptor reflect immune activation and are independent predictors of mortality in HIV-1-infected patients. *J. Acquir. Immune Defic. Syndr.* **2005**, *39*, 23–31. [CrossRef]

48. Lawn, S.D.; Myer, L.; Bangani, N.; Vogt, M.; Wood, R. Plasma levels of soluble urokinase-type plasminogen activator receptor (suPAR) and early mortality risk among patients enrolling for antiretroviral treatment in South Africa. *Bmc Infect. Dis.* **2007**, *7*, 41. [CrossRef]

49. Florquin, S.; Berg, J.G.V.D.; Olszyna, D.P.; Claessen, N.; Opal, S.M.; Weening, J.J.; Van Der Poll, T. Release of urokinase plasminogen activator receptor during urosepsis and endotoxemia. *Kidney Int.* **2001**, *59*, 2054–2061. [CrossRef] [PubMed]

50. Lomholt, A.F.; Christensen, I.J.; Høyer-Hansen, G.; Nielsen, H.J. Prognostic value of intact and cleaved forms of the urokinase plasminogen activator receptor in a retrospective study of 518 colorectal cancer patients. *Acta Oncol.* **2010**, *49*, 805–811. [CrossRef]

51. Wittenhagen, P.; Kronborg, G.; Weis, N.; Nielsen, H.; Obel, N.; Pedersen, S.; Eugen-Olsen, J. The plasma level of soluble urokinase receptor is elevated in patients with Streptococcus pneumoniae bacteraemia and predicts mortality. *Clin. Microbiol. Infect.* **2004**, *10*, 409–415. [CrossRef] [PubMed]

52. Eugen-Olsen, J.; Andersen, O.; Linneberg, A.; Ladelund, S.; Hansen, T.; Langkilde, A.; Petersen, J.; Pielak, T.; Møller, L.N.; Jeppesen, J.; et al. Circulating soluble urokinase plasminogen activator receptor predicts cancer, cardiovascular disease, diabetes and mortality in the general population. *J. Intern. Med.* **2010**, *268*, 296–308. [CrossRef] [PubMed]

53. Geboers, D.G.P.J.; De Beer, F.M.; Boer, A.M.T.-D.; Van Der Poll, T.; Horn, J.; Cremer, O.L.; Bonten, M.J.M.; Ong, D.; Schultz, M.J.; Bos, L.D.J. Plasma suPAR as a prognostic biological marker for ICU mortality in ARDS patients. *Intensiv. Care Med.* **2015**, *41*, 1281–1290. [CrossRef]

54. Koch, A.; Voigt, S.; Kruschinski, C.; Sanson, E.; Dückers, H.; Horn, A.; Yagmur, E.; Zimmermann, H.; Trautwein, C.; Tacke, F. Circulating soluble urokinase plasminogen activator receptor is stably elevated during the first week of treatment in the intensive care unit and predicts mortality in critically ill patients. *Crit. Care* **2011**, *15*, R63. [CrossRef] [PubMed]

55. Kofoed, K.; Eugen-Olsen, J.; Petersen, J.; Larsen, K.; Andersen, O. Predicting mortality in patients with systemic inflammatory response syndrome: An evaluation of two prognostic models, two soluble receptors, and a macrophage migration inhibitory factor. *Eur. J. Clin. Microbiol.* **2008**, *27*, 375–383. [CrossRef]

56. Donadello, K.; Scolletta, S.; Covajes, C.; Vincent, J.-L. suPAR as a prognostic biomarker in sepsis. *Bmc Med.* **2012**, *10*, 2. [CrossRef]

57. Emsley, H.C.; Smith, C.J.; Gavin, C.M.; Georgiou, R.F.; Vail, A.; Barberan, E.M.; Hallenbecke, J.M.; del Zoppof, G.J.; Rothwellg, N.J.; Tyrrellab, P.J.; et al. An early and sustained peripheral inflammatory response in acute ischaemic stroke: Relationships with infection and atherosclerosis. *J. Neuroimmunol.* **2003**, *139*, 93–101. [CrossRef]

58. Rost, N.S.; Wolf, P.A.; Kase, C.S.; Kelly-Hayes, M.; Silbershatz, H.; Massaro, J.; D'Agostino, R.B.; Franzblau, C.; Wilson, P.W. Plasma Concentration of C-Reactive Protein and Risk of Ischemic Stroke and Transient Ischemic Attack: The Framingham Study. *Stroke* **2001**, *32*, 2575–2579. [CrossRef]

59. Anuk, T.; Assayag, E.B.; Rotstein, R.; Fusman, R.; Zeltser, D.; Berliner, S.; Avitzour, D.; Shapira, I.; Arber, N.; Bornstein, N.M. Prognostic implications of admission inflammatory profile in acute ischemic neurological events. *Acta Neurol. Scand.* **2002**, *106*, 196–199. [CrossRef]

60. Arenillas, J.F.; Alvarez-Sabin, J.; Molina, C.A.; Chacoón, P.; Montaner, J.; Rovira, A.; Ibarra, B.; Quintana, M. C-Reactive Protein Predicts Further Ischemic Events in First-Ever Transient Ischemic Attack or Stroke Patients With Intracranial Large-Artery Occlusive Disease. *Stroke* **2003**, *34*, 2463–2468. [CrossRef]

61. Christensen, H.; Boysen, G. C-Reactive Protein and White Blood Cell Count Increases in the First 24 Hours after Acute Stroke. *Cereb. Dis.* **2004**, *18*, 214–219. [CrossRef]

62. Di Napoli, M.; Papa, F.; Bocola, V. C-reactive protein in ischemic stroke: An independent prognostic factor. *Stroke* **2001**, *32*, 917–924. [CrossRef]

63. Elkind, M.S.V.; Tai, W.; Coates, K.; Paik, M.C.; Sacco, R.L. High-Sensitivity C-Reactive Protein, Lipoprotein-Associated Phospholipase A2, and Outcome After Ischemic Stroke. *Arch. Intern. Med.* **2006**, *166*, 2073–2080. [CrossRef] [PubMed]

64. Danesh, J.; Whincup, P.; Walker, M.; Lennon, L.; Thomson, A.; Appleby, P.; Gallimore, J.R.; Pepys, M.B. Low grade inflammation and coronary heart disease: Prospective study and updated meta-analyses. *BMJ* **2000**, *321*, 199–204. [CrossRef] [PubMed]

65. Ridker, P.M.; Danielson, E.; Fonseca, F.A.; Genest, J.; Gotto, A.M., Jr.; Kastelein, J.J.; Koenig, W.; Libby, P.; Lorenzatti, A.J.; MacFadyen, J.G.; et al. Rosuvastatin to Prevent Vascular Events in Men and Women with Elevated C-Reactive Protein. *N. Engl. J. Med.* **2008**, *359*, 2195–2207. [CrossRef] [PubMed]

66. Redgrave, J.; Lovett, J.; Gallagher, P.; Rothwell, P. Histological Assessment of 526 Symptomatic Carotid Plaques in Relation to the Nature and Timing of Ischemic Symptoms. *Circulation* **2006**, *113*, 2320–2328. [CrossRef] [PubMed]

67. Golledge, J.; Cuming, R.; Beattie, D.K.; Davies, A.H.; Greenhalgh, R.M. Influence of patient-related variables on the outcome of carotid endarterectomy. *J. Vasc. Surg.* **1996**, *24*, 120–126. [CrossRef]

68. Benavente, O.; Eliasziw, M.; Streifler, J.Y.; Fox, A.J.; Barnett, H.J.; Meldrum, H. Prognosis after Transient Monocular Blindness Associated with Carotid-Artery Stenosis. *N. Engl. J. Med.* **2001**, *345*, 1084–1090. [CrossRef]

69. Olson, F.J.; Thurison, T.; Ryndel, M.; Høyer-Hansen, G.; Fagerberg, B. Soluble urokinase-type plasminogen activator receptor forms in plasma as markers of atherosclerotic plaque vulnerability. *Clin. Biochem.* **2010**, *43*, 124–130. [CrossRef]

70. Elkind, M.S.V.; Luna, J.M.; McClure, L.A.; Zhang, Y.; Coffey, C.S.; Roldan, A.; Del Brutto, O.H.; Pretell, E.J.; Pettigrew, L.C.; Meyer, B.C.; et al. C-reactive protein as a prognostic marker after lacunar stroke: Levels of inflammatory markers in the treatment of stroke study. *Stroke* **2014**, *45*, 707–716. [CrossRef]

71. Ross, R. Atherosclerosis is an inflammatory disease. *N. Engl. J. Med.* **1999**, *340*, 115–126. [CrossRef] [PubMed]

72. Elias-Smale, S.E.; Kardys, I.; Oudkerk, M.; Hofman, A.; Witteman, J.C. C-reactive protein is related to extent and progression of coronary and extra-coronary atherosclerosis; results from the Rotterdam study. *Atherosclerosis* **2007**, *195*, e195–e202. [CrossRef] [PubMed]

73. Musunuru, K.; Kral, B.G.; Blumenthal, R.S.; Fuster, V.; Campbell, C.Y.; Gluckman, T.J.; A Lange, R.; Topol, E.; Willerson, J.T.; Desai, M.Y.; et al. The use of high-sensitivity assays for C-reactive protein in clinical practice. *Nat. Clin. Pr. Cardiovasc. Med.* **2008**, *5*, 621–635. [CrossRef]

74. Idicula, T.T.; Brøgger, J.C.; Naess, H.; Waje-Andreassen, U.; Thomassen, L. Admission C—Reactive protein after acute ischemic stroke is associated with stroke severity and mortality: The 'Bergen stroke study'. *Bmc Neurol.* **2009**, *9*, 18. [CrossRef] [PubMed]

75. Vogelgesang, A.; Grunwald, U.; Langner, S.; Jack, R.; Bröker, B.; Kessler, C.; Dressel, A. Analysis of Lymphocyte Subsets in Patients With Stroke and Their Influence on Infection After Stroke. *Stroke* **2008**, *39*, 237–241. [CrossRef] [PubMed]

76. Stoll, G.; Jander, S.; Schroeter, M. Detrimental and beneficial effects of injury-induced inflammation and cytokine expression in the nervous system. *Adv. Exp. Med. Biol.* **2002**, *513*, 87–113.

77. Sallusto, F.; Geginat, J.; Lanzavecchia, A. Central Memory and Effector Memory T Cell Subsets: Function, Generation, and Maintenance. *Annu. Rev. Immunol.* **2004**, *22*, 745–763. [CrossRef]

78. Haupt, T.; Kallemose, T.; Ladelund, S.; Rasmussen, L.J.H.; Thorball, C.W.; Andersen, O.; Pisinger, C.; Eugen-Olsen, J. Risk Factors Associated with Serum Levels of the Inflammatory Biomarker Soluble Urokinase Plasminogen Activator Receptor in a General Population. *Biomark. Insights* **2014**, *9*, 91–100. [CrossRef]

79. Rallidis, L.S.; Vikelis, M.; Panagiotakos, D.B.; Rizos, I.; Zolindaki, M.G.; Kaliva, K.; Kremastinos, D.T. Inflammatory markers and in-hospital mortality in acute ischaemic stroke. *Atherosclerosis* **2006**, *189*, 193–197. [CrossRef]
80. Andersen, O.; Eugen-Olsen, J.; Kofoed, K.; Iversen, J.; Haugaard, S.B. Soluble urokinase plasminogen activator receptor is a marker of dysmetabolism in HIV-infected patients receiving highly active antiretroviral therapy. *J. Med. Virol.* **2008**, *80*, 209–216. [CrossRef]

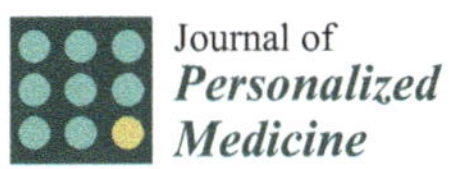

Journal of
Personalized
Medicine

Article

Assessment of Sleep among Patients with Chronic Liver Disease: Association with Quality of Life

Oana-Mihaela Plotogea [1,2], Gina Gheorghe [1,2], Madalina Stan-Ilie [1,2], Gabriel Constantinescu [1,2], Nicolae Bacalbasa [3], Simona Bungau [4] and Camelia Cristina Diaconu [1,5,*]

1   Department 5, "Carol Davila" University of Medicine and Pharmacy, 050474 Bucharest, Romania; plotogea.oana@gmail.com (O.-M.P.); gheorghe_gina2000@yahoo.com (G.G.); drmadalina@gmail.com (M.S.-I.); gabrielconstantinescu63@gmail.com (G.C.)
2   Department of Gastroenterology, Clinical Emergency Hospital of Bucharest, 105402 Bucharest, Romania
3   Department of Visceral Surgery, "Carol Davila" University of Medicine and Pharmacy, Center of Excellence in Translational Medicine, "Fundeni" Clinical Institute, 022328 Bucharest, Romania; nicolae_bacalbasa@yahoo.ro
4   Department of Pharmacy, Faculty of Medicine and Pharmacy, University of Oradea, 410028 Oradea, Romania; simonabungau@gmail.com
5   Department of Internal Medicine, Clinical Emergency Hospital of Bucharest, 105402 Bucharest, Romania
*   Correspondence: drcameliadiaconu@gmail.com; Tel.: +40-726-377-300

Abstract: The present study aims to assess the sleep characteristics and health-related quality of life (HRQOL) among patients with chronic liver diseases (CLDs), as well as the relationship between them. We conducted a prospective cross-sectional study, over a period of eight months, on patients with CLDs. Sleep was assessed by subjective tools (self-reported validated questionnaires), semi-objective methods (actigraphy), and HRQOL by using the 36-Item Short Form Survey (SF-36) and Chronic Liver Disease Questionnaire (CLDQ). The results indicated that 48.21% of patients with CLDs had a mean Pittsburgh Sleep Quality Index (PSQI) score higher than five, suggestive of poor sleep; 39.29% of patients had a mean Epworth Sleepiness Scale (ESS) score ≥ 11, indicative of daytime sleepiness. Actigraphy monitoring showed that patients with cirrhosis had significantly more delayed bedtime hours and get-up hours, more awakenings, and more reduced sleep efficacy when compared to pre-cirrhotics. The CLDQ and SF-36 questionnaire scores were significantly lower in cirrhotics compared to pre-cirrhotics within each domain. Moreover, we identified significant correlations between the variables from each questionnaire, referring to HRQOL and sleep parameters. In conclusion, sleep disturbances are commonly encountered among patients with CLDs and are associated with impaired HRQOL. This is the first study in Romania that assesses sleep by actigraphy in a cohort of patients with different stages of CLD.

Keywords: sleep; chronic liver disease; quality of life

Citation: Plotogea, O.-M.; Gheorghe, G.; Stan-Ilie, M.; Constantinescu, G.; Bacalbasa, N.; Bungau, S.; Diaconu, C.C. Assessment of Sleep among Patients with Chronic Liver Disease: Association with Quality of Life. *J. Pers. Med.* **2021**, *11*, 1387. https://doi.org/10.3390/jpm11121387

Academic Editors: Fábio G. Teixeira, Catarina Godinho and Júlio Belo Fernandes

Received: 17 October 2021
Accepted: 16 December 2021
Published: 20 December 2021

Publisher's Note: MDPI stays neutral with regard to jurisdictional claims in published maps and institutional affiliations.

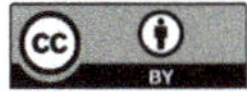

1. Introduction

Quality of life (QOL) represents an important endpoint in healthcare and has been extensively studied in the past decades, especially among patients with chronic diseases [1,2]. Health-related QOL (HRQOL) is a complex concept that was described in various ways, "generally considered to reflect the impact of disease and treatment on disability and daily functioning" (Mayo's dictionary, 2016) [3].

Sleep health is less frequently defined in the literature compared to HRQOL, and it is mostly expressed in association with its outcomes. There are five main indicators of sleep health, measured either by self-reported and/or objective methods [4,5]:

- Quality (subjectively assessed and divided into "good" or "poor" sleep);
- Duration (time slept over 24 h);
- Efficacy (sleep latency, wake after sleep onset);
- Timing (chronotype—morning vs. evening type);

- Alertness vs. sleepiness.

Based on these indicators, Buysse [5] defined sleep health as "a multidimensional pattern of sleep-wake-fulness, characterized by subjective satisfaction, appropriate timing, adequate duration, high efficiency, and sustained alertness during waking hours" (Buysse DJ, 2014).

Worldwide, in 2017, chronic liver diseases (CLDs) were estimated to affect 1.5 billion persons, whose diagnoses included non-alcoholic fatty liver disease, viral hepatitis B and C, and alcoholic liver disease [6]. Apart from addressing the morbidity derived from major complications (e.g., liver cirrhosis and cancer), a deep focus has lately been oriented toward sleep disturbances/disorders (SDs) in patients with chronic liver disease (CLD) [7–10]. It was observed that sleep indicators are impaired in more than half of these patients and that these are independently associated with reduced HRQOL [11].

The current study aimed to assess sleep characteristics and HRQOL among patients with CLDs, starting from the hypothesis that patients with more severe liver disease have poorer sleep indicators and reduced QOL. Second, we intended to examine the relationship between sleep alterations and HRQOL in this population.

2. Materials and Methods

2.1. Study Design

We conducted a prospective cross-sectional study over a period of 8 months (December 2020–July 2021) in the Clinical Emergency Hospital of Bucharest, Romania, both in ambulatory and hospitalized patients. Convenience sampling was applied as we recruited patients with CLDs who presented for regular follow-ups, or patients who presented for de-compensation of their liver disease, taking into consideration the including and excluding criteria which are mentioned below.

2.2. Subjects

We included in the study 56 adult patients (older than 18 years) who had been previously diagnosed with a CLD, namely steatosis, hepatitis, or cirrhosis. All patients underwent clinical assessment and laboratory and imaging investigations to establish the diagnosis and differentiate pre-cirrhotic stages from cirrhotic ones. Based on transient elastographic (FibroScan) evaluation, we divided the patients into two subgroups: group 1 (pre-cirrhosis)—including patients diagnosed with CLD who had no/mild/moderate fibrosis ($F = 0/F = 1/F = 2-3$), and group 2 (cirrhosis)—including patients with cirrhosis and severe fibrosis ($F = 4$).

The sociodemographic and clinical variables obtained were the following: gender, age, etiology, and comorbidities (diabetes and cardiovascular disease).

We decided to exclude from the study analysis, due to foreseeable bias/influence, acute hepatitis or acute liver failure, overt hepatic encephalopathy (WEST HAVEN score ≥ 2), known sleep disorders or ongoing treatment with sleep medication, unstable cardiovascular/hemodynamic status (e.g., coma), night-shift workers, patients who did not complete the questionnaires/answer all questions, and patients who did not wear the device 24 h/7 days. There were 9 patients who either answered incompletely (3 patients) or who did not wear the actiwatch at all times for the required period (6 patients), resulting in a dropout rate of 13.84%. Patients who did not complete all the questionnaires argued that the tests were exhaustive, with no personal benefit. Patients who took off the watch either misunderstood the instructions for wearing it or felt uncomfortable with the watch during sleep at night.

2.3. Sleep Health Assessment

Sleep was assessed by both subjective (self-reported validated questionnaires) and semi-objective methods (actigraphy) to increase diagnosis specificity and sensitivity. All patients completed the Pittsburgh Sleep Quality Index (PSQI), developed by Buysse et al. from the University of Pittsburgh, using National Institute of Mental Health funding [12].

In addition, the participants completed the Epworth Sleepiness Scale (ESS) [13]. These questionnaires were distributed in the Romanian version by Mapi Research Trust, and were also used before this study in patients with other conditions [14,15]. The PSQI is used to evaluate sleep quality in the previous month and separates "good" sleepers from "poor" sleepers. It comprises 19 items grouped in 7 components: sleep quality, sleep latency, sleep duration, sleep efficacy, sleep disturbances, sleep medication, and daytime dysfunction, each component being evaluated from 0 (no impairment) to 3 (severe impairment). The total score is obtained by summing and it ranges from 0 to 21. Scores higher than 5 points are considered suggestive of "poor" sleepers. ESS identifies patients with daytime sleepiness according to the likelihood of falling asleep in 8 different situations. The scores range from 0 to 24 and, the higher the score, the sleepier the subject. Scores ≥ 11 are considered abnormal [8,16].

Actigraphy is an alternative to polysomnography, being similarly cost-effective but less invasive and easier to use. The actigraph is a wristwatch incorporating an accelerometer that detects subject's movements [8]. In the present study, the patients were instructed to wear for 7 days an actigraphy wrist device (Actiwatch Philips Respironics; Spectrum Pro, manufactured by Philips Healthcare USA, purchased via LAG MedTech, Kolmar, Sweden). Data were recorded and analyzed by automated Philips Actiware software with standardized reports of bedtime, get-up time, time in bed, total sleep time, onset latency, sleep efficacy, wake time after sleep onset (WASO), and number of awakenings per night.

2.4. HRQOL Assessment

HRQOL was assessed using the 36-Item Short Form Survey (SF-36) and Chronic Liver Disease Questionnaire (CLDQ). SF-36 is a self-related questionnaire which contains 36 multiple-choice questions indicating overall physical and mental health status. The questions are grouped into 8 domains: physical functioning, role limitations because of physical health, role limitations because of emotional problems, body pain, general health, energy/fatigue, social functioning, and emotional well-being. The scores can range from 0 to 100 and the lower the score, the more altered the HRQOL [17]. CLDQ is a self-reported questionnaire which assesses the HRQOL of patients with CLDs. It comprises 29 questions grouped in 6 domains: abdominal symptoms, fatigue, systemic symptoms, emotional function, worry, and activity. CLDQ evaluates the symptoms which occurred over the last two weeks before completion, each domain being scored from 1 to 7. The total score is obtained as the mean value of the six domains and a higher score corresponds to a better QOL [18].

2.5. Ethics

The study was approved by the Research Ethics Committee of the Clinical Emergency Hospital of Bucharest, Romania (approval no. 3928/12.04.2021) and all participants provided written, informed consent for wearing the actigraph, while completing the questionnaires was considered implied consent to participate. The study was conducted according to the Declaration of Helsinki (1975), as revised in 2008, for medical research involving human subjects [19].

2.6. Statistical Analysis

Data were collected in Microsoft Excel and statistically analyzed with the IBM SPSS v.20 software package program. Descriptive analysis was performed for the prevalence of poor sleep and reduced HRQOL in the study groups and comparison of demographic and clinical variables between groups. Continuous variables were expressed as means ± standard deviations and ranges or as medians and ranges. Categorical variables were expressed as frequencies/absolute numbers with percentages. A two-sided p-value of <0.05 was indicative of statistical significance.

3. Results

3.1. Background Patients' Caracteristics

A total of 56 patients were enrolled during the study period and their baseline characteristics are depicted in Table 1. There were 41 males and 15 females, with a mean age of 59.75 ± 10.06 years. Alcoholic liver disease was the most predominant etiology (37.50%), followed by chronic viral hepatitis (30.40%). There were 11 patients with mixed etiology, both viral and alcoholic, and 7 patients who had been diagnosed with non-alcoholic fatty liver disease (NAFLD). Regarding comorbidities, we interviewed patients whether or not they had diabetes mellitus and/or cardiovascular disease. An important number of patients were known to have cardiovascular disease (19 patients) and diabetes (17 patients).

Table 1. Demographic and clinical data of patients with CLDs.

Demographic and Clinical Data	All Patients ($n = 56$)	Pre-Cirrhosis ($n =23$)	Cirrhosis		
			Total ($n = 33$)	Compensated ($n = 11$)	Decompensated ($n = 22$)
Age (mean $\pm$ SD)	59.75 ± 10.06	55.96 ± 11.50 *	62.39 ± 8.05 *	59.27 ± 7.24	63.95 ± 8.13
Gender (males), n (%)	41 (73.20%)	16 (69.60%)	25 (75.80%)	8 (72.70%)	17 (77.30%)
Etiology, n (%)					
Alcoholic	21 (37.50%)	7 (30.40%)	14 (42.40%)	5 (45.40%)	9 (40.90%)
Viral hepatitis	17 (30.40%)	9 (39.10%)	8 (24.20%)	4 (36.30%)	4 (18.20%)
Alcoholic + Viral Hepatitis	11 (19.60%)	2 (8.70%)	9 (27.30%)	2 (18.20%)	7 (31.80%)
NAFLD	7 (12.50%)	5 (21.70%)	2 (6.10%)	0 (0%)	2 (9.10%)
Diabetes, n (%)	17 (30.40%)	6 (26.10%)	11 (33.30%)	2 (18.20%)	9 (40.90%)
Cardiovascular disease, n (%)	19 (33.90%)	9 (39.10%)	10 (30.30%)	2 (18.20%)	8 (36.40%)

NAFLD = non-alcoholic fatty liver disease; * $p < 0.05$, ANOVA.

We further divided the entire group in two groups:

- Group 1: 23 patients with pre-cirrhosis (patients with steatosis and chronic hepatitis with Fibro Scan results that revealed no/mild/moderate fibrosis (F $\leq$ 3);
- Group 2: 33 patients with cirrhosis (F = 4).

Patients with cirrhosis had a significantly higher mean age than pre-cirrhotic patients (62.39 ± 8.05 vs. 55.96 ± 11.50 years, $p < 0.05$, ANOVA). There were 11 cases with compensated cirrhosis and 22 with decompensated stages, comprising ascites, jaundice, and upper gastrointestinal bleeding, and none had clinical hepatic encephalopathy, as this represented an exclusion criterion.

3.2. Sleep Assessment–Patients' Characteristics

We evaluated sleep characteristics of the patients included in the study through self-administered questionnaires (PSQI and ESS) and also by a semi-objective method: actigraphy (Table 2). The overall results showed that 48.21% of patients with CLD had a mean PSQI score higher than 5, suggestive of poor sleep. Moreover, 39.29% of all patients included in the study had a mean ESS score $\geq$ 11, which indicates that daytime sleepiness is also frequent.

When comparing the PSQI and ESS mean scores between the two groups, we noticed that cirrhotic patients had a significantly higher prevalence of daytime sleepiness evaluated by ESS score (9.73 ± 4.80 vs. 6.30 ± 5.14, $p = 0.014$, ANOVA). Poor sleepers (PSQI score > 5) were more prevalent among cirrhotic patients (54.55%), but without statistical significance compared to pre-cirrhotics (39.13%).

Table 2. Sleep assessment among patients with CLDs.

Sleep Parameters	All Patients (*n* = 56)	Pre-Cirrhosis (*n* = 23)	Cirrhosis (*n* = 33)	*p*-Value
PSQI (mean ± SD)	6.50 ± 3.90	5.65 ± 3.57	7.09 ± 4.06	0.177
Good sleepers (≤5), *n* (%)	29 (51.79%)	14 (60.87%)	15 (45.45%)	0.194
Poor sleepers (>5), *n* (%)	27 (48.21%)	9 (39.13%)	18 (54.55%)	
ESS (mean ± SD)	8.32 ± 5.18	6.30 ± 5.14	9.73 ± 4.80	0.014 *
≥11, *n* (%)	22 (39.29%)	7 (30.43%)	15 (45.45%)	0.197
<11, *n* (%)	34 (60.71%)	16 (69.57%)	18 (54.55%)	
Bed time (hour: minutes ± SD)	22:26 ± 0:48	22:09 ± 0:47	22:38 ± 0:45	0.025 *
Get-up time (hour: minutes ± SD)	7:46 ± 0:55	7:04 ± 0:37	8:15 ± 0:45	<0.001 *
Time in bed (hour: minutes ± SD)	9:19 ± 0:51	8:54 ± 0:47	9:36 ± 0:46	0.002 *
Total sleep time (hour: minutes ± SD)	7:36 ± 0:40	7:34 ± 0:40	7:38 ± 0:40	0.752
Onset latency (minutes ± SD)	19.43 ± 8.27	17.91 ± 9.09	20.49 ± 7.61	0.253
Sleep efficacy (% ± SD)	80.85 ± 4.67	84.20 ± 4.55	78.51 ± 3.11	<0.001 *
WASO (minutes ± SD)	38.69 ± 8.22	38.74 ± 9.60	38.65 ± 7.27	0.966
Number of awakenings per night (mean ± SD)	35.42 ± 12.33	28.18 ± 11.88	40.47 ± 10.01	<0.001 *

PSQI = Pittsburgh Sleep Quality Index; ESS = Epworth Sleepiness Scale; WASO = Wake time After Sleep Onset; * $p < 0.05$, ANOVA.

Actigraphy monitoring showed that patients with cirrhosis had a significantly more delayed bedtime hour and also get-up hour when compared to pre-cirrhotics. Consequently, they also spent more time in bed, even though sleep time was similar between the two groups. Sleep efficacy, evaluated as a mean percentage of the entire group of patients with CLD, was 80.85 ± 4.67%, considered as normal (the cut-off being 80%). However, we observed a statistically significant difference when we compared the results in the two groups: 78.51 ± 3.11% in cirrhotics vs. 84.20 ± 4.55% in pre-cirrhotics ($p < 0.001$, ANOVA). The number of awakenings per night was additionally registered and it revealed a significantly higher mean number among cirrhotic patients compared to pre-cirrhotic patients (40.47 ± 10.01 vs. 28.18 ± 11.88, $p < 0.001$, ANOVA). There was no significant difference between groups regarding the total sleep time, onset latency, or WASO.

By comparing patients with compensated cirrhosis with those with decompensated cirrhosis, we noticed a significant difference regarding PSQI and ESS scores, with 72.73% of the decompensated cirrhotics having a poor sleep quality and 63.64% of them having severe daytime sleepiness (Table 3). Moreover, actigraphic monitoring demonstrated that decompensated stages were associated with significantly more awakenings during night (44.93 ± 6.80), compared to compensated stages (31.55 ± 9.60), and reduced overall sleep efficacy (77.36 ± 2.29 vs. 80.82 ± 3.33).

Table 3. Comparison between compensated and decompensated cirrhosis regarding sleep assessment.

Sleep Parameters	Compensated (*n* = 11)	Decompensated (*n* = 22)	*p*-Value
PSQI (mean ± SD)	4 ± 2	8.64 ± 3.97	0.001 *
Good sleepers (≤5), *n* (%)	9 (81.82%)	6 (27.27%)	0.004 **
Poor sleepers (>5), *n* (%)	2 (18.18%)	16 (72.73%)	
ESS (mean ± SD)	6 ± 3	11.59 ± 4.46	0.001 *

Table 3. *Cont.*

Sleep Parameters	Compensated ($n = 11$)	Decompensated ($n = 22$)	*p*-Value
≥11, *n* (%)	1 (9.10%)	14 (63.64%)	0.004 **
<11, *n* (%)	10 (90.90%)	8 (36.36%)	
Bedtime (hour: minutes ± SD)	22:35 ± 0:45	22:40 ± 0:45	0.811
Get-up time (hour: minutes ± SD)	8:05 ± 0:39	8:20 ± 0:48	0.391
Time in bed (hour: minutes ± SD)	9:29 ± 0:40	9:40 ± 0:50	0.544
Total sleep time (hour: minutes ± SD)	7:46 ± 0:38	7:34 ± 0:42	0.421
Onset latency (minutes ± SD)	18.34 ± 5.83	21.57 ± 8.26	0.256
Sleep efficacy (%± SD)	80.82 ± 3.33	77.36 ± 2.29	0.001 *
WASO (minutes)	37.48 ± 7.11	39.23 ± 7.44	0.524
Number of awakenings per night (mean ± SD)	31.55 ± 9.60	44.93 ± 6.80	<0.001 *

PSQI = Pittsburgh Sleep Quality Index; ESS = Epworth Sleepiness Scale; WASO =Wake time After Sleep Onset; * $p < 0.05$, ANOVA; ** $p < 0.05$, Pearson Chi-square.

3.3. Predictors of Poor Sleep and Daytime Sleepiness

In order to determine the predictors of poor sleep and daytime somnolence, we used simple and multiple logistic regression analysis. Age, etiology, diabetes, and cardiovascular disease were included as variables in the multiple regression; however, only age was an independent predictor of a poor sleep (PSQI < 5). Therefore, with every year, a patient with CLD has an 18% chance to be categorized as a poor sleeper (Table 4).

Table 4. Logistic regression analysis for predictors of poor sleep (PSQI > 5).

	Logistic Regression Analysis for Predictors of Poor Sleep (PSQI > 5)					
	Simple Regression			Multiple Regression		
Variables	Poor Sleepers ($n = 27$)	Good Sleepers ($n = 29$)	*p*-Value	OR [95% CI]	β Coef.	*p*-Value
Age (mean ± SD)	66.59 ± 7.02	53.38 ± 8.13	<0.001 *	0.828 [0.725–0.945]	−0.189	0.003 ***
Gender (males), *n* (%)	19 (70.40%)	22 (75.90%)	0.765	-	-	-
Etiology, *n* (%)						
Alcoholic	10 (37%)	11 (37.90%)		REF		
Viral Hepatitis	4 (14.80%)	13 (44.80%)	0.027 **	2.687 [0.096−75.017]	0.988	0.561
Alcoholic+Viral Hepatitis	7 (25.90%)	4 (13.80%)		3.913 [0.156–98.37]	1.364	0.407
NAFLD	6 (22.20%)	1 (3.40)		3.024 [0.101–90.437]	1.107	0.523
Diabetes, *n* (%)	15 (55.60%)	2 (6.90%)	<0.001 **	4.531 [0.458–42.354]	1.511	0.185
Cardiovascular disease, *n* (%)	16 (59.30%)	3 (10.30%)	<0.001 **	0.930 [0.103–8.419]	−0.073	0.948

NAFLD = non-alcoholic fatty liver disease; * $p < 0.05$, ANOVA; ** $p < 0.05$, Pearson Chi-square; *** $p < 0.05$, ANOVA.

Furthermore, using the same multivariate analysis of variance as above, we included the variables age, diabetes, and cardiovascular disease to evaluate the predictors of daytime somnolence. Both age and diabetes were independently associated with ESS $\geq$ 11 (Table 5).

Table 5. Logistic regression analysis for predictors of daytime somnolence (ESS $\geq$ 11).

	Logistic Regression Analysis for Predictors of Daytime Somnolence (ESS $\geq$ 11)					
	Simple			Multiple		
Variables	ESS $\geq$ 11 (*n* = 22)	ESS < 11 (*n* = 34)	*p*-Value	OR [95% CI]	β Coef.	*p*-Value
Age (mean ± SD)	68.32 ± 5.28	54.21 ± 8.40	<0.001 *	0.776 [0.641–0.940]	−0.254	0.009 ***
Gender (males), *n* (%)	15 (68.20%)	26 (76.50%)	0.351	-	-	-
Etiology, *n* (%)						
Alcoholic	8 (36.20%)	13 (38.20%)		-	-	-
Viral hepatitis	3 (13.60%)	14 (41.20%)	0.059	-	-	-
Alcoholic+Viral Hepatitis	6 (27.30%)	5 (14.70%)		-	-	-
NAFLD	5 (22.70%)	2 (5.90%)		-	-	-
Diabetes, *n* (%)	15 (68.20%)	2 (5.90%)	<0.001 **	13,311 [1.253–141.4]	2.589	0.032 ***
Cardiovascular disease, *n* (%)	16 (59.30%)	3 (10.30%)	<0.001 **	2.525 [0.321–19.86]	0.926	0.379

NAFLD = non-alcoholic fatty liver disease; * $p < 0.05$, ANOVA; ** $p < 0.05$, Pearson Chi-square; *** $p < 0.05$, ANOVA.

3.4. HRQOL Assessment—Patients' Characteristics

We administered two questionnaires to investigate the HRQOL among patients with CLDs (Table 6). The CLDQ total score was 3.90 ± 1.59 for all patients, with significantly lower scores in cirrhotics compared to pre-cirrhotics, both in total score and within each domain. Abdominal symptoms were the lowest rated items (2.77 ± 1.10) of complaint in patients with cirrhosis, followed by systemic symptoms (3.04 ± 1.03) and worry (3.07 ± 1.28).

For the SF-36 questionnaire, the subdomain "general health" registered the lowest score, with noticeable differences between the two groups. Cirrhotic patients experienced significantly more body pain and physical functioning limitations because of physical health problems than pre-cirrhotic patients.

Table 6. Assessment of QOL among patients with CLDs.

HRQOL Parameters	All Patients (*n* = 56)	Pre-Cirrhosis (*n* = 23)	Cirrhosis (*n* = 33)	*p*-Value
CLDQ (mean ± SD)				
Total score	3.90 ± 1.59	4.98 ± 1.64	3.15 ± 1.06	<0.001 *
Abdominal symptoms	3.55 ± 1.66	4.67 ± 1.71	2.77 ± 1.10	<0.001 *
Fatigue	3.86 ± 1.70	4.96 ± 1.81	3.09 ± 1.10	<0.001 *
Systemic symptoms	3.93 ± 1.76	5.21 ± 1.81	3.04 ± 1.03	<0.001 *
Activity	4.03 ± 1.81	5.27 ± 1.71	3.17 ± 1.33	<0.001 *
Emotional function	4.35 ± 1.53	5.18 ± 1.56	3.78 ± 1.24	<0.001 *
Worry	3.70 ± 1.71	4.60 ± 1.86	3.07 ± 1.28	0.001 *

Table 6. *Cont.*

HRQOL Parameters	All Patients (*n* = 56)	Pre-Cirrhosis (*n* = 23)	Cirrhosis (*n* = 33)	*p*-Value
SF-36 (%, mean ± SD)				
Physical functioning	74.10 ± 21.76	85.00 ± 21.05	66.51 ± 19.10	0.001 *
Role limitations due to physical health problems	65.71 ± 26.10	75.00 ± 23.83	59.24 ± 25.98	0.025 *
Role limitations due to emotional problems	61.91 ± 23.30	66.67 ± 24.63	58.59 ± 22.11	0.205
Energy fatigue	61.16 ± 23.58	65.21 ± 21.76	58.33 ± 24.70	0.287
Emotional wellbeing	67.76 ± 15.46	70.26 ± 15.10	66.03 ± 15.70	0.318
Social functioning	73.97 ± 21.37	79.34 ± 20.50	70.22 ± 21.46	0.117
Pain	72.63 ± 19.50	82.50 ± 18.01	65.75 ± 17.67	0.001 *
General health	51.07 ± 24.13	60.86 ± 21.51	44.24 ± 23.78	0.010 *

HRQOL = Health-Related Quality of Life; CLDQ = Chronic Liver Disease Questionnaire; SF-36 = Short Form-36; * *p* < 0.05, ANOVA.

We further investigated the HRQOL, comparing compensated cirrhotics with decompensated stages and observed significantly lower scores in all subdomains completed by patients with a more severe disease (Table 7). From the specific questionnaire (CLDQ), the deepest impact was given by abdominal symptoms, followed by worry, while SF-36 revealed the lowest score in the general health section, followed by limitations because of physical health problems.

Table 7. Assessment of HRQOL among patients with cirrhosis.

HRQOL Parameters	Compensated (*n* = 11)	Decompensated (*n* = 22)	*p*-Value
CLDQ (mean ± SD)			
Total score	4.19 ± 0.89	2.63 ± 0.69	<0.001 *
Abdominal symptoms	3.87 ± 1.03	2.22 ± 0.63	<0.001 *
Fatigue	4.07 ± 1.09	2.60 ± 0.73	<0.001 *
Systemic symptoms	3.91 ± 0.92	2.61 ± 0.79	<0.001 *
Activity	4.35 ± 1.09	2.58 ± 1.01	<0.001 *
Emotional function	4.89 ± 1.14	3.22 ± 0.87	<0.001 *
Worry	4.07 ± 1.20	2.57 ± 1.01	0.001 *
SF-36 (%, mean ± SD)			
Physical functioning	84.09 ± 7.68	57.72 ± 16.88	<0.001 *
Role limitations due to physical health problems	84.09 ± 12.61	46.81 ± 21.63	<0.001 *
Role limitations due to emotional problems	75.78 ± 15.55	49.99 ± 19.94	0.001 *
Energy fatigue	76.36 ± 14.33	49.31 ± 24.01	0.002 *
Emotional wellbeing	78.81 ± 12.71	59.63 ± 13.05	<0.001 *
Social functioning	90.22 ± 10.33	60.22 ± 18.35	<0.001 *
Pain	83.40 ± 11.02	56.93 ± 13.15	<0.001 *
General health	61.36 ± 18.31	35.68 ± 21.72	0.001 *

HRQOL = Health-Related Quality of Life; CLDQ = Chronic Liver Disease Questionnaire; SF-36 = Short Form-36; * *p* < 0.05, ANOVA.

3.5. Associations between Sleep Characteristics and HRQOL among Enrolled Patients

We identified significant correlations between variables from each questionnaire, both the HRQOL and sleep assessment (Table 8). We included the PSQI and ESS scores as well as two parameters recorded by actigraphy: sleep efficacy and episodes of awakenings/night. Patients with CLDs who expressed low scores on the two questionnaires about HRQOL also experienced high scores for PSQI and ESS, indicative of poor night-time sleep and daytime sleepiness. The sleep efficacy proved to be good in patients with high HRQOL parameters, while a high number of awakenings was associated with a reduced HRQOL. The strongest effect was observed with physical functioning, which was the lowest for patients who experienced the highest PSQI and ESS scores. Moreover, high activity scores—a subdomain of CLDQ—were strongly correlated with good sleep efficacy and reduced episodes of awakenings.

Table 8. Correlations between sleep assessment and HRQOL among enrolled patients.

HRQOL	PSQI	ESS	Sleep Efficacy	Number of Awakenings/Nights
CLDQ (mean ± SD)				
Total score	−0.671	−0.729	0.785	−0.769
Abdominal symptoms	−0.608	−0.671	0.724	−0.735
Fatigue	−0.670	−0.711	0.763	−0.768
Systemic symptoms	−0.644	−0.705	0.746	−0.741
Activity	−0.691	−0.751	0.819	−0.753
Emotional function	−0.571	−0.625	0.688	−0.674
Worry	−0.597	−0.650	0.689	−0.665
SF-36 (mean %)				
Physical functioning	−0.804	−0.809	0.711	−0.693
Role limitations due to physical health problems	−0.741	−0.825	0.634	−0.732
Role limitations due to emotional problems	−0.653	−0.669	0.566	−0.565
Energy fatigue	−0.667	−0.632	0.488	−0.502
Emotional wellbeing	−0.648	−0.595	0.517	−0.519
Social functioning	−0.735	−0.732	0.637	−0.63
Pain	−0.735	−0.752	0.716	−0.612
General health	−0.690	−0.682	0.585	−0.635

Values are correlation coefficients (Spearman's r); HRQOL = Health-Related Quality of Life; CLDQ = chronic liver disease questionnaire; SF-36 = Short Form-36; PSQI = Pittsburgh Sleep Quality Index; ESS = Epworth Sleepiness Scale.

Figures 1 and 2 show the relationship between total CLDQ score and results obtained by sleep questionnaires and actigraphic monitoring. Most patients with high CLDQ scores had low PSQI and ESS scores (Figure 1A,B), while patients with the lowest sleep efficacy and most frequent awakenings reported the greatest impairment in HRQOL (Figure 2A,B).

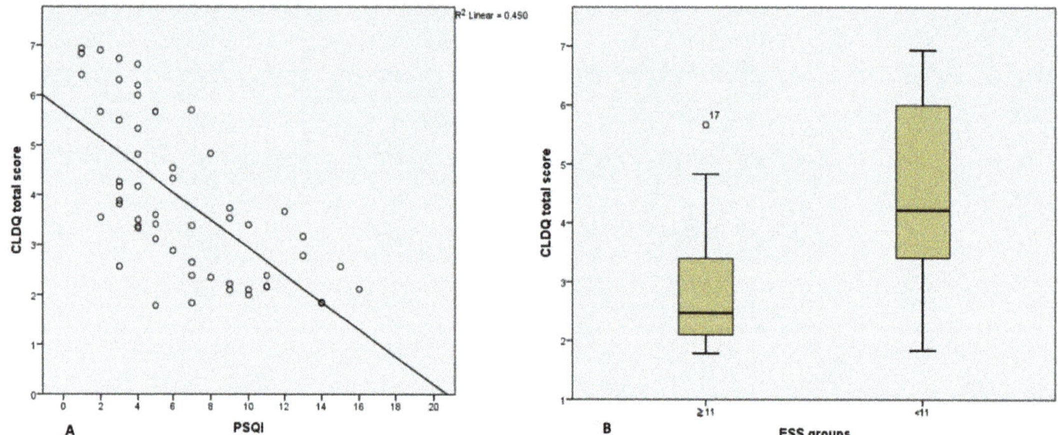

Figure 1. Scatter Plot representing the relationship between PSQI scores and CLDQ scores (**A**) and Box Plot representing the relationship between ESS scores and CLDQ scores (**B**); Abbreviations: PSQI = Pittsburgh Sleep Quality Index, CLDQ = chronic liver disease questionnaire, ESS = Epworth Sleepiness Scale.

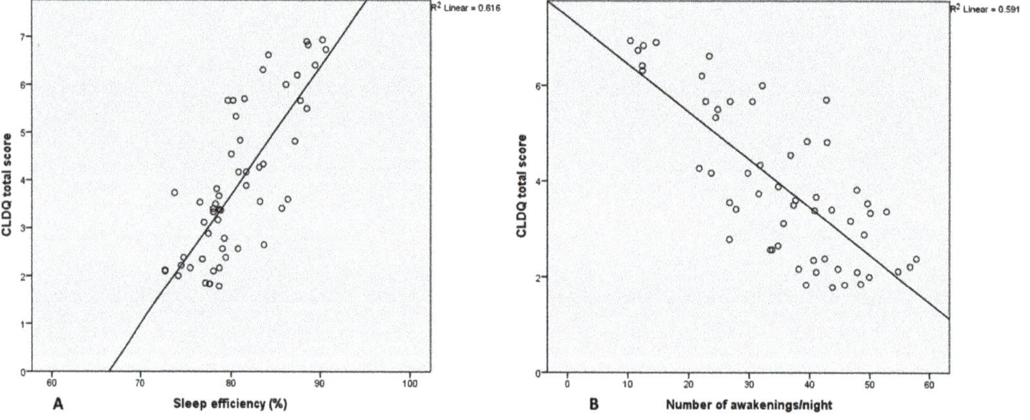

Figure 2. Scatter Plot representing the relationship between sleep efficacy (**A**) and number of awakenings per night (**B**) and CLDQ scores. Abbreviations: CLDQ = chronic liver disease questionnaire.

4. Discussion

This prospective ongoing study is the first to assess sleep disorders among Romanian patients with CLDs by using actigraphy and correlate its results with subjective tools for sleep quality and HRQOL.

Sleep disorders have been previously described in patients with CLDs in several studies [8,10,11,20–22], where their prevalence varies widely from 47% to 81%, mainly due to different assessment methods, heterogenous population, and cumulative influencing/bias factors (e.g., coffee intake, alcohol, sleep medication, presence of hepatic encephalopathy, associated comorbidities, etc.). We reported in our study, among CLD patients, a prevalence of 48.21% of nighttime disturbances and 39.29% of daytime sleepiness, evaluated by PSQI and ESS, respectively. The scores for both questionnaires were significantly higher in decompensated patients, showing a direct relationship between impaired sleep quality and daytime somnolence, and complicated, severe liver disease. Excessive daytime sleepiness has been considered a feature of hepatic encephalopathy, since ESS score has been shown to correlate with the degree of hepatic encephalopathy [16,23–25]. Still, we demonstrated that daytime somnolence is present in a high percentage even in pre-cirrhotic patients. This finding may indicate a possible early minimal hepatic encephalopathy (HE) before becoming clinically evident in patients with cirrhosis, however, of course, further prospective studies are needed to confirm this hypothesis.

In addition to the subjective data of sleep quality, we added objective measures of sleep characteristics by using actigraphy. Studies from the literature show that patients with cirrhosis, in particular, experience "delayed sleep phase syndrome" [26], with prolonged onset latency, poor sleep efficacy, and fragmented sleep with frequent awakenings [16,20,26]. This information is also supported by our study, which showed delayed bedtime and get-up hours, lower sleep efficacy, and also more awakenings in patients with cirrhosis compared to pre-cirrhotic ones. Controversially, our study failed to reveal significant differences of onset latency and total sleep time between pre-cirrhotic and cirrhotic patients, as the periods were similar. Moreover, our evidence shows that the difference in sleep parameters is even more important when comparing decompensated stages with compensated forms.

HRQOL in patients with CLDs is influenced by various factors. On one hand, patients experience multiple symptoms related to liver disease, such as itching, fatigue, weight loss, and "fuzzy-thinking", which can also interfere with their social life. On the other hand, psychological distress strains on patients with advanced stages, when concerns regarding disease progression tremendously impact their QOL [27]. All these factors are also contributors to sleep abnormalities. However, researchers investigated the relationship between sleep impairment in patients with cirrhosis and HRQOL independently of other factors [11,16]. An important finding of our study showed that, besides cirrhotics, patients in pre-cirrhotic stages also experience reduced QOL, directly influenced by poor sleep quality.

The study has a series of limitations. First of all, it has been conducted in an emergency hospital, where decompensated cirrhosis represented a high percentage of the patients enrolled. Secondly, the study was based on a single assessment and exclusively among patients with a diagnosis of CLD, lacking a normal control group. However, the aim of the study was to investigate sleep and HRQOL in a population with presumed abnormalities. Third, the study did not track either the medication, nor the reasons of decompensation, which might have explained the significant difference between compensated and decompensated patients regarding sleep parameters and HRQOL scores. Further studies are needed to elucidate the contributing factors and their pathogenesis.

Finally, we need to mention the limits given by the subjective and semi-objective methods (questionnaires and actigraphy) that we used to assess sleep and HRQOL. These evaluations, especially questionnaires, are predisposed to bias as they might be overestimated by the patients. Therefore, an objective method is advisable to support the evidence, namely polysomnography, which would definitely offer a valuable extension of our work into future prospective studies.

5. Conclusions

Sleep disturbances are commonly encountered among patients with CLDs and are associated with impaired HRQOL. In the present study, we demonstrated that the more severe the liver disease, the poorer that sleep and QOL are. Moreover, this is the first study in Romania that assessed sleep by actigraphy in a cohort of patients with different stages of CLDs.

Author Contributions: Conceptualization, O.-M.P. and C.C.D.; methodology, G.G.; software, O.-M.P. and G.G.; validation, N.B., S.B. and C.C.D.; formal analysis, G.C.; investigation, G.G. and M.S.-I.; resources, G.C.; data curation, S.B. and C.C.D.; writing—original draft preparation O.-M.P.; writing—review and editing, M.S.-I. and C.C.D.; visualization, N.B.; supervision, C.C.D. All authors have read and agreed to the published version of the manuscript.

Funding: This research received no external funding.

Institutional Review Board Statement: The study was conducted according to the guidelines of the Declaration of Helsinki, and approved by the Research Ethics Committee of the Clinical Emergency Hospital of Bucharest, Romania (no. 3928/12.04.2021).

Informed Consent Statement: Informed consent was obtained from all subjects involved in the study.

Data Availability Statement: Study data are available from the first author (O.-M.P.) upon request.

Conflicts of Interest: The authors declare no conflict of interest.

References

1. Haraldstad, K.; Wahl, A.; Andenæs, R.; Andersen, J.R.; Andersen, M.H.; Beisland, E.; Borge, C.R.; Engebretsen, E.; Eisemann, M.; Halvorsrud, L.; et al. A systematic review of quality of life research in medicine and health sciences. *Qual. Life Res.* **2019**, *28*, 2641–2650. [CrossRef]
2. Megari, K. Quality of life in chronic disease patients. *Health Psychol. Res.* **2013**, *1*, e27. [CrossRef]
3. Mayo, N. *Dictionary of Quality of Life and Health Outcomes Measurement*; International Society for Quality of Life Research: Milwaukee, WI, USA, 2015.
4. Katulka, E.K.; Berube, F.R.; D'Agata, M.N. Dreaming of better health: Quantifying the many dimensions of sleep. *Sleep* **2019**, *43*, 275. [CrossRef] [PubMed]
5. Buysse, D.J. Sleep Health: Can We Define It? Does It Matter? *Sleep* **2014**, *37*, 9–17. [CrossRef] [PubMed]
6. Moon, A.M.; Singal, A.G.; Tapper, E.B. Contemporary Epidemiology of Chronic Liver Disease and Cirrhosis. *Clin. Gastroenterol. Hepatol.* **2019**, *18*, 2650–2666. [CrossRef]
7. Plotogea, O.-M.; Ilie, M.; Bungau, S.; Chiotoroiu, A.; Stanescu, A.; Diaconu, C. Comprehensive Overview of Sleep Disorders in Patients with Chronic Liver Disease. *Brain Sci.* **2021**, *11*, 142. [CrossRef] [PubMed]
8. Formentin, C.; Garrido, M.; Montagnese, S. Assessment and Management of Sleep Disturbance in Cirrhosis. *Curr. Hepatol. Rep.* **2018**, *17*, 52–69. [CrossRef]
9. Shah, N.M.; Malhotra, A.M.; Kaltsakas, G. Sleep disorder in patients with chronic liver disease: A narrative review. *J. Thorac. Dis.* **2020**, *12* (Suppl. S2), S248–S260. [CrossRef] [PubMed]
10. Umbro, I.; Fabiani, V.; Fabiani, M.; Angelico, F.; Del Ben, M. Association between non-alcoholic fatty liver disease and obstructive sleep apnea. *World J. Gastroenterol.* **2020**, *26*, 2669–2681. [CrossRef]
11. Ghabril, M.; Jackson, M.; Gotur, R.; Weber, R.; Orman, E.; Vuppalanchi, R.; Chalasani, N. Most Individuals with Advanced Cirrhosis Have Sleep Disturbances, Which Are Associated with Poor Quality of Life. *Clin. Gastroenterol. Hepatol.* **2017**, *15*, 1271–1278.e6. [CrossRef] [PubMed]
12. Buysse, D.J.; Reynolds, C.F., 3rd; Monk, T.H.; Berman, S.R.; Kupfer, D.J. The Pittsburgh Sleep Quality Index: A new instrument for psychiatric practice and research. *Psychiatry Res.* **1989**, *28*, 193–213. [CrossRef]
13. Johns, M.W. A New Method for Measuring Daytime Sleepiness: The Epworth Sleepiness Scale. *Sleep* **1991**, *14*, 540–545. [CrossRef]
14. Rosca, L.E.; Todea, A.A.; Rusu, A. Reliability and validity of the Romanian version of the Epworth sleepiness scale. *Eur. Respir. J.* **2011**, *38* (Suppl. S55), 3924.
15. Blanariu, G.-E.G.; Ștefănescu, G.; Trifan, A.V.; Moscalu, M.; Dimofte, M.-G.; Ștefănescu, C.; Drug, V.L.; Afrăsânie, V.-A.; Ciocoiu, M. Sleep Impairment and Psychological Distress among Patients with Inflammatory Bowel Disease—Beyond the Obvious. *J. Clin. Med.* **2020**, *9*, 2304. [CrossRef] [PubMed]
16. Montagnese, S.; Middleton, B.; Skene, D.; Morgan, M.Y. Night-time sleep disturbance does not correlate with neuropsychiatric impairment in patients with cirrhosis. *Liver Int.* **2009**, *29*, 1372–1382. [CrossRef]
17. Brazier, J.; Harper, R.; Jones, N.M.; O'Cathain, A.; Thomas, K.J.; Usherwood, T.; Westlake, L. Validating the SF-36 health survey questionnaire: New outcome measure for primary care. *BMJ* **1992**, *305*, 160–164. [CrossRef]
18. Taru, V.; Indre, M.G.; Ignat, M.D.; Forgione, A.; Racs, T.; Olar, B.A.; Farcau, O.; Chereches, R.; Stefanescu, H.; Procopet, B. Validation and Performance of Chronic Liver Disease Questionnaire (CLDQ-RO) in the Romanian Population. *J. Gastrointest. Liver Dis.* **2021**, *30*, 240–246. [CrossRef]
19. World Medical Association. World Medical Association Declaration of Helsinki: Ethical principles for medical research in-volving human subjects. *JAMA* **2013**, *310*, 2191–2194. [CrossRef] [PubMed]
20. Córdoba, J.; Cabrera, J.; Lataif, L.; Penev, P.; Zee, P.; Blei, A.T. High prevalence of sleep disturbance in cirrhosis. *Hepatology* **1998**, *27*, 339–345. [CrossRef] [PubMed]
21. AL-Jahdali, H.; Al Enezi, A.; Anwar, A.E.; AL-Harbi, A.; Baharoon, S.; Aljumah, A.; Shimemeri, A.; Abudallah, K. Preva-lence of insomnia and sleep patterns among liver cirrhosis patients. *J. Circadian Rhythm.* **2014**, *12*, 1–6. [CrossRef]
22. Abdullah, A.E.; Al-Jahdali, F.; Ahmed, A.E.; Shirbini, N.; Salim, B.; Ali, Y.Z.; Abdulrahman, A.; Khan, M.; Khaleid, A.; Hamdan, A.-J. Symptoms of Daytime Sleepiness and Sleep Apnea in Liver Cirrhosis Patients. *Ann. Hepatol.* **2017**, *16*, 591–598. [CrossRef]
23. Samanta, J.; Dhiman, R.K.; Khatri, A.; Thumburu, K.K.; Grover, S.; Duseja, A.; Chawla, Y. Correlation between degree and quality of sleep disturbance and the level of neuropsychiatric impairment in patients with liver cirrhosis. *Metab. Brain Dis.* **2013**, *28*, 249–259. [CrossRef] [PubMed]

24. De Rui, M.; Schiff, S.; Aprile, D.; Angeli, P.; Bombonato, G.; Bolognesi, M.; Sacerdoti, D.; Gatta, A.; Merkel, C.; Amodio, P.; et al. Excessive daytime sleepiness and hepatic encephalopathy: It is worth asking. *Metab. Brain Dis.* **2013**, *28*, 245–248. [CrossRef]
25. Mostacci, B.; Ferlisi, M.; Antognini, A.B.; Sama, C.; Morelli, C.; Mondini, S.; Cirignotta, F. Sleep Disturbance and Daytime Sleepiness in Patients with Cirrhosis: A Case Control Study. *Neurol. Sci.* **2008**, *29*, 237–240. [CrossRef] [PubMed]
26. Montagnese, S.; Middleton, B.; Mani, A.R.; Skene, D.J.; Morgan, M.Y. Sleep and circadian abnormalities in patients with cir-rhosis: Features of delayed sleep phase syndrome? *Metab. Brain Dis.* **2009**, *24*, 427–439. [CrossRef] [PubMed]
27. Loria, A.; Escheik, C.; Gerber, L.; Younossi, Z.M. Quality of Life in Cirrhosis. *Curr. Gastroenterol. Rep.* **2012**, *15*, 301. [CrossRef] [PubMed]

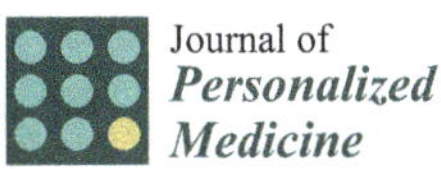

Journal of
*Personalized
Medicine*

Article

Stigma towards People with Mental Illness among Portuguese Nursing Students

Júlio Belo Fernandes [1,2,3,*], Carlos Família [1,2,3,4], Cidália Castro [1,3] and Aida Simões [1,3]

[1] Escola Superior de Saúde Egas Moniz, Caparica, 2829-511 Almada, Portugal; carlosfamilia@egasmoniz.edu.pt (C.F.); ccastro@egasmoniz.edu.pt (C.C.); aidasimoes@gmail.com (A.S.)
[2] Grupo de Patologia Médica, Nutrição e Exercício Clínico (PaMNEC)—Centro de Investigação Interdisciplinar Egas Moniz (CiiEM), 2829-511 Almada, Portugal
[3] Centro de Investigação Interdisciplinar Egas Moniz (CiiEM), 2829-511 Almada, Portugal
[4] Molecular Pathology and Forensic Biochemistry Laboratory (MPFBL), Centro de Investigação Interdisciplinar Egas Moniz (CiiEM), Monte de Caparica, 2829-511 Caparica, Portugal
[*] Correspondence: juliobelo01@gmail.com

Abstract: Stigma is a substantial obstacle when caring for people with mental illness. Nursing students' negative attitudes towards people with mental illness may impact the quality of care delivered and consequentially patient outcomes. In this study, we assessed the stigmatising attitudes and beliefs of nursing students towards people with mental illness and examined its relationship with several psycho-socio-demographic variables. This was a quantitative, cross-sectional descriptive correlational study, which was developed with a non-probabilistic convenience sample of 110 nursing students. Stigmatising attitudes and beliefs were assessed using the Portuguese version of the Attribution Questionnaire AQ-27. Results show that the dimensions of stigma with higher scores were help, pity, coercion and avoidance. However, significant differences were only observed depending on the year of study (fourth-year students, who already had clinical placements in this area, are less likely to show stigma), the relationship (family is less prone to show coercion), the history of mental health treatment (students with a history of mental health treatment have more tendency to help) and whether they considered working in the mental health field (students who have considered working in this field are less prone to show anger, avoidance and think of patients as dangerous). Therefore, we conclude that education in a classroom setting alone is not enough to reduce stigma in nursing students, clinical placement in the area is required to achieve such results. It is thus essential to improve nursing curricula worldwide so that students are exposed to both psychiatric nursing theory and clinical practice in the first years of the nursing degree.

Keywords: mental disorders; mental illness; social stigma; nursing; students

Citation: Fernandes, J.B.; Família, C.; Castro, C.; Simões, A. Stigma towards People with Mental Illness among Portuguese Nursing Students. *J. Pers. Med.* **2022**, *12*, 326. https://doi.org/10.3390/jpm12030326

Academic Editor: Alessio Gori and Igor Elman

Received: 7 January 2022
Accepted: 17 February 2022
Published: 22 February 2022

Publisher's Note: MDPI stays neutral with regard to jurisdictional claims in published maps and institutional affiliations.

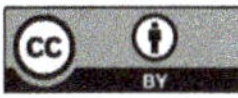

1. Introduction

Mental illness emerges as a consequence of mental disorders and is usually manifested by abnormal thoughts, emotions, perceptions, behaviours and relationships with others. Mental illness is a highly heterogeneous group of disorders, which include depression, psychosis, dementia and developmental disorders, among others [1]. Mental illness is presently recognised as a severe health problem that affects the life of one in every three Europeans [2] and is one of the leading causes of disease-related burden worldwide [3].

The knowledge and attitude of the general public towards people with mental illness differs depending on the type of illness. For example, several studies described a higher propensity for people to maintain a greater social distance from a person with schizophrenia when compared with someone with an anxiety disorder or depression [4–6]. This tendency was also verified in a study that compared physicians' attitudes towards people with schizophrenia and depression [7].

When a stigma towards a specific population is identified, it is vital to develop interventions to mitigate distress and shift harmful behaviours that may compromise this population's wellbeing [8]. To interrupt the stigmatisation process, it is essential to assess the presence of stigma and promote educational anti-stigma campaigns, presenting factual information about the stigmatised condition, and to develop contact-based strategies aimed to facilitate the interaction and connection between groups [9–11].

According to the Health Stigma and Discrimination Framework, stigma spans across the socio-ecological spectrum in the form of stereotyping, prejudice and discrimination [11]. Stigma is, therefore, a multidimensional concept that includes different dimensions (cognitive, affective and behavioural) that operate at the micro-level (singular person), meso-level (social networks), macro-level (cultural or institutional) and that can occur consciously (explicitly) or unconsciously (implicitly) [11,12].

The stigmatisation process can unfold into different domains, including drivers and facilitators, stigma marking and stigma manifestations, all of which have a direct effect on several outcomes among populations targeted by stigma [11]. The first domain includes factors that drive or facilitate the stigmatisation process and are usually conceptualised as inherently negative and might diverge according to the targeted population's health condition [11]. Stigma marking and manifestations are usually displayed as a series of stigma experiences (i.e., experienced stigma and discrimination) and practices (i.e., stereotypes, prejudice and discriminatory attitudes) [11]. In addition, these experiences can also induce self-stigma, which occurs when stigmatised group members internalise the negative societal beliefs and feelings and suffer numerous negative consequences as a result [11–13].

Stigmatisation experiences and the inherent associated labelling, usually result from the lack of knowledge about mental illnesses and contact with cases of discrimination and negative attitudes from society [6]. These negative attitudes towards people with mental illness, can lead to social isolation and delay or prevent these persons from getting help and treatment or even interacting with essential community services [7,8]. In fact, recently, the Health Stigma and Discrimination Framework postulated that stigma manifestations will have an impact on several outcomes for affected populations. These might include access to essential services like justice and healthcare services and influence outcomes for organisations, including the availability and quality of health services [11].

Healthcare professionals, contrary to expectations, are also prone to display negative and stigmatising attitudes and behaviours towards people with mental illness [9], which leads to mismanagement and low attention to patients, undoubtedly affecting their interaction, and ultimately leading to a lack of support, acceptance and of an appropriate and adequate care of these patients [7,8,14,15]. Positive attitudes toward people with mental illness are thus a prerequisite healthcare professionals must demonstrate in order to provide quality care to these patients. For example, having adequate expectations about the behaviours and traits of the disease and being able to correctly identify and avoid incorrect messages and societal misconceptions [14,16].

Nursing students share the same misconceptions towards people with mental illness as the general public, and those with a high level of stigma often display discomfort, anxiety and fear when caring for people with mental illness [17,18]. In fact, a recent study identified stigmatised misconceptions about people with mental illness in nursing students, such as the assumption of them being dangerous and having worse prognoses [19]. Other studies also identify that nursing students believed that people with mental illness needed to be segregated from the community [20,21] and had more difficulty expressing compassion for those patients [20].

Current evidence indicates that theoretical preparation and clinical placements in mental health units, effectively reduce the stigma of nursing students towards people with mental illness [22,23]. Furthermore, it can represent an opportunity to attract students into this field [22]. In fact, presently, there is a severe shortage of qualified professionals, trained to provide timely and effective treatment for mental health patients, roughly less than 9 workers per 100,000 population [24]. For these reasons, it is crucial to deconstruct nursing students' misconceptions regarding people with mental illness as their attitudes and beliefs will certainly have a major impact on the career path they will take after graduation [17,25]. Educational institutions are thus in a privileged position to address this problem by elucidating these misconceptions and promoting the idea that people with mental illness are not entirely responsible for their condition and cannot control it [17].

Considering that the first action to intervene in order to mitigate the stigmatisation process is the assessment of the situation, with this study, we aim to assess the stigma nursing students have towards people with mental illness and examine the relationship between stigma and psycho-socio-demographic variables, so that intervention actions that allow changing this panorama can be developed.

2. Methods

2.1. Design

This is a quantitative study that was conducted using a cross-sectional descriptive correlational web-based survey design.

2.2. Study Setting

The study took place in a Portuguese private Higher School of Health in the region of Lisbon and Tagus Valley. A non-probabilistic convenience sample was used where all undergraduate students attending the nursing degree course were invited to participate in the study through their school e-mail address.

2.3. Data Collection

The data collection instrument was written in Portuguese and included the study information page, psycho-socio-demographic questionnaire and Attribution Questionnaire (AQ-27) [26]. All questions were transcribed into Google Forms™ and were applied from May to July 2020.

The psycho-socio-demographic questionnaire collected background information such as age, sex, religion, place of residence, year of study, prior contact with mental illness, history of mental health treatment and if the student ever considered working in the field of mental health.

The AQ-27 [26] questionnaire was used to assess stigma towards people with mental illness. For this study, we used the Portuguese version of the AQ-27, which was previously translated and validated for the Portuguese population by Sousa, Queirós, Marques, Rocha and Fernandes [27], having previous studies performed on the Portuguese population with this questionnaire yielded Cronbach alpha values of reliability of 0.88 [28], 0.76 [29] and 0.83 [30]. The AQ-27 is a self-administered questionnaire that consists of a brief vignette about a hypothetical person with schizophrenia, chosen among the provided vignettes, specifically not to influence emotional reactions from the participants. This vignette was followed by a set of 27 questions addressing one of nine subscales or dimensions of stigmatising attitudes and beliefs towards people with mental illness (Anger, Avoidance, Blame, Coercion, Dangerousness, Fear, Help, Pity and Segregation). The score for each subscale is obtained by the sum of the three questions corresponding to that subscale. Each question is answered on a Likert-type scale that ranges from 1 to 9. The AQ-27 has no defined threshold score for levels of stigma, for this reason, the score obtained in each dimension of stigma should be interpreted comparatively [26].

2.4. Data Analysis

The statistical analysis of the questionnaires was performed using the R language and environment for statistical computing v. 4.1.2 [31], with RStudio v.2021.09.0 [32] as the integrated development environment. Only surveys with all questions answered were analysed.

Descriptive statistic measures of count, mean, standard deviation, median, minimum, maximum and range were computed for sample characterisation, using the function table1 from the table1 v.1.4.2 library [33] for R. Values of minimum, maximum, mean and standard deviation were also computed for each question, and each dimension of stigma existing in the questionnaire, which was summarised in a table using the kable function from knitr v.1.36 library [34–36] for R.

Linear models were developed for each dimension of stigma with the categorical variables of Year of study, Sex, Religion, Residence, Relationship (know someone with mental illness and their relationship to that person), History of mental health treatment and Considered working in the mental health field as predictors, using the lm function provided by the R base library. The Year of study included four levels (first, second, third and fourth years), as well as Relationship (None, Acquaintance, Friend or Family), Sex consisted of two levels (Male or Female), as well as Religion (Yes or No), Residence (Rural or Urban), History of mental health treatment (Yes or No) and Considered working in the mental health field (Yes or No).

Model assumptions were verified through the visual observation of the residuals plot, Q-Q plot, Index plot and Histogram provided by the resid_panel function of the ggResidpanel v.0.3.0 library [37] for R. In addition, assumptions of normality and homoscedasticity of the standardised residuals were also formally evaluated with the Shapiro–Wilk and the Breush–Pagan tests, respectively. The former is provided by the shapiro.test function of the R stats v. 4.1.2 library, and the latter was provided by the bptest function of the lmtest v. 0.9.38 library [38] for R. Whenever these assumptions were violated, the dimension of stigma in question was transformed with the Box-Cox transformation, with a lambda value determined computationally by the powerTransform function of the car v.3.0.11 library [39] for R, after which a new linear model was developed and assumptions reverified as previously described.

Subsequently, a factorial analysis of variance (ANOVA) of type 2 was performed using the Anova function from the car library for R, and the results were summarised in a table using the apa.aov.table function from the apaTables v.2.0.8 library [40] for R. Multiple comparisons with Tuckey contrasts were performed for each main effect identified to have at least two groups with significant differences, using the glht function of the multcomp v.1.4.17 library [41] for R. For all statistical tests a level of significance of 0.05 was considered.

2.5. Ethical Considerations

Ethics approval was obtained from the Board of Directors and the Institutional Ethical Review Committee of the Education Institution involved (Date: April 2020 ID: 884). The survey's first page contained a clarification of the objectives and procedures of the study and the guarantee that confidentiality and anonymity of the data were assured by the researchers. Participants would need to accept and agree to the online informed consent in order to complete the survey. The survey was set up so that participants had to answer "Yes" or "No" indicating that they had read the consent information and agreed to participate. Only the participants who answered "Yes" to the informed consent question were directed to the research survey. Participants who answered "No" to the informed consent question were directed to the end of the survey. Participants were free to decide not to answer any question, change or review their responses, or voluntarily quit at any time. To comply with the ethical principles of anonymity and confidentiality, all data collected were free of any personally identifying information, including any form of electronic identifiers.

3. Results

A total of 110 nursing students have participated in this study, obtaining a response rate of 51.2%. Most participants were female (91.8%), with a mean age was 22 years (SD = 4.47). From these, 90.9% lived in a predominantly urban environment, 50.9% knew or had direct contact with people with mental illness, 33.6% had a history of mental health treatment and 52.7% had already considered the possibility of working in the mental health field after graduating (Table 1).

Table 1. Socio-demographic characteristics of the sample.

	1st Year (N = 36)	2nd Year (N = 24)	3rd Year (N = 29)	4th Year (N = 21)	Overall (N = 110)
			Sex		
Female	33 (91.7%)	24 (100%)	26 (89.7%)	18 (85.7%)	101 (91.8%)
Male	3 (8.3%)	0 (0%)	3 (10.3%)	3 (14.3%)	9 (8.2%)
			Age		
Mean (SD)	21.5 (5.61)	21.1 (1.54)	21.8 (1.64)	24.4 (6.34)	22.0 (4.47)
Median	20.0	21.0	21.0	22.0	21.0
[Min, Max]	[18.0, 48.0]	[19.0, 24.0]	[19.0, 25.0]	[21.0, 47.0]	[18.0, 48.0]
			Religious		
Yes	7 (19.4%)	11 (45.8%)	8 (27.6%)	7 (33.3%)	33 (30.0%)
No	29 (80.6%)	13 (54.2%)	21 (72.4%)	14 (66.7%)	77 (70.0%)
			Residence		
Rural	2 (5.6%)	1 (4.2%)	5 (17.2%)	2 (9.5%)	10 (9.1%)
Urban	34 (94.4%)	23 (95.8%)	24 (82.8%)	19 (90.5%)	100 (90.9%)
		Knows someone with mental illness			
False	18 (50.0%)	12 (50.0%)	10 (34.5%)	14 (66.7%)	54 (49.1%)
True	18 (50.0%)	12 (50.0%)	19 (65.5%)	7 (33.3%)	56 (50.9%)
			Relationship		
None	18 (50.0%)	12 (50.0%)	10 (34.5%)	14 (66.7%)	54 (49.1%)
Acquaintance	5 (13.9%)	1 (4.2%)	5 (17.2%)	3 (14.3%)	14 (12.7%)
Friend	2 (5.6%)	5 (20.8%)	8 (27.6%)	2 (9.5%)	17 (15.5%)
Family	11 (30.6%)	6 (25.0%)	6 (20.7%)	2 (9.5%)	25 (22.7%)
			Frequency		
Not applicable	18 (50.0%)	12 (50.0%)	10 (34.5%)	14 (66.7%)	54 (49.1%)
Never	1 (2.8%)	1 (4.2%)	2 (6.9%)	1 (4.8%)	5 (4.5%)
Occasionally	6 (16.7%)	4 (16.7%)	10 (34.5%)	4 (19.0%)	24 (21.8%)
Monthly	4 (11.1%)	3 (12.5%)	1 (3.4%)	0 (0%)	8 (7.3%)
Weekly	3 (8.3%)	1 (4.2%)	5 (17.2%)	1 (4.8%)	10 (9.1%)
Daily	4 (11.1%)	3 (12.5%)	1 (3.4%)	1 (4.8%)	9 (8.2%)
		History of mental health treatment			
False	21 (58.3%)	14 (58.3%)	21 (72.4%)	17 (81.0%)	73 (66.4%)
True	15 (41.7%)	10 (41.7%)	8 (27.6%)	4 (19.0%)	37 (33.6%)
		Consider working in mental health field			
False	17 (47.2%)	13 (54.2%)	14 (48.3%)	8 (38.1%)	52 (47.3%)
True	19 (52.8%)	11 (45.8%)	15 (51.7%)	13 (61.9%)	58 (52.7%)

Table 2, presents the mean and standard deviation obtained for each dimension of stigma, divided by each level of the various psycho-socio-demographics under study, as well as the overall measures for these dimensions. In addition, values of minimum, maximum, mean and standard deviation, obtained for each of the AQ-27 items are presented in Table A1.

Table 2. Values of means and standard deviation for each subclass or dimension of stigmatising attitudes or behaviours of AQ-27 according to the participants' socio-demographic characteristics.

	Anger		Avoidance		Blame		Coercion		Dangerousness		Fear		Help		Pity		Segregation	
	M	SD	M	SD	M	SD	M	SD	M	SD	M	SD	M	SD	M	SD	M	SD
Year of study																		
1st (N = 36)	10.47	5.15	14.64	6.15	8.64	5.05	16.58	4.05	11.75	5.6	10.44	5.75	21.69	3.98	17.78	3.99	10.83	6.06
2nd (N = 24)	11.83	7.28	15.92	6.42	13.54	6.87	18.46	5.36	13.88	6.74	15.08	7.55	21.33	3.61	20.96	4.48	12.83	6.93
3rd (N = 29)	8.79	5.83	12.97	7.27	10.66	5.36	17.24	4.89	11.9	5.14	10.38	6.06	22.48	4.04	18.14	4.21	10.59	6.12
4th (N = 21)	6	2.68	8.43	3.44	4.67	2.96	15.57	4.01	6.57	3.22	6.05	2.97	24.76	2.83	12.33	7.84	5	2.66
Sex																		
Female (N = 101)	9.33	5.72	13.18	6.59	9.38	5.92	16.76	4.7	11.24	5.79	10.59	6.46	22.49	3.95	17.63	5.59	10.12	6.25
Male (N = 9)	11.11	6.85	14.56	6.77	10.67	6.93	19.33	2.78	11.56	6.93	10.67	7.19	21.56	2.88	16.33	7.62	9.78	7.29
Religious																		
No (N = 77)	9.56	5.95	13.25	6.73	9.44	5.91	17.44	4.26	11.34	5.92	10.29	6.46	22.74	3.76	17.55	5.51	9.9	6.21
Yes (N = 33)	9.27	5.54	13.39	6.32	9.58	6.27	15.88	5.28	11.09	5.78	11.33	6.6	21.64	4.07	17.48	6.36	10.55	6.59
Residence																		
Rural (N = 10)	8.5	8.44	12	8.79	9.5	7.43	15.6	6.38	11.2	7.64	8.9	8.63	24.1	4.33	16.1	6.66	8.6	8.57
Urban (N = 100)	9.57	5.53	13.42	6.36	9.48	5.87	17.11	4.43	11.27	5.7	10.77	6.27	22.24	3.81	17.67	5.67	10.24	6.07
Relationship																		
None (N = 54)	10.26	6.71	13.31	7.44	9.91	7.15	18.02	4.88	11.5	6.99	10.98	7.2	22.56	4.42	17.19	6.82	10.65	7.5
Acquaintance (N = 14)	8.71	4.81	16.5	5.71	8.57	4.62	15.71	4.39	10.29	4.53	9.93	4.18	21.07	4.03	14.79	5.54	10.36	4.94
Friend (N = 17)	10.12	6.07	11.41	6.7	11.65	5.67	18.18	4.3	12.53	4.98	11.71	6.73	23.06	3.11	19.35	3.06	11.24	6.11
Family (N = 25)	7.76	3.41	12.72	4.23	7.6	3	14.6	3.37	10.44	4.2	9.4	5.86	22.4	2.87	18.56	4.05	7.96	3.42
History of mental health treatment																		
No (N = 73)	10.15	6	14.1	6.49	10.07	6.44	17.9	4.35	11.59	6.18	11.05	6.45	21.71	3.97	17.63	5.73	10.6	6.51
Yes (N = 37)	8.14	5.22	11.7	6.55	8.32	4.86	15.14	4.65	10.62	5.19	9.7	6.56	23.78	3.32	17.32	5.87	9.08	5.83
Consider working in mental health field																		
No (N = 52)	11.79	6.23	16	6.56	10.88	7.24	18.06	4.99	12.96	6.31	12.29	6.88	21.5	3.98	18.31	5.53	11.94	6.97
Yes (N = 58)	7.4	4.53	10.86	5.62	8.22	4.28	16	4.07	9.74	5	9.09	5.77	23.22	3.61	16.83	5.9	8.43	5.16
Overall (N = 110)	9.47	5.81	13.29	6.58	9.48	5.99	16.97	4.62	11.26	5.86	10.6	6.49	22.41	3.87	17.53	5.75	10.09	6.3

A factorial ANOVA of type 2 was performed to compare the main effects of Year of study, Sex, Religion, Residence, Relationship, History of mental health treatment and Considered working in the mental health field on the score of each subscale or dimension of the stigmatising attitudes and beliefs towards mental illness defined in AQ-27 (Anger, Avoidance, Blame, Coercion, Dangerousness, Fear, Help, Pity and Segregation), detailed ANOVA tables can be found in the Appendix A (Tables A2–A10).

The main effect for Year of study showed to significantly affect all dimensions, Anger, Avoidance, Blame, Coercion, Dangerousness, Fear, Help, Pity and Segregation ($F(3.98) = 6.27$, $p = 0.001$, partial $\eta^2 = 0.16$; $F(3.98) = 7.97$, $p \leq 0.001$, partial $\eta^2 = 0.20$; $F(3.98) = 22.29$, $p \leq 0.001$, partial $\eta^2 = 0.41$; $F(3.98) = 3.18$, $p = 0.027$, partial $\eta^2 = 0.09$; $F(3.98) = 7.04$, $p \leq 0.001$, partial $\eta^2 = 0.18$; $F(3.98) = 7.94$, $p \leq 0.001$, partial $\eta^2 = 0.20$; $F(3.98) = 6.22$, $p \leq 0.001$, partial $\eta^2 = 0.16$; $F(3.98) = 8.01$, $p \leq 0.001$, partial $\eta^2 = 0.20$; and $F(3.98) = 8.87$, $p \leq 0.001$, partial $\eta^2 = 0.21$, respectively). Subsequent multiple comparisons showed significant differences between the 1st and 2nd Year for Blame ($t = 3.18$, $p = 0.010$). Borderline significant differences between the 1st and the 3rd Year for Anger ($t = -2.40$, $p = 0.084$) were shown. Significant differences between the 1st and 4th year for Anger, Avoidance, Blame, Dangerousness, Fear, Help, Pity and Segregation ($t = -3.91$, $p = 0.001$; $t = -4.05$, $p \leq 0.001$; $t = -5.56$, $p \leq 0.001$; $t = -3.70$, $p = 0.002$; $t = -3.31$, $p = 0.007$; $t = 3.89$, $p \leq 0.001$; $t = -3.34$, $p = 0.006$; and $t = -4.32$, $p \leq 0.001$, respectively) were shown. Borderline differences between the 2nd and 3rd Year for Fear ($t = -2.59$, $p = 0.053$) were shown. Significant differences between the 2nd and 4th year for Anger, Avoidance, Blame, Coercion, Dangerousness, Fear, Help, Pity and Segregation ($t = -3.34$, $p = 0.007$; $t = -4.56$, $p \leq 0.001$; $t = -7.80$, $p \leq 0.001$; $t = -3.08$, $p = 0.014$; $t = -4.31$, $p \leq 0.001$; $t = -4.83$, $p \leq 0.001$; $t = 3.78$, $p = 0.002$; $t = -4.84$, $p \leq 0.001$; and $t = -4.78$, $p \leq 0.001$, respectively) were shown. There were also significant differences between the 3rd and 4th year for Avoidance, Blame, Dangerousness, Fear, Help, Pity and Segregation ($t = -2.80$, $p = 0.031$; $t = -6.45$, $p \leq 0.001$; $t = -3.43$, $p = 0.005$; $t = -2.63$, $p = 0.048$; $t = 2.59$, $p = 0.053$; $t = -3.28$, $p = 0.008$; and $t = -3.73$, $p = 0.002$, respectively).

The main effect for Religion was shown to significantly affect the dimension Help ($F(3.98) = 6.01$, $p = 0.016$, partial $\eta^2 = 0.06$) and to borderline significantly affect Coercion ($F(3.98) = 3.60$, $p = 0.061$), indicating significant or borderline significant differences between students who are religious and those who are not for these dimensions.

The main effect of Relationship was shown to significantly affect the dimension Coercion ($F(3.98) = 4.73$, $p = 0.004$, partial $\eta^2 = 0.13$). Subsequent multiple comparisons showed significant differences between the None and Family and borderline significant differences between Friend and Family ($t = -3.37$, $p = 0.006$; and $t = -2.49$, $p = 0.066$, respectively) for this dimension.

The main effect of Considered working in the mental health field was shown to significantly affect the dimensions of Anger, Avoidance and Dangerousness ($F(1.98) = 14.39$, p-value $= 0.001$, partial $\eta^2 = 0.13$; $F(1.98) = 11.59$, $p = 0.001$, partial $\eta^2 = 0.11$; and $F(1.98) = 5.25$, $p = 0.024$, partial $\eta^2 = 0.05$, respectively) and to borderline significantly affect Segregation ($F(1.98) = 3.01$, p-value $= 0.086$, partial $\eta^2 = 0.03$), which indicates significant differences between the group of students who had considered working in mental health and the group of students who did not for these dimensions.

The main effect for History of mental health treatment was shown to significantly affect the dimension Help ($F(3.98) = 10.18$, $p = 0.002$, partial $\eta^2 = 0.09$) and to borderline significantly affect Coercion ($F(1.98) = 4.73$, p-value $= 0.092$, partial $\eta^2 = 0.03$), which indicates significant differences between students who had previously received treatment for any mental illness and those who did not for these dimensions.

4. Discussion

The overall results from this study show that some level of stigma towards people with mental illness is present across all dimensions of stigma, which is in line with previous studies that also found explicit stigma in nursing students regarding people with mental illness [19–23].

Nursing students that participated in the present study showed higher scores in the stigmatisation attitudes and behaviours subclasses of Help, Pity and Coercion. This agrees with what was observed in a previous study with Portuguese students from different healthcare courses, which also revealed a high level of Pity, especially among nursing students [21]. These high scores obtained for Help and Pity may imply that students have the tendency to aid and demonstrate kindness towards people with mental illness. However, as reported in previous studies, this result may also point to a paternalistic view of people with mental illness because they portray them as not competent and in the need of help [42–44]. In addition, the high scores obtained for Coercion may indicate that the students prioritise the compliance to pharmacological treatments and routine medical appointments on the person's wellbeing, as they do not see these patients as having the capability of making healthcare-related decisions, and thus students tend to avoid empowering these patients and to ignore their involvement in the process, similarly to what was observed in previous studies [20,21,45]. In particular, this was observed by Querido et al. [21], with Portuguese students from different healthcare courses, who also revealed a high level of Pity, especially among nursing students.

Another dimension of stigmatisation with high scores was Avoidance, which is interesting, considering that high scores were also observed for Help and that low scores were observed for Dangerousness and Segregation. This may imply that despite the students do not fear or perceive people with mental illness as dangerous or necessary to be segregated and though they recognise these patients need help, they still try to avoid them. Interestingly, fourth-year students which were exposed to a second curricular unit of psychiatric nursing theory and the clinical placement and with a formal theory training, show a considerably lower score for avoidance than colleges from different class years. These findings show that contrary to most nursing curricula, the inclusion of a clinical placement prior to the beginning of the 4th year which puts the students in direct contact with these patients, is extremely important to mitigate some of the preconceptions they might have, leading to Avoidance attitudes and behaviours.

However, our respondents, regardless of the year, reported lower scores in the dimensions of Anger, Blame, Segregation, Fear and Dangerousness than in the remaining dimensions, which contrast with the findings of Querido et al. [21], where students showed similar scores across all dimensions of stigma. Exposure to psychiatric nursing theory in their first year of the degree may explain the low scores obtained in these factors, which allows them to perceive people with mental illness differently, since the very beginning of their academic path. These results are consistent with data from current and previous studies that identified that a higher load of theoretical preparation in the nursing curricula was usually associated with fewer stigmatising attitudes towards people with mental illness [22,46].

Significant differences, with considerable effect sizes, were only identified in the stigmatisation attitudes and behaviours between different class years. It is important to emphasise that first-year students were only exposed to a curricular unit of psychiatric nursing theory, and only the fourth-year students were exposed to a second curricular unit of psychiatric nursing theory and a practical clinical placement in the psychiatric-mental health field. As suggested by the American Psychiatric Nurses Association Education Council [47], this theoretical class curriculum has several vital contents for student nurses' skill development, required to provide quality care for people with mental illness, namely: principles of cognitive, emotional and psychological growth; therapeutic interventions for patients and families experiencing, or at risk for, psychiatric disorders; appropriate affective and cognitive responses to patients; communication with patients experiencing common psychiatric symptoms; and de-escalation of aggressive behaviour. However, at our institution, we decided to complement the students' formation of this area by introducing a second curricular unit focused on the concepts of psychopathology, neurological basis of psychiatric-mental health practice, pharmacotherapeutics and basic principles of pharmacology, clinical decision-making and health promotion and illness prevention in a second curricular unit. This exposure to a complementary theoretical curricular unit and to the clinical placement practise seems to be the differentiating factor that impacts the overall stigma scores for our students. This is consistent with prior literature that revealed that, in nursing students, practical experience with mental illness patients is related to fewer stigma attitudes and behaviours [22,48]. Interestingly, stigma scores obtained from first-year students are generally lower than the scores obtained from second and third-year students, which indicates that exposure to psychiatric nursing theory alone does not have a long-standing impact on the students' attitudes towards people with mental illness, and thus by itself is not the key factor to eliminate or reduce stigma in the long term.

In the analysis of the dimension Coercion, even though the present study did not assess kinship, it is essential to emphasise that the score of Coercion was lower among students who have a family member with mental illness.

In the Avoidance dimension, it was identified that students who have considered working in the mental health field show less tendency to avoid people with mental illness. This trend was also identified in the dimensions Anger and Dangerousness. This result seems logical as by choosing to work in the mental health field, students opt for a nursing field where they think they will feel comfortable providing their care and establishing a nurse–patient relationship. Therefore, they are more available to interact with people with mental illness [49].

This study also shows that students who have a history of mental health treatment are less prone to show anger and tend to help people with mental illness, probably because students can empathise easier with these patients. In addition, by experiencing the need to undergo psychiatric or psychological treatment, students become more aware of the difficulties patients are experiencing, so they can show less anger and demonstrate more willingness to help. This is in sharp contrast with a previous study conducted among Indonesian nursing students, which showed that having experienced a mental illness was not correlated with the students' attitudes toward mental illness [46].

Nonetheless, this study has some limitations that deserve to be mentioned: (i) the sample limited size and composition; (ii) its limitation to only one nursing school, which limits possible generalisations to other contexts and settings [50]; (iii) the use of a self-report survey as opposed to direct behavioural observations, as the participants' answers may not represent their actual behaviours due to social desirability [51] (however, due to the online nature of the survey and since no identifying data were collected, we believe that this imitation might have been mitigated); and (iv) even though the survey's first page clarified that the study aimed to assess the stigma of nursing students towards people with mental illness, the AQ-27 contains a brief vignette about a hypothetical person with schizophrenia. Therefore, the findings from this study may need to be interpreted as being attitudes towards people with schizophrenia rather than mental illnesses in general.

5. Conclusions

This study assessed stigma towards people with mental illness among nursing students and examined the relationship between nursing students' stigma and psycho-socio-demographic variables.

Findings revealed that nursing students mainly show stigmatising attitudes in the form of help, pity, coercion and avoidance. Findings also indicate that clinical placement may play a more vital role than acquired theoretical knowledge alone. All students received formal training in their first year of study, but only the students who completed the clinical placement showed decreased stigmatisation attitudes and behaviours. Hence it is clear that combining theoretical education with the practice of clinical placement is one possible and effective approach to help reduce nursing students' stigma towards these patients. By being exposed to psychiatric nursing theory, students are expected to increase their knowledge about mental illness, treatment and nursing care. Associating this knowledge to the practise of the clinical placement can increase a positive attitude towards people with mental illness. These findings have important implications for academic education, reinforcing the need to develop effective strategies to help advance the fight against stigma towards people with mental illness. The improvement in nursing curricula with the development of psychiatric nursing theory and clinical placement in the first years of study can be an effective strategy, as shown by this work. Nonetheless, further investigations focused on the effect of this strategy are essential for a better comprehension of their impact on the nursing students' stigmatisation attitudes and behaviours towards people with mental illness.

Author Contributions: Conceptualisation; Formal analysis; Investigation; Methodology; Writing and Reviewing; writing—original draft preparation; Project administration, J.B.F.; Conceptualisation; Formal analysis; Methodology; Writing and Reviewing; writing—original draft preparation, C.F.; Conceptualisation; Data curation; Formal analysis; Investigation; Methodology; Writing—Reviewing and Editing, C.C.; Formal analysis; Investigation; Methodology; Writing and Reviewing, A.S. All authors have read and agreed to the published version of the manuscript.

Funding: This research received no external funding.

Institutional Review Board Statement: The study was conducted according to the guidelines of the Declaration of Helsinki and approved by the Institutional Review Board and Ethics Committee of Egas Moniz CRL (ID: 884, Date: April 2020).

Data Availability Statement: The data presented in this study are available on request from the first author.

Acknowledgments: This publication is financed by national funds through the FCT—Foundation for Science and Technology, I.P., under the project UIDB/04585/2020. The researchers would like to thank the Centro de Investigação Interdisciplinar Egas Moniz (CiiEM) for the support provided for the publication of this article.

Conflicts of Interest: The authors declare no conflict of interest.

Appendix A

Table A1. Values of minimum, maximum, mean and standard deviation, obtained for each of the AQ-27 items.

Question	Stereotype	Min	Max	Mean	SD
I would feel aggravated by Joseph.	Anger	1	9	3.74	2.07
How angry would you feel at Joseph?	Anger	1	9	4.25	2.19
How irritated would you feel by Joseph?	Anger	1	9	3.81	2.25
If I were an employer, I would interview Joseph for a job.	Avoidance	1	9	2.72	2.08
I would share a car pool with Joseph every day.	Avoidance	2	9	7.94	1.52
If I were a landlord, I probably would rent an apartment to Joseph.	Avoidance	1	9	3.95	2.37
I would think that it was Joseph's own fault that he is in the present condition.	Blame	1	9	5.73	2.48
How controllable, do you think, is the cause of Joseph's present condition?	Blame	2	9	7.54	1.75
How responsible, do you think, is Joseph for his present condition?	Blame	1	9	5.62	2.42
If I were in charge of Joseph's treatment, I would require him to take his medication.	Coercion	1	9	2.18	2.18
How much do you agree that Joseph should be forced into treatment with his doctor even if he does not want to?	Coercion	1	9	4.65	2.36
If I were in charge of Joseph's treatment, I would force him to live in a group home.	Coercion	1	8	3.02	2.14
I would feel unsafe around Joseph.	Dangerousness	1	9	3.86	2.28
How dangerous would you feel Joseph is?	Dangerousness	1	9	5.92	2.57
I would feel threatened by Joseph.	Dangerousness	1	9	3.45	2.27
Joseph would terrify me.	Fear	1	9	4.93	2.49
How scared of Joseph would you feel?	Fear	1	9	2.69	2.35
How frightened of Joseph would you feel?	Fear	1	9	3.15	2.09
I would be willing to talk to Joseph about his problems.	Help	1	9	3.35	2.27
How likely is it that you would help Joseph?	Help	4	9	7.75	1.29
How certain would you feel that you would help Joseph?	Help	3	9	7.13	1.55
I would feel pity for Joseph.	Pity	1	9	4.85	2.59
How much sympathy would you feel for Joseph?	Pity	1	8	2.65	2.29

Table A1. *Cont.*

Question	Stereotype	Min	Max	Mean	SD
How much concern would you feel for Joseph?	Pity	1	9	3.44	2.23
I think Joseph poses a risk to his neighbors unless he is hospitalised.	Segregation	1	9	3.12	2.32
I think it would be best for Joseph's community if he were put away in a psychiatric hospital.	Segregation	1	9	6.05	2.38
How much do you think an asylum, where Joseph can be kept away from his neighbors, is the best place for him?	Segregation	1	9	7.06	2.01

Appendix A.1. Anger

A Factorial ANOVA type 2 was performed to compare the main effects of Year of study, Sex, Religion, Residence, Relationship, History of mental health treatment and Consider working in the mental health field on the Box-Cox transformed score of Anger ($\lambda = -0.1060$) (Table A2). Analysis of the standardised residuals diagnostic plots, the Shapiro–Wilk normality test ($W = 0.98$, $p = 0.092$) and the Breusch–Pagan test ($BP(11) = 13.21$, $p = 0.102$), showed no clear violations of the normality and homoscedasticity assumptions of this model.

Table A2. Fixed-Effects ANOVA results using linkfun (Anger) as the criterion, where p values lower than the significance level of 0.05 are highlighted in bold, and LL and UL represent the lower-limit and upper-limit of the partial η^2 confidence interval, respectively.

Predictor	Sum of Squares	df	Mean Square	F	P	Partial η^2	Partial η^2 95% CI [LL, UL]
(Intercept)	21.40	1	21.40	126.66	0.000		
Year of study	3.18	3	1.06	6.27	0.001	0.16	[0.03, 0.27]
Sex	0.19	1	0.19	1.10	0.297	0.01	[0.00, 0.08]
Religion	0.04	1	0.04	0.27	0.608	0.00	[0.00, 0.06]
Residence	0.08	1	0.08	0.48	0.488	0.00	[0.00, 0.07]
Relationship	0.40	3	0.13	0.78	0.506	0.02	[0.00, 0.08]
History of mental health treatment	0.25	1	0.25	1.50	0.223	0.01	[0.00, 0.09]
Consider working in mental health field	2.43	1	2.43	14.39	0.000	0.13	[0.03, 0.25]
Error	16.56	98	0.17				

Appendix A.2. Avoidance

A Factorial ANOVA type 2 was performed to compare the main effects of the Year of study, Sex, Religion, Residence, Relationship, Treatment and Psychiatry on the score of Avoidance (Table A3). Analysis of the standardised residuals diagnostic plots, the Shapiro–Wilk normality test ($W = 0.90$, $p = 0.39$) and the Breusch–Pagan test ($BP(11) = 19.48$, $p = 0.05$), showed no clear violations of the normality and homoscedasticity assumptions of this model.

Table A3. Fixed-Effects ANOVA results using Avoidance as the criterion, where p values lower than the significance level of 0.05 are highlighted in bold, and LL and UL represent the lower-limit and upper-limit of the partial η^2 confidence interval, respectively.

Predictor	Sum of Squares	df	Mean Square	F	P	partial η^2	Partial η^2 95% CI [LL, UL]
(Intercept)	1420.71	1	1420.71	45.49	0.000		
Year of study	747.13	3	249.04	7.97	0.000	0.20	[0.06, 0.31]
Sex	52.12	1	52.12	1.67	0.199	0.02	[0.00, 0.10]
Religion	8.66	1	8.66	0.28	0.600	0.00	[0.00, 0.06]
Residence	0.43	1	0.43	0.01	0.907	0.00	[0.00, 0.02]
Relationship	185.49	3	61.83	1.98	0.122	0.06	[0.00, 0.14]
History of mental health treatment	31.95	1	31.95	1.02	0.314	0.01	[0.00, 0.08]
Consider working in mental health field	361.89	1	361.89	11.59	0.001	0.11	[0.02, 0.23]
Error	3060.54	98	31.23				

Appendix A.3. Blame

A Factorial ANOVA type 2 was performed to compare the main effects of the Year of study, Sex, Religion, Residence, Relationship, History of mental health treatment and Consider working in the mental health field on the Box-Cox transformed score of Blame ($\lambda = -0.2011$) (Table A4). Analysis of the standardised residuals diagnostic plots, the Shapiro–Wilk normality test ($W = 0.99$, $p = 0.445$) and the Breusch–Pagan test ($BP(11) = 6.09$, $p = 0.867$), showed no clear violations of the normality and homoscedasticity assumptions of this model.

Table A4. Fixed-Effects ANOVA results using linkfun (Blame) as the criterion, where p values lower than the significance level of 0.05 are highlighted in bold, and LL and UL represent the lower-limit and upper-limit of the partial η^2 confidence interval, respectively.

Predictor	Sum of Squares	Df	Mean Square	F	P	Partial η^2	Partial η^2 95% CI [LL, UL]
(Intercept)	13.24	1	13.24	134.05	0.000		
Year of study	6.60	3	2.20	22.29	0.000	0.41	[0.24, 0.51]
Sex	0.17	1	0.17	1.74	0.191	0.02	[0.00, 0.10]
Religion	0.03	1	0.03	0.27	0.605	0.00	[0.00, 0.06]
Residence	0.00	1	0.00	0.00	0.994	0.00	[0.00, 1.00]
Relationship	0.48	3	0.16	1.61	0.193	0.05	[0.00, 0.13]
History of mental health treatment	0.17	1	0.17	1.70	0.195	0.02	[0.00, 0.10]
Consider working in mental health field	0.02	1	0.02	0.20	0.657	0.00	[0.00, 0.05]
Error	9.68	98	0.10				

Appendix A.4. Coercion

Factorial ANOVA type 2 was performed to compare the main effects of the Year of study, Sex, Religion, Residence, Relationship, History of mental health treatment and Consider working in the mental health field on the score of Coercion (Table A5). Analysis of the standardised residuals diagnostic plots, the Shapiro–Wilk normality test ($W = 0.99$, $p = 0.413$) and the Breusch–Pagan test ($BP(11) = 15.20$, $p = 0.174$), showed no clear violations of the normality and homoscedasticity assumptions for this model.

Table A5. Fixed-Effects ANOVA results using Coercion as the criterion, where p values lower than the significance level of 0.05 are highlighted in bold, and LL and UL represent the lower-limit and upper-limit of the partial η^2 confidence interval, respectively.

Predictor	Sum of Squares	df	Mean Square	F	p	Partial η^2	Partial η^2 95% CI [LL, UL]
(Intercept)	1377.96	1	1377.96	81.65	0.000		
Year of study	160.97	3	53.66	3.18	0.027	0.09	[0.00, 0.19]
Sex	50.13	1	50.13	2.97	0.088	0.03	[0.00, 0.12]
Religion	60.78	1	60.78	3.60	0.061	0.04	[0.00, 0.13]
Residence	0.29	1	0.29	0.02	0.897	0.00	[0.00, 0.03]
Relationship	239.45	3	79.82	4.73	0.004	0.13	[0.02, 0.23]
History of mental health treatment	48.91	1	48.91	2.90	0.092	0.03	[0.00, 0.12]
Consider working in mental health field	21.58	1	21.58	1.28	0.261	0.01	[0.00, 0.09]
Error	1653.83	98	16.88				

Appendix A.5. Dangerousness

A Factorial ANOVA type 2 was performed to compare the main effects of the Year of study, Sex, Religion, Residence, Relationship, History of mental health treatment and Consider working in the mental health field on the score of Box-Cox transformed score of Dangerousness ($\lambda = 0.3453$) (Table A6). Analysis of the standardised residuals diagnostic plots, the Shapiro–Wilk normality test ($W = 0.99$, $p = 0.325$) and the Breusch–Pagan test ($BP(11) = 15.69$, $p = 0.153$), showed no clear violations of the normality and homoscedasticity assumptions of these models.

Table A6. Fixed-Effects ANOVA results using linkfun (Dangerousness) as the criterion, where p values lower than the significance level of 0.05 are highlighted in bold, and LL and UL represent the lower-limit and upper-limit of the partial η^2 confidence interval, respectively.

Predictor	Sum of Squares	Df	Mean Square	F	p	Partial η^2	Partial η^2 95% CI [LL, UL]
(Intercept)	75.70	1	75.70	60.88	0.000		
Year of study	26.26	3	8.75	7.04	0.000	0.18	[0.05, 0.29]
Sex	0.21	1	0.21	0.17	0.682	0.00	[0.00, 0.05]
Religion	0.03	1	0.03	0.03	0.870	0.00	[0.00, 0.03]
Residence	0.04	1	0.04	0.03	0.866	0.00	[0.00, 0.03]
Relationship	2.29	3	0.76	0.62	0.607	0.02	[0.00, 0.07]
History of mental health treatment	0.23	1	0.23	0.18	0.668	0.00	[0.00, 0.05]
Consider working in mental health field	6.53	1	6.53	5.25	0.024	0.05	[0.00, 0.15]
Error	121.86	98	1.24				

Appendix A.6. Fear

A Factorial ANOVA type 2 was performed to compare the main effects of the Year of study, Sex, Religion, Residence, Relationship, History of mental health treatment and Consider working in the mental health field on the Box-Cox transformed score of Fear ($\lambda = 0.0169$) (Table A7). Analysis of the standardised residuals diagnostic plots, the Shapiro–Wilk normality test (W = 0.99, $p = 0.325$) and the Breusch–Pagan test (BP(11) = 15.69, $p = 0.153$) showed no clear violations of the normality and homoscedasticity assumptions of these models.

Table A7. Fixed-Effects ANOVA results using linkfun (Fear) as the criterion, where p values lower than the significance level of 0.05 are highlighted in bold, and LL and UL represent the lower-limit and upper-limit of the partial η^2 confidence interval, respectively.

Predictor	Sum of Squares	Df	Mean Square	F	p	Partial η^2	Partial η^2 95% CI [LL, UL]
(Intercept)	23.65	1	23.65	69.49	0.000		
Year of study	8.11	3	2.70	7.94	0.000	0.20	[0.06, 0.31]
Sex	0.01	1	0.01	0.04	0.841	0.00	[0.00, 0.04]
Religion	0.35	1	0.35	1.04	0.311	0.01	[0.00, 0.08]
Residence	0.57	1	0.57	1.68	0.198	0.02	[0.00, 0.10]
Relationship	0.45	3	0.15	0.45	0.721	0.01	[0.00, 0.06]
History of mental health treatment	0.52	1	0.52	1.54	0.218	0.02	[0.00, 0.09]
Consider working in mental health field	1.02	1	1.02	2.99	0.087	0.03	[0.00, 0.12]
Error	33.36	98	0.34				

Appendix A.7. Help

A Factorial ANOVA type 2 was performed to compare the main effects of the Year of study, Sex, Religion, Residence, Relationship, History of mental health treatment and Consider working in the mental health field on the Box-Cox transformed score of Help ($\lambda = 2.9852$) (Table A8). Analysis of the standardised residuals diagnostic plots, the Shapiro–Wilk normality test (W = 0.97, $p = 0.014$) and the Breusch–Pagan test (BP(11) = 14.73, $p = 0.195$), showed no clear violations of the normality and homoscedasticity assumptions for this model.

Table A8. Fixed-Effects ANOVA results using linkfun (Help) as the criterion, where *p* values lower than the significance level of 0.05 are highlighted in bold, and LL and UL represent the lower-limit and upper-limit of the partial η^2 confidence interval, respectively.

Predictor	Sum of Squares	Df	Mean Square	F	P	Partial η^2	Partial η^2 95% CI [LL, UL]
(Intercept)	45,425,647.47	1	45,425,647.47	20.06	0.000		
Year of study	42,269,057.61	3	14,089,685.87	6.22	0.001	0.16	[0.03, 0.27]
Sex	2,235,687.98	1	2,235,687.98	0.99	0.323	0.01	[0.00, 0.08]
Religion	13,598,139.32	1	13,598,139.32	6.01	0.016	0.06	[0.00, 0.16]
Residence	3,332,818.29	1	3,332,818.29	1.47	0.228	0.01	[0.00, 0.09]
Relationship	8,811,066.04	3	2,937,022.01	1.30	0.280	0.04	[0.00, 0.11]
History of mental health treatment	23,047,423.51	1	23,047,423.51	10.18	0.002	0.09	[0.01, 0.21]
Consider working in mental health field	2,653,178.32	1	2,653,178.32	1.17	0.282	0.01	[0.00, 0.08]
Error	221,909,016.33	98	2,264,377.72				

Appendix A.8. Pity

A Factorial ANOVA type 2 was performed to compare the main effects of Year of study, Sex, Religion, Residence, Relationship, History of mental health treatment and Consider working in the mental health field on the score of Box-Cox transformed score of Pity ($\lambda = 1.3199$) (Table A9). Analysis of the standardised residuals diagnostic plots, the Shapiro–Wilk normality test ($W = 0.98$, $p = 0.256$) showed no clear violations of the normality and homoscedasticity assumptions of these models, and though the Breusch–Pagan test ($BP(11) = 23.18$, $p = 0.016$) indicated a deviation to homoscedasticity, this was not clear in the residuals plot.

Table A9. Fixed-Effects ANOVA results using linkfun (Pity) as the criterion, where *p* values lower than the significance level of 0.05 are highlighted in bold, and LL and UL represent the lower-limit and upper-limit of the partial η^2 confidence interval, respectively.

Predictor	Sum of Squares	df	Mean Square	F	P	Partial η^2	Partial η^2 95% CI [LL, UL]
(Intercept)	5501.05	1	5501.05	36.36	0.000		
Year of study	3635.74	3	1211.91	8.01	0.000	0.20	[0.06, 0.31]
Sex	0.55	1	0.55	0.00	0.952	0.00	[0.00, 1.00]
Religion	0.25	1	0.25	0.00	0.968	0.00	[0.00, 1.00]
Residence	10.26	1	10.26	0.07	0.795	0.00	[0.00, 0.04]
Relationship	643.75	3	214.58	1.42	0.242	0.04	[0.00, 0.12]
History of mental health treatment	174.15	1	174.15	1.15	0.286	0.01	[0.00, 0.08]
Consider working in mental health field	69.37	1	69.37	0.46	0.500	0.00	[0.00, 0.06]
Error	14,826.02	98	151.29				

Appendix A.9. Segregation

A Factorial ANOVA type 2 was performed to compare the main effects of the Year of study, Sex, Religion, Residence, Relationship, History of mental health treatment and Consider working in the mental health field on the score of Box-Cox transformed score of Segregation ($\lambda = 0.0987$) (Table A10). Analysis of the standardised residuals diagnostic plots, the Shapiro–Wilk normality test ($W = 0.98$, $p = 0.270$) and the Breusch–Pagan test ($BP(11) = 15.09$, $p = 0.178$), showed no clear violations of the normality and homoscedasticity assumptions of these models.

Table A10. Fixed-Effects ANOVA results using linkfun (Segregation) as the criterion, where *p* values lower than the significance level of 0.05 are highlighted in bold, and LL and UL represent the lower-limit and upper-limit of the partial η^2 confidence interval, respectively.

Predictor	Sum of Squares	*df*	Mean Square	*F*	*P*	Partial η^2	Partial η^2 95% CI [LL, UL]
(Intercept)	26.86	1	26.86	50.83	0.000		
Year of study	14.05	3	4.68	8.87	0.000	0.21	[0.07, 0.33]
Sex	0.03	1	0.03	0.05	0.816	0.00	[0.00, 0.04]
Religion	0.04	1	0.04	0.07	0.786	0.00	[0.00, 0.04]
Residence	0.94	1	0.94	1.78	0.185	0.02	[0.00, 0.10]
Relationship	1.92	3	0.64	1.21	0.310	0.04	[0.00, 0.11]
History of mental health treatment	0.60	1	0.60	1.14	0.287	0.01	[0.00, 0.08]
Consider working in mental health field	1.59	1	1.59	3.01	0.086	0.03	[0.00, 0.12]
Error	51.78	98	0.53				

References

1. World Health Organization. Available online: https://www.who.int/news-room/fact-sheets/detail/mental-disorders (accessed on 20 December 2021).
2. European Social Network. *(Mental Health and Wellbeing in Europe. Person Centred Community Approach) Salud Mental y Bienestar en Europa. Un Enfoque Comunitario Centrado en la Persona*; European Social Network: Brighton, UK, 2011.
3. Feigin, V.L.; Nichols, E.; Alam, T.; Bannick, M.S.; Beghi, E.; Blake, N.; Culpepper, W.J.; Dorsey, E.R.; Elbaz, A.; Ellenbogen, R.G.; et al. Global, regional, and national burden of neurological disorders, 1990–2016: A systematic analysis for the Global Burden of Disease Study 2016. *Lancet Neurol.* **2019**, *18*, 459–480. [CrossRef]
4. Pescosolido, B.A.; Halpern-Manners, A.; Luo, L.; Perry, B. Trends in Public Stigma of Mental Illness in the US, 1996–2018. *JAMA Netw. Open* **2021**, *4*, e2140202. [CrossRef] [PubMed]
5. Schomerus, G.; Schwahn, C.; Holzinger, A.; Corrigan, P.; Grabe, H.; Carta, M.; Angermeyer, M. Evolution of public attitudes about mental illness: A systematic review and meta-analysis. *Acta Psychiatr. Scand.* **2012**, *125*, 440–452. [CrossRef] [PubMed]
6. Zhang, Z.; Sun, K.; Jatchavala, C.; Koh, J.; Chia, Y.; Bose, J.; Li, Z.; Tan, W.; Wang, S.; Chu, W.; et al. Overview of Stigma against Psychiatric Illnesses and Advancements of Anti-Stigma Activities in Six Asian Societies. *Int. J. Environ. Res. Public Health* **2019**, *17*, 280. [CrossRef]
7. Lam, T.P.; Lam, K.F.; Lam, E.W.W.; Ku, Y.S. Attitudes of primary care physicians towards patients with mental illness in Hong Kong. *Asia-Pac. Psychiatry* **2012**, *5*, E19–E28. [CrossRef]
8. Stangl, A.L.; Lloyd, J.K.; Brady, L.M.; Holland, C.E.; Baral, S. A systematic review of interventions to reduce HIV-related stigma and discrimination from 2002 to 2013: How far have we come? *J. Int. AIDS Soc.* **2013**, *16*, 18734. [CrossRef]
9. Committee on the Science of Changing Behavioral Health Social Norms; Board on Behavioral, Cognitive, and Sensory Sciences; Division of Behavioral and Social Sciences and Education; National Academies of Sciences, Engineering, and Medicine. *Ending Discrimination against People with Mental and Substance Use Disorders: The Evidence for Stigma Change*; National Academies Press (US): Washington, DC, USA, 2016.
10. Rüsch, N.; Xu, Z. Strategies to reduce mental illness stigma. In *The Stigma of Mental Illness—End of the Story?* Gaebel, W., Rössler, W., Sartorius, N., Eds.; Springer International Publishing: Berlin/Heidelberg, Germany, 2017; pp. 451–467. [CrossRef]
11. Stangl, A.L.; Earnshaw, V.A.; Logie, C.H.; Van Brakel, W.; Simbayi, L.C.; Barré, I.; Dovidio, J.F. The Health Stigma and Discrimination Framework: A global, crosscutting framework to inform research, intervention development, and policy on health-related stigmas. *BMC Med.* **2019**, *17*, 1–13. [CrossRef]
12. Pescosolido, B.A.; Martin, J.K. The Stigma Complex. *Annu. Rev. Sociol.* **2015**, *41*, 87–116. [CrossRef]
13. Corrigan, P.W.; Rao, D. On the Self-Stigma of Mental Illness: Stages, Disclosure, and Strategies for Change. *Can. J. Psychiatry* **2012**, *57*, 464–469. [CrossRef]
14. Lien, Y.-Y.; Lin, H.-S.; Tsai, C.-H.; Wu, T.-T.; Lien, Y.-J. Changes in Attitudes toward Mental Illness in Healthcare Professionals and Students. *Int. J. Environ. Res. Public Health* **2019**, *16*, 4655. [CrossRef]
15. Da Silva, A.G.; Baldaçara, L.; Cavalcante, D.A.; Fasanella, N.A.; Palha, A.P. The Impact of Mental Illness Stigma on Psychiatric Emergencies. *Front. Psychiatry* **2020**, *11*, 573. [CrossRef] [PubMed]
16. Hsiao, C.-Y.; Lu, H.-L.; Tsai, Y.-F. Factors influencing mental health nurses' attitudes towards people with mental illness. *Int. J. Ment. Health Nurs.* **2015**, *24*, 272–280. [CrossRef] [PubMed]
17. Hunter, L.; Weber, T.; Shattell, M.; Harris, B.A. Nursing Students' Attitudes about Psychiatric Mental Health Nursing. *Issues Ment. Health Nurs.* **2014**, *36*, 29–34. [CrossRef] [PubMed]
18. Thongpriwan, V.; Leuck, S.E.; Powell, R.L.; Young, S.; Schuler, S.G.; Hughes, R.G. Undergraduate nursing students' attitudes toward mental health nursing. *Nurse Educ. Today* **2015**, *35*, 948–953. [CrossRef] [PubMed]

19. Masedo, A.; Grandón, P.; Saldivia, S.; Vielma-Aguilera, A.; Castro-Alzate, E.S.; Bustos, C.; Romero-López-Alberca, C.; Pena-Andreu, J.M.; Xavier, M.; Moreno-Küstner, B. A multicentric study on stigma towards people with mental illness in health sciences students. *BMC Med. Educ.* **2021**, *21*, 324. [CrossRef]

20. Palou, R.G.; Vigué, G.P.; Tort-Nasarre, G. Attitudes and stigma toward mental health in nursing students: A systematic review. *Perspect. Psychiatr. Care* **2020**, *56*, 243–255. [CrossRef]

21. Querido, A.; Tomás, C.; Carvalho, D. (Mental health stigma in health care students) O Estigma face à doença mental nos estudantes de saúde. *Rev. Port. Enferm. Saúde Ment.* **2016**, *3*, 67–72. [CrossRef]

22. Foster, K.; Withers, E.; Blanco, T.; Lupson, C.; Steele, M.; Giandinoto, J.; Furness, T. Undergraduate nursing students' stigma and recovery attitudes during mental health clinical placement: A pre/post-test survey study. *Int. J. Ment. Health Nurs.* **2019**, *28*, 1065–1077. [CrossRef]

23. Happell, B.; Gaskin, C. The attitudes of undergraduate nursing students towards mental health nursing: A systematic review. *J. Clin. Nurs.* **2012**, *22*, 148–158. [CrossRef]

24. World Health Organization. *Mental Health Atlas 2017*; World Health Organization: Geneva, Switzerland, 2018.

25. Martensson, G.; Jacobsson, J.W.; Engström, M. Mental health nursing staff's attitudes towards mental illness: An analysis of related factors. *J. Psychiatr. Ment. Health Nurs.* **2014**, *21*, 782–788. [CrossRef]

26. Corrigan, P.; Markowitz, F.; Watson, A.; Rowan, D.; Kubiak, M.A. An Attribution Model of Public Discrimination towards Persons with Mental Illness. *J. Health Soc. Behav.* **2003**, *44*, 162–179. [CrossRef] [PubMed]

27. Sousa, S.; Queirós, C.; Marques, A.; Rocha, N.; Fernandes, A. (*Portuguese Preliminary version of the Attribution Questionnaire AQ-27*) *Versão preliminar portuguesa do Attribution Questionnaire AQ-27*; Faculty of Psychology and Educational Sciences, University of Porto: Porto, Portugal, 2008.

28. De Sousa, S.; Marques, A.; Rosário, C.; Queirós, C. Stigmatizing attitudes in relatives of people with schizophrenia: A study using the Attribution Questionnaire AQ-27. *Trends Psychiatry Psychother.* **2012**, *34*, 186–197. [CrossRef] [PubMed]

29. Marques, A.; Barbosa, T.; Queiros, C. Stigma in mental health: Perceptions of students who will be future health professionals. *Eur. Psychiatry* **2011**, *26*, 1439. [CrossRef]

30. Barrantes, F.J. O Estigma na Esquizofrenia: Atitude dos Profissionais da Saúde Mental. Master's Thesis, Universidade Católica Portuguesa, Porto, Portugal, 2010.

31. R Core Team. *R: A Language and Environment for Statistical Computing*; R Foundation for Statistical Computing: Vienna, Austria, 2021; Available online: https://www.R-project.org/ (accessed on 5 December 2021).

32. R Studio Team. *RStudio: Integrated Development Environment for R*; RStudio: Boston, MA, USA, 2021; Available online: http://www.rstudio.com/ (accessed on 5 December 2021).

33. Rich, B. Table1: Tables of Descriptive Statistics in HTML. 2021. Available online: https://cran.r-project.org/package=table1 (accessed on 5 December 2021).

34. Xie, Y. knitr: A General-Purpose Package for Dynamic Report Generation in R, R Package Version 1.36. 2021. Available online: https://cran.r-project.org/web/packages/knitr/index.html (accessed on 5 December 2021).

35. Xie, Y. *Dynamic Documents with R and Knitr*, 2nd ed.; Chapman and Hall/CRC: Boca Raton, FL, USA, 2015; ISBN 978-1498716963.

36. Xie, Y. Knitr: A Comprehensive Tool for Reproducible Research in R. In *Implementing Reproducible Computational Research*; Stodden, V., Leisch, F., Peng, R.D., Eds.; Chapman and Hall/CRC: Boca Raton, FL, USA, 2014; ISBN 978-1466561595.

37. Goode, K.; Rey, K. ggResidpanel: Panels and Interactive Versions of Diagnostic Plots Using 'ggplot2'; R Package Version 0.3.0. 2019. Available online: https://CRAN.R-project.org/package=ggResidpanel (accessed on 5 December 2021).

38. Zeileis, A.; Hothorn, T. Diagnostic Checking in Regression Relationships. *R News* **2002**, *2*, 7–10. Available online: https://CRAN.R-project.org/doc/Rnews/ (accessed on 5 December 2021).

39. Fox, J.; Weisberg, S. *An {R} Companion to Applied Regression*, 3rd ed.; Sage: Thousand Oaks, CA, USA, 2019; Available online: https://socialsciences.mcmaster.ca/jfox/Books/Companion/ (accessed on 6 December 2021).

40. Stanley, D. apaTables: Create American Psychological Association (APA) Style Tables, R Package Version 2.0.8. 2021. Available online: https://CRAN.R-project.org/package=apaTables (accessed on 7 December 2021).

41. Hothorn, T.; Bretz, F.; Westfall, P. Simultaneous Inference in General Parametric Models. *Biom. J.* **2008**, *50*, 346–363. [CrossRef] [PubMed]

42. Barney, L.J.; Griffiths, K.M.; Christensen, H.; Jorm, A.F. Exploring the nature of stigmatising beliefs about depression and help-seeking: Implications for reducing stigma. *BMC Public Health* **2009**, *9*, 61. [CrossRef]

43. Hamilton, S.; Pinfold, V.; Cotney, J.; Couperthwaite, L.; Matthews, J.; Barret, K.; Warren, S.; Corker, E.; Rose, D.; Thornicroft, G.; et al. Qualitative analysis of mental health service users' reported experiences of discrimination. *Acta Psychiatr. Scand.* **2016**, *134*, 14–22. [CrossRef]

44. Reeves, S.L.; Tse, C.; Logel, C.; Spencer, S.J. When seeing stigma creates paternalism: Learning about disadvantage leads to perceptions of incompetence. *Group Process. Intergroup Relat.* **2021**. [CrossRef]

45. Larsen, I.B.; Terkelsen, T.B. Coercion in a locked psychiatric ward. *Nurs. Ethic.* **2013**, *21*, 426–436. [CrossRef]

46. Sari, S.P.; Yuliastuti, E. Investigation of attitudes toward mental illness among nursing students in Indonesia. *Int. J. Nurs. Sci.* **2018**, *5*, 414–418. [CrossRef]

47. American Psychiatric Nurses Association Education Council, Undergraduate Branch. Crosswalk Toolkit: Defining and Using Psychiatric-Mental Health Nursing Skills in Undergraduate Nursing Education. 2016. Available online: https://www.apna.org/resources/undergraduate-education-toolkit/ (accessed on 20 December 2021).
48. Happell, B.; Platania-Phung, C.; Bocking, J.; Scholz, B.; Horgan, A.; Manning, F.; Doody, R.; Hals, E.; Granerud, A.; Lahti, M.; et al. Nursing Students' Attitudes Towards People Diagnosed with Mental Illness and Mental Health Nursing: An International Project from Europe and Australia. *Issues Ment. Health Nurs.* **2018**, *39*, 829–839. [CrossRef] [PubMed]
49. Abrahamsen, B. A longitudinal study of nurses' career choices: The importance of career expectations on employment in care of older people. *J. Adv. Nurs.* **2018**, *75*, 348–356. [CrossRef] [PubMed]
50. Kukull, W.A.; Ganguli, M. Generalizability: The trees, the forest, and the low-hanging fruit. *Neurology* **2012**, *78*, 1886–1891. [CrossRef] [PubMed]
51. Caputo, A. Social desirability bias in self-reported well-being measures: Evidence from an online survey. *Univ. Psychol.* **2017**, *16*, 245–255. [CrossRef]

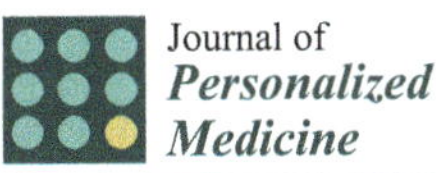

Journal of
*Personalized
Medicine*

Review

Bibliometric Analysis of the Informal Caregiver's Scientific Production

Bruno Ferreira [1],* , Ana Diz [2], Paulo Silva [3], Luís Sousa [4,5], Lara Pinho [4,5], César Fonseca [4,5] and Manuel Lopes [4,5]

1   Hospital Beatriz Ângelo, 2674-514 Loures, Portugal
2   Centro Hospitalar de Setúbal, EPE, 2900-182 Setubal, Portugal; ananfdiz@gmail.com
3   Unidade Local de Saúde do Baixo Alentejo, EPE, 7801-849 Beja, Portugal; paulocesarlopessilva@gmail.com
4   São João de Deus School of Nursing, University of Évora, 7000-811 Evora, Portugal; lmms@uevora.pt (L.S.); lmgp@uevora.pt (L.P.); cfonseca@uevora.pt (C.F.); mjl@uevora.pt (M.L.)
5   Comprehensive Health Research Centre (CHRC), 7000-811 Evora, Portugal
*   Correspondence: brunoamferreira@gmail.com

Abstract: (1) Background: Due to the increase in care needs, especially in the elderly, the concept of caregiver has emerged. This concept has undergone changes over the years due to new approaches and new research in the area. It is in this context that the concept of informal caregiver emerged. (2) Objectives: To analyse the evolution of the caregiver concept. (3) Methods: Bibliometric analysis, data collection (Web of Science Core Collection) and analysis (Excel; CiteSpace; VOSviewer). (4) Results: Obtained 22,326 articles. The concept emerged in 1990, being subjected to changes, mostly using the term "informal caregiver" since 2016, frequently related to the areas of Gerontology and Nursing. The following research boundaries emerged from the analysis: "Alzheimer's Disease", "Elderly" and "Institutionalization". (5) Conclusions: The informal caregiver emerges as a useful care partner, being increasingly studied by the scientific community, particularly in the last 5 years. Registration number from Open Science Framework: osf.io/84e5v.

Keywords: informal caregiver; caregiver; bibliometrics; data analysis

Citation: Ferreira, B.; Diz, A.; Silva, P.; Sousa, L.; Pinho, L.; Fonseca, C.; Lopes, M. Bibliometric Analysis of the Informal Caregiver's Scientific Production. *J. Pers. Med.* **2022**, *12*, 61. https://doi.org/10.3390/jpm12010061

Academic Editors: Fábio G. Teixeira, Catarina Godinho and Júlio Belo Fernandes

Received: 24 November 2021
Accepted: 6 January 2022
Published: 6 January 2022

Publisher's Note: MDPI stays neutral with regard to jurisdictional claims in published maps and institutional affiliations.

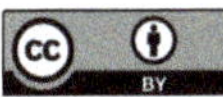

1. Introduction

The average life expectancy at birth, worldwide, increased from 66.8 years in 2000 to 73.3 years in 2021; there was also an increase in the average healthy life expectancy in the same period of time, from 58.3 years to 63.7 years respectively [1]. Countries with lesser economic power have seen a growth of about 11 years in average life expectancy at birth in the period between 2000 and 2016 [2], but between 2015 and 2019 the speed of this growth slowed. The African region had an average life expectancy of 64.5 years in 2019 and an average healthy life expectancy of 56 years. Europe had presented an average life expectancy in 2019 of 78.2 years and 68.3 years for average healthy life expectancy [1]. In Portugal, in the triennium 2017−2019, the average life expectancy at birth was 80.93 years, while the ageing index was 163.2 elderly per 100 young people in the year 2019, and this index is expected to double by 2080 [3]. Maintaining the quality of life of the elderly population has proved to be a pressing challenge, a consequence of the increase in the number of years with some degree of dependency, allied to the need for support or differentiated care, inherent to the increase in average life expectancy [4].

The aging process brings with it an increase in the degree of dependence of the elderly person, requiring care which brings family changes [4], which lead to the need to adapt to the new life situation. In this readjustment process, the specialist nurse in rehabilitation nursing is a facilitator in the management of the transition to the new reality, implementing interventions aimed not only at the individual, but also at the family/caregivers [5,6].

Within the scope of the caregiver's role, a transition which is commonly seen is the transition of roles or transition of functions. In this type of transition there is a change in the role played, often within the family, which generates a reformulation of expectations and changes in the definition of agents as individuals and their role in the social context [5]. This transition requires an adaptation that includes the acquisition of knowledge, skills and abilities to deal with the problems that arise at the self-care level and that affect the well-being and, in this sense, the nurse plays a key role in promoting the person's functional readaptation [7].

As the better positioned professionals to help the person in these transitions, nurses assess psychosocial needs and direct their intervention according to individual needs, empowering the informal caregiver to perform their role, allowing for greater adherence to the therapeutic regimen of the person in a situation of chronic disease [5,8].

The informal caregiver presents himself as an ally of the health team [8]. Person-centred care is a partnership between the person and their caregivers, whether family, neighbours or friends, who provide emotional, physical or practical support in response to illness, disability or age-related need [9]. This type of approach implies that the specific needs, preferences and expectations of the person and their caregivers are continuously assessed, respected and considered in care planning, implementation and adaptation of care over time [10,11].

Based on the approaches mentioned above, informal caregivers should be seen as an integral part of the health system, due to their high relevance in today's society, in order to maintain the quality of care and quality of life of both the person receiving care and their own. The care developed should be centred on the person and the caregiver, who is considered in several countries as a critical component of high-quality care, respecting their needs, preferences and expectations when implementing and adapting the care plan for adherence to the therapeutic regime [12,13]. In this sense, the caregiver is the main focus of attention, which justifies the development of this research.

In the preparation of this research, it was found that there are several terms related to the informal caregiver/family caregiver and not all terms are part of the Descriptors in Health Sciences (DeCS) and Medical Subject Headings (MESH). On the other hand, it becomes important to identify the researchers who stand out for the quality and peer recognition of their contributions, as well as the pattern of publications and their behaviour over time. Thus, with this bibliometric analysis of published studies related to the concept of informal caregiver/family caregiver, we intended to answer the following research question: How is the scientific production on the concept of informal caregiver characterized? The general objective was to present the characteristics of the scientific production on the topic, specifically regarding the aspects of authorship, cited work, co-authorship networks and bibliographic coupling.

2. Materials and Methods

2.1. Type of Research

This is a bibliometric analysis, which essentially consists of a statistical and quantitative technique that allows the measuring of the production and dissemination rates of knowledge, monitoring of the development of the concept under study in the various scientific areas and areas of interest, and analysis of publication patterns [14]. This type of analysis aims to quantify and analyse the processes of written communication through mathematical and statistical analysis to determine the nature and historical evolution of a particular discipline or concept [15].

This analysis assumes significant importance since it deciphers and maps scientific knowledge as well as established nuances, responding to large volumes of data in a consistent manner, building solid bases for scientific advancement, identifying gaps in knowledge and positioning scientific contributions according to their respective fields of action. Thus, bibliometric analysis can reveal emerging development areas of scientific knowledge in a respective field, contributing to the evolution of scientific knowledge and generating research opportunities [16,17].

This methodology has been a rapidly growing academic interest among researchers due to the increased availability of databases and software used [16,18].

This analysis was conducted following four steps: (1) Definition of the study objective; (2) Choice of the analysis technique; (3) Collection of data for analysis; (4) Performance of the bibliometric analysis and exposure of the respective results [16].

2.2. Research Strategy, Study Selection and Data Extraction

For data extraction, a previous search was conducted in the Virtual Health Library (VHL), and the following DeCS/MeSH descriptors were found: "Care Giver", "Care Givers", "Caregiver", "Caregiver, Family", "Caregiver, Spouse", "Caregivers, Family", "Caregivers, Spouse", "Family Caregiver", "Family Caregivers", "Spouse Caregivers", "Informal Caregiver". Criteria for their selection were also established, and included review and empirical studies, publications in newspapers and scientific journals in article format, with no chronological limit of publication, published in English, Spanish, French and Portuguese and which addressed or referred to the informal caregiver or any of the descriptors found. A search in Web of Science (Clarivate Analytics) was then performed with the following search equation: AK = ((Care Giver) OR (Care Givers) OR (Caregiver) OR (Caregiver, Family) OR (Caregiver, Spouse) OR (Caregivers, Family) OR (Caregivers, Spouse) OR (Family Caregiver) OR (Family Caregivers) OR (Spouse Caregivers) OR (informal Caregiver)) OR KP = ((Care Giver) OR (Care Givers) OR (Caregiver) OR (Caregiver, Family) OR (Caregiver, Spouse) OR (Caregivers, Family) OR (Caregivers, Spouse) OR (Family Caregiver) OR (Family Caregivers) OR (Spouse Caregiver) OR (Spouse Caregivers) OR (informal Caregiver)), refined by: Document Types: (ARTICLE) and Languages: (ENGLISH OR SPANISH OR FRENCH OR PORTUGUESE). Indexes: SCI-EXPANDED, SSCI, A&HCI, CPCI-S, CPCI-SSH, ESCI, CCR-EXPANDED, IC.

The search was performed on 25 June 2021 at 17:33 GMT+1, reserving any bias arising from the constant updating of the databases. After the search in the Web of Science, data collection began, and this was carried out in the form of a file compatible with the bibliometric analysis software used, these being Excel 2020 (Redmond, WA, USA), CiteSpace 5.7.R2 (Drexel University, Philadelphia, PA, USA), and VOSviewer (Leiden University, The Netherlands).

The search and data extraction were validated by three independent researchers, and in occasional cases, with any doubt or inconsistency of results, these were analysed by two other researchers, and discussed by the team of researchers in order to correct and eliminate duplicate data.

2.3. Statistical Analysis of the Data

The bibliometric analysis was carried out simultaneously to the extraction of the bibliometric data and took into consideration its two main techniques: performance analysis, which allows examining the contributions of research to a given field in a descriptive way and which reveals itself as the initial phase of bibliometric studies; and scientific mapping, which examines the relationships between the constituents of research, where analysis relates to the intellectual interaction and structural connections between the constituents of research [16].

The description of the data is based on graphs, figures and tables that were produced by analysis software such as VOSviewer [16], CiteSpace and Excel.

3. Results
3.1. Trend in the Annual Evolution of Publications

After applying the inclusion criteria described above, a sample of 22,326 articles was obtained. Since 1990, when the first articles on the subject were published, the number of publications has been increasing annually, with a more accentuated growth being noted from 2006 (Figure 1). Of the 22,326 articles, 1055 articles were published in the year 2021, up to the date of this research. This shows a growing interest in the subject, which has been increasing every year, without there ever having been a decrease in the number of publications from 2006 to the present day.

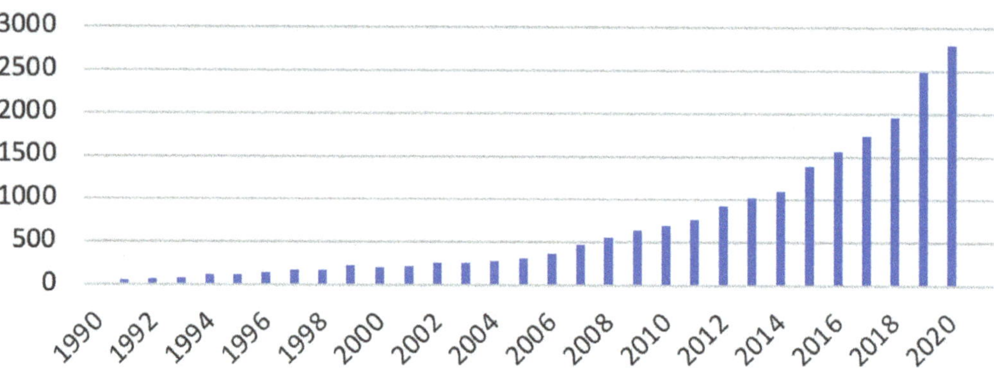

Figure 1. Annual number of publications on the informal caregiver (1990–2021); Source: elaborated by the author based on VOSviewer and CiteSpace data.

3.2. Distribution of Articles by Journal and Area of Publication

The 25 scientific journals or magazines with the highest number of published articles (n = 5130) were identified, corresponding to 22.98% of the total. The top three are: Aging Mental Health (n = 388) (1.74%), with a 2020 impact factor (2020 IF) of 3.66; Gerontologist (n = 358) (1.6%), with a 2020 IF of 5.27 and International Journal of Geriatric Psychiatry (n = 321) (1.44%), with a 2020 IF of 12.38. It is noteworthy that the Journal of Clinical Nursing appears in sixth place (n = 254) (1.14%), with an IF 2020 of 16.92, and in fifteenth place is the journal Disability and Rehabilitation, with (n = 162) (0.73%) and IF 2020 of 14.88.

Using the data from CiteSpace and VOSViewer, it is possible to identify the 25 research areas with the highest number of publications identified (Figure 2); the 10 with the highest number of publications on the topic are, in descending order: Geriatrics and Gerontology; Nursing; Psychology; Psychiatry; Health and Social Services; Public, Occupational and Environmental Health; Neurology and Neurosciences; Rehabilitation; Oncology; General and Family Medicine.

3.3. Distribution of Articles by Language and Country of Publication

With regard to the language chosen for publication and taking into account the selected languages for data extraction, the prevalence of the English language is evident, for 97% of the articles published (n = 21,664), with the remaining 3% represented by Spanish (n = 345), French (n = 194) and Portuguese (n = 123).

When analysing the data collected by VOSViewer and CiteCpace, and concerning the countries of origin of the publications (Figure 3), the United States of America (USA) appears with the largest presentation of publications (40.4%), followed by England, Canada, Australia and Spain, with Portugal occupying the 25th place (1.1%).

3.4. Authors Profile

Regarding scientific contribution to the subject of informal caregivers, the following authors stand out in descending order as those with more scientific contributions: Richard Schulz followed by Laura Gitlin, Steven Zarit, George Demiris, Debra Parker Oliver, among others, as can be verified in Figure 4.

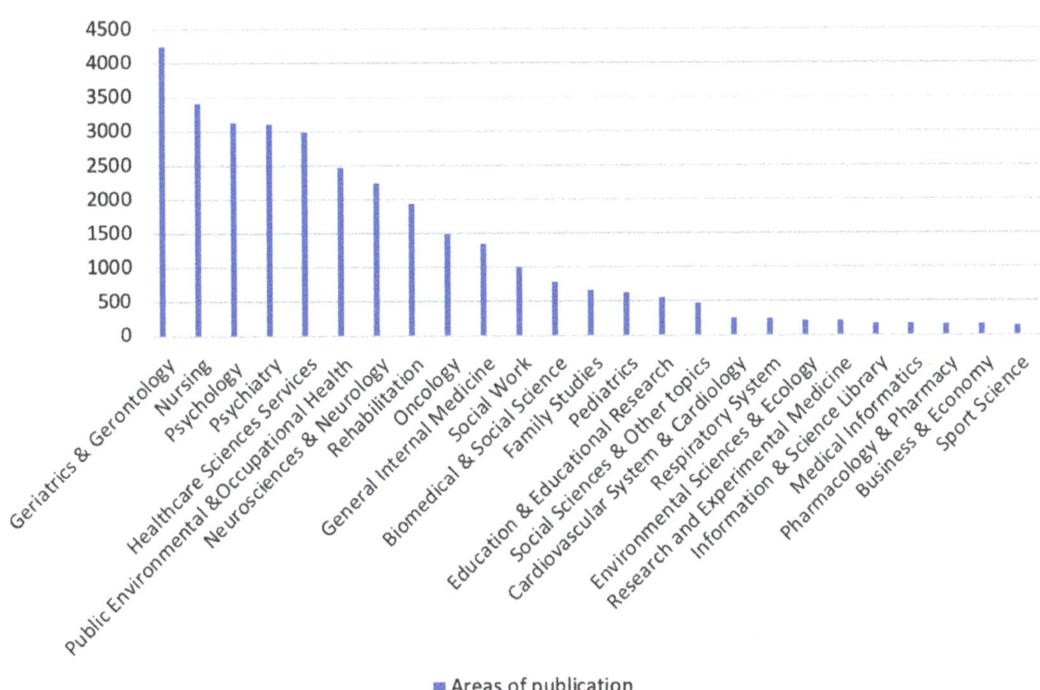

Figure 2. Number of publications by research area. Source: elaborated by the author based on VOSviewer and CiteSpace data.

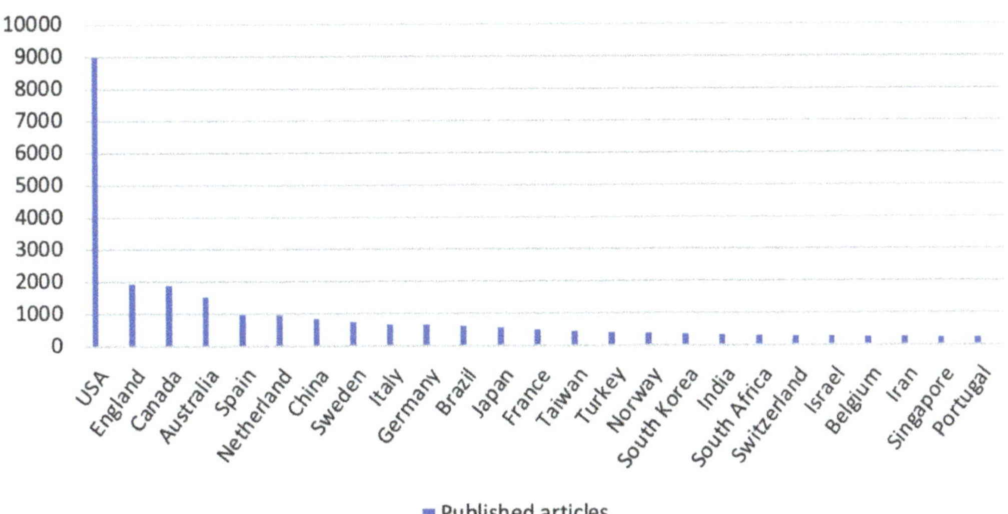

Figure 3. Number of published articles per country; Source: elaborated by the author based on VOSviewer and CiteSpace data.

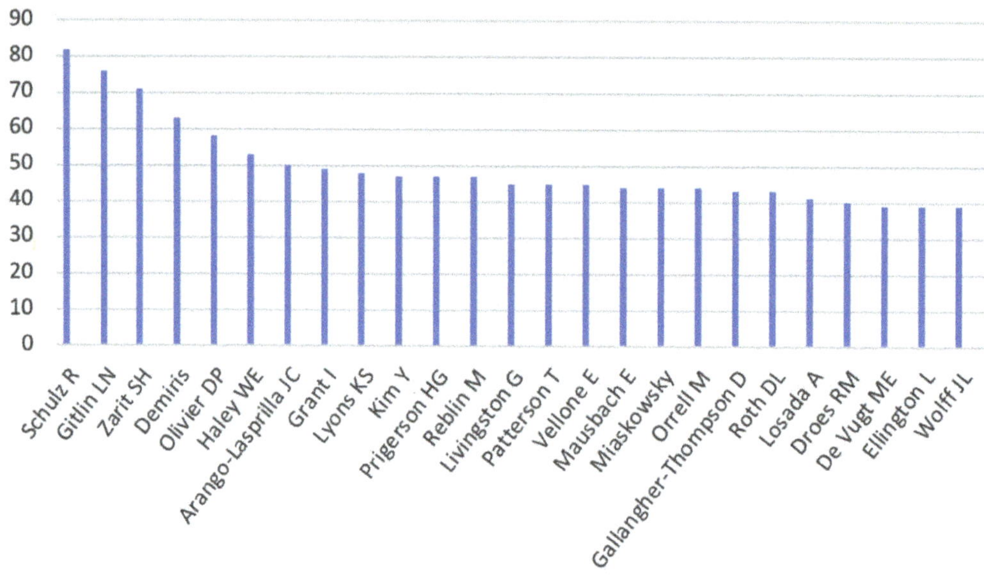

Figure 4. Distribution of articles per author. Source: Elaborated by the author based on VOSviewer and CiteSpace data.

3.5. Network and Density of Co-Citations by Author

Regarding the co-citation density of authors, this is represented by colour density, demonstrating the incidence of relevant authors. The hotter the colour (yellow) the greater the number of publications and citations of the author; at the other extreme, the colder the colour (blue) the lower the number of publications and citations of the author [19]. Thus, through the interpretation of the density network, a greater expressiveness of authors such as: Zarit; Folstein; Pearlin; Radloff and Schulz can be verified (Figure 5).

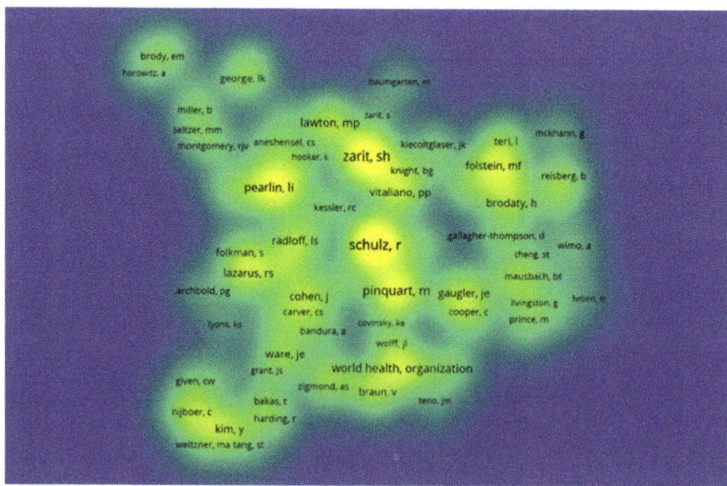

Figure 5. Density of author co-citations.

Regarding the network of author co-citations, this concerns documents in which authors are jointly cited, allowing understanding of grouping of authorship content [17]. The larger the cluster, the greater the number of citations that the author received; the same colour reflects a cooperative relationship between authors [19]; the closer the clusters, the stronger the relationship between them [17]. Taking such evidence as support and using the data in Table 1 and Figure 6, it was possible to identify 10 clusters. The first cluster is formed by 20 authors, highlighting Zarit with 1449 citations. The second cluster is formed by 12 authors, highlighting Folstein with 1397 citations. The third cluster with the most citations also stands out, with Pearlin appearing at its top with 1296 citations. The cluster led by Schulz, despite visually representing a cluster of larger dimensions, appears in fifth place with 977 citations and 282 authors.

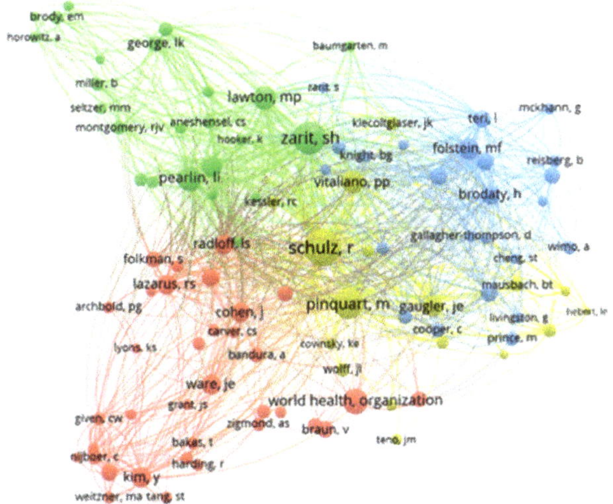

Figure 6. Authors' co-citation network.

Table 1. Ranking of citation counts and centrality; Source: elaborated by the author based on VOSviewer and CiteSpace data.

Citation Counts	Centrality	References	Cluster
1449	1738	ZARIT SH, … , GERONTOLOGIST, 20	33.5
1397	1729	FOLSTEIN MF, … , J PSYCHIATRES, 12	37.5
1296	1723	PEARLIN LI, … , GERONTOLOGIST, 30	22.5
1098	1723	RADLOFF L S, … , APPLIED PSYCH MEASUREMENT, 1	35.5
977	1615	SCHULZ R, … , JAMA-J AM MED ASSOC, 282	13.5
837	1455	LAZARUS RS, … , STRESS APPRAISAL COP, 0	28.5
796	1453	BRAUN V, … , QUALITATIVE RES PSYC, 3	12.5
781	1432	PINQUART M, … , PSYCHOL AGING, 18	12.5
629	1388	ZIGMOND AS, … , ACTA PSYCHIAT SCAND, 67	32.5
612	1385	SCHULZ R, … , GERONTOLOGIST, 35	12.5

The degree of centrality refers to the number of established ties that an author has in a co-authorship network [16]. Thus, Zarit, presents himself as the author with the highest centrality, followed by Folstein and Perlin (Table 1).

3.6. Network and Density of Bibliographic Coupling

Bibliographic coupling represents a scientific mapping technique and is associated with the relationships between citing publications and themes. Assuming that two publications that share the same bibliographic references are similar in their content, bibliographic coupling divides the publications into thematic groups based on the shared references [16].

Thus, regarding bibliographic coupling, it was possible to determine, through the interpretation of the graphic representations produced by the VosViewer tool, the most cited articles, these being "2013 Alzheimer's disease facts and figures" by Thies (2013); "Cancer and caregiving: the impact on the caregiver's health" by Nijboer et al. (1998); "Differences between caregivers and non-caregivers in psychological health and physical health: A meta-analysis" by Pinquart (2011); "Introduction to the special section on Resources for Enhancing Alzheimer's Caregiver Health (REACH)" by Gitlin et al. (2003); and "Predicting Caregiver Burden and Depression in Alzheimer's Disease" by Clyburn et al. (2000) (Figure 7).

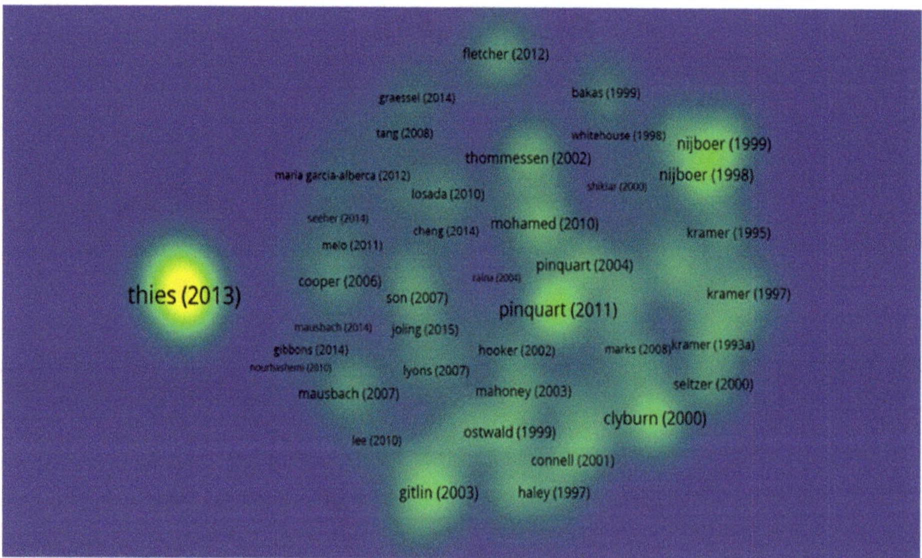

Figure 7. Density of bibliographic coupling.

It was also possible to determine the clusters of articles that cite each other (Figure 8), as well as the temporal evolution of these same citations (Figure 9). Thus, we were able to trace some networks of links between references in order to highlight them: Thies (2013) appears with a cluster of large dimensions and in isolation from the other references; Nijboer (1998) appears with a cluster and very close to Nijboer (1999); Pinquart (2011) also appears with a cluster of significant dimensions with some proximity to Pinquart (2004); Gitlin (2003) appears in isolation and Clyburn (2000) appears with some proximity to Seltzer (2000) (Figure 8).

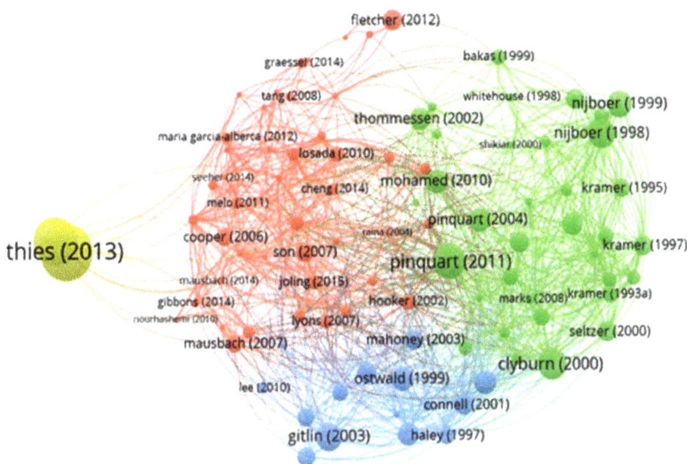

Figure 8. Bibliographic coupling network.

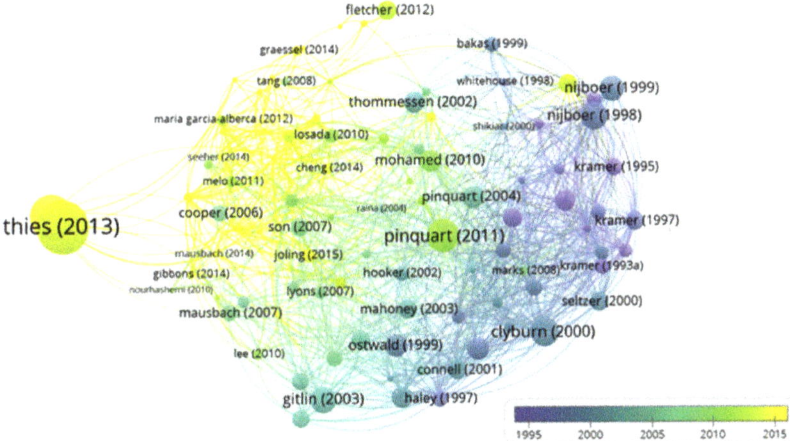

Figure 9. Chronological network of bibliographic coupling.

By date, it can be gauged that the greatest density of scientific production occurs from 2005 onwards, with Thies (2013) being a work of great relevance, followed by Pinquart (2011) (Figure 9).

3.7. Analysis of Bursts

Using CiteSpace IV, it was possible to analyse the most commonly used keywords in citations in the period between 1995 and 2025, most relevant being: Alzheimer's disease, family caregiver, elderly, institutionalization and stress (Table 2). The same process was carried out to ascertain the references with stronger citation bursts, with George (1986); Braun (2006); Stone (1987); Adelman (2014); Cantor (1983) standing out in these (Table 3).

Table 2. Top 15 keywords with strongest citation bursts; Source: elaborated by the author based on VOSviewer and CiteSpace data.

Keywords	Year	Strength	Begin	End	1995–2025
Alzheimer's disease	1995	54.33	1995	2025	
Family caregiver	1995	21.18	1995	2025	
Elderly	1995	21.02	1995	2025	
Institutionalization	1995	16.37	1995	2025	
Stress	1995	16.29	1995	2025	
HIV/AID	1995	13.68	1995	2025	
Assessment	1995	11.77	1995	2025	
Elder care	1995	11.76	1995	2025	
Ethnicity	1995	10.23	1995	2025	
Alzheimer disease	1995	9.93	1995	2025	
Aging	1995	8.32	1995	2025	
Support group	1995	7.28	1995	2025	
African American	1995	6.76	1995	2025	
Respite	1995	6.14	1995	2025	
Women	1995	5.84	1995	2025	

The red line represents the time line related to the keywords with strongest citation bursts.

3.8. Keyword Network and Co-Occurrence Density

The interpretation of the graphical representations obtained by the VosViewer allows the co-occurrence density of the keywords to be ascertained through the evaluation of the colour of the density diagram, keywords which appear most frequently being perceptible. The higher the occurrence of the keywords, the warmer the colour becomes (yellow) and the lower the occurrence, the colder the colour becomes (blue) [19]. Thus, it could be perceived that the keywords that appear with greater frequency are: caregivers; family caregivers; dementia; burden and depression (Figure 10). In the following figure (Figure 11), we were able to interpret the co-occurrence network of the key words, where the larger the cluster, the greater the frequency with which the key word appears, and the colour of the clusters represents the relationship between the key words: family caregivers, dementia and burden may be associated to the same cluster, while caregivers and depression are found in distinct clusters.

Table 3. Top 15 references with strongest citation bursts; Source: elaborated by the author based on VOSviewer and CiteSpace data. (All links in this table have been accessed on 25 June 2021.)

Keywords	Year	Strength	Begin	End	1995–2025
GEORGE LK, 1986, GERONTOLOGIST, V26, P253, https://doi.org/10.1093/geront/26.3.253	1986	158.39	1995	2025	
Braun V, 2006, QUALITATIVE RES PSYC, V3, P77, https://www.tandfonline.com/doi/abs/10.1191/1478088706qp063oa	2006	145.1	2006	2025	
STONE R, 1987, GERONTOLOGIST, V27, P616, https://doi.org/10.1093/geront/27.5.616	1987	139.14	1995	2025	
Adelman RD, 2014, JAMA-J AM MED ASSOC, V311, P1052, https://doi:10.1001/jama.2014.304	2014	95.38	2014	2025	
CANTOR MH, 1983, GERONTOLOGIST, V23, P597, https://doi.org/10.1093/geront/23.6.597	1983	91.62	1995	2025	
SCHULZ R, 1995, GERONTOLOGIST, V35, P771, https://doi.org/10.1093/geront/35.6.771	1995	89.76	1995	2025	
ZARIT SH, 1986, GERONTOLOGIST, V26, P260, https://doi.org/10.1093/geront/26.3.260	1986	81.06	1995	2025	
BRODY EM, 1985, GERONTOLOGIST, V25, P19, https://doi.org/10.1093/geront/25.1.19	1985	69.16	1995	2025	
POULSHOCK SW, 1984, J GERONTOL, V39, P230, https://doi.org/10.1093/geronj/39.2.230	1984	64.39	1995	2025	
Tong A, 2007, INT J QUAL HEALTH C, V19, P349, https://doi.org/10.1093/intqhc/mzm042	2007	61.1	2007	2025	
DEIMLING GT, 1986, J GERONTOL, V41, P778, https://doi.org/10.1093/geronj/41.6.778	1986	59.18	1995	2025	
LAWTON MP, 1969, GERONTOLOGIST, V9, P9, https://doi.org/10.1093/geront/9.1.9	1969	58.41	1995	2025	
COLERICK EJ, 1986, J AM GERIATR SOC, V34, P493, https://doi.org/10.1111/j.1532-5415.1986.tb04239.x	1986	57.51	1995	2025	
CHENOWETH B, 1986, GERONTOLOGIST, V26, P267, https://doi.org/10.1093/geront/26.3.267	1986	57.35	1995	2025	
Mittelman MS, 1996, JAMA-J AM MED ASSOC, V276, P1725, http://doi:10.1001/jama.1996.035402100330	1996	56.38	1996	2025	

The red line represents the time line related to the references with strongest citation bursts.

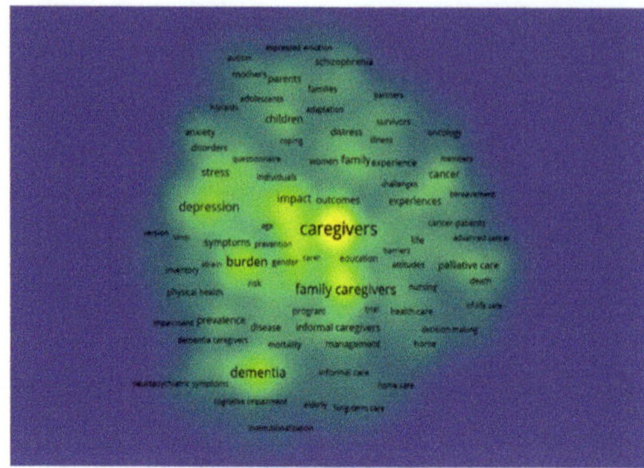

Figure 10. Co-occurrence density of the keywords.

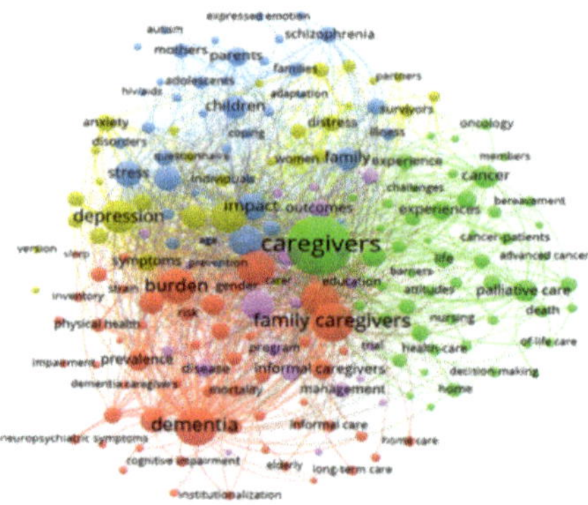

Figure 11. Co-occurrence network of the keywords.

The chronology of occurrence of these keywords can also be inferred (Figure 12), with the terms caregivers and family caregivers appearing in 2013 and informal caregivers in 2016, and no new terms appearing after 2016. In 2013, the terms burden and depression appeared in addition to the terms caregivers and family caregivers; in 2016, the terms anxiety, experiences and oncology appeared in addition to the term informal caregivers.

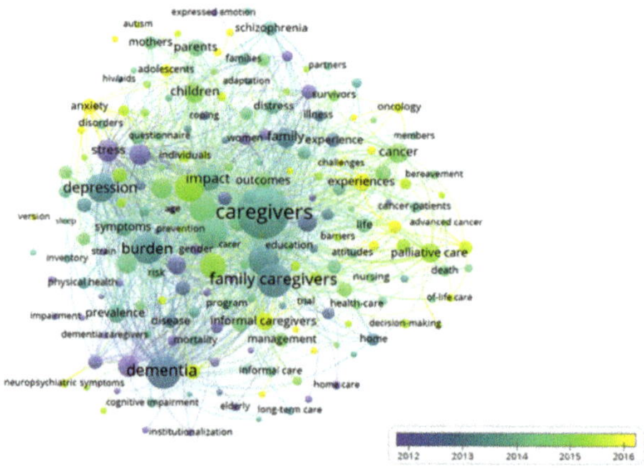

Figure 12. Chronological network of co-occurrence of keywords.

3.9. Analysis of Keyword Clusters

Through Citespace it was possible to carry out a network analysis of clusters by keywords. This procedure will allow us to verify if the works under analysis have been homogeneous in the use of descriptors. The Silhouette score is an indicator of the homogeneity or consistency of the cluster under analysis and Silhouette score values close to 1 confirm this homogeneity [20]. The largest keyword clusters present a Silhouette score above 0.77, revealing moderate to high consistency and homogeneity (Table 4).

Table 4. Silhouette indexes by cluster, year and size; Source: elaborated by the author based on VOSviewer and CiteSpace data.

Cluster	Silhouette Index	Mean (Year)	Size
0	0.829	1990	746
1	0.771	2006	649
2	0.809	2005	517
3	0.782	2001	409

4. Discussion

In this study, a bibliometric analysis of global trends on the concept of informal/family caregiver was conducted. The timeframe was determined based on the first publication on the topic (1990) until today (2021).

The analysis shows a steady increase in the number of publications over the years.

English is the most widely used language and the United States of America is the country that has contributed the most to research on the subject, with Portugal occupying 25th place in terms of number of publications.

After data analysis and as previously mentioned, it is possible to state that the use of the term informal caregiver began in 1990, with an exponential and constant growth from 2006 onwards, an evolving use of the term being currently perceptible.

Among the 25 scientific journals with the largest number of publications, the following journals stand out: "Aging and Mental Health", "Gerontologist" and "International Journal of Geriatric Psychiatry", with impact factors of 3.66, 5.27 and 12.38, respectively.

The largest number of publications appears in journals or magazines dedicated to Gerontology & Geriatrics, Nursing and Psychology. The largest number of co-citations belongs to Schulz, Gitlin and Zarit, the latter being the author the author with the most published articles on the topic, followed by Folstein and Pearlin, Alzheimer's disease", "institutionalization" and "family caregiver" appearing as the keywords with the strongest citation bursts. With the support of Table 2, it is possible to indicate that these keywords appear with the strongest citation bursts since the beginning of the 1990s until currently, suggesting that they are themes still discussed by the authors. Eom & Fortunato (2011) [21], when studying the dynamic properties of citation flows, found that the first years after the publication of articles are characterized by citations bursts that work as an indicator of the popularity dynamics of the evidence produced and that have different durability over time.

The most commonly used terms in the publications are "caregivers" and "family caregivers", which appeared in 2013, with the term "informal caregivers" gaining greater relevance from 2016 onwards, maintaining its expression to date.

Given this lexometric change, and in order to avoid ambiguity in the applicability of the concept, it will be important to analyze it in a future study. According to Tofthagen & Fagerstrøm (2010) [22], nursing research should focus on the unambiguous use of concepts, for which Rodgers' method is a possible method.

4.1. Research Frontiers

The citation bursts of the keywords were identified using CiteSpace, in order to predict research frontiers. Through the analysis of Table 2, it is concluded that the keywords with strongest citation bursts are "Alzheimer's Disease", "Elderly" and "Institutionalization", thus revealing the most relevant research frontiers.

4.2. Alzheimer's Disease

Alzheimer's disease is a progressive, disabling and long-term neurodegenerative disease, characterised by cognitive impairment, progressive loss of autonomy and behavioural disorders, often manifesting with memory loss and subsequent progression to an inability to perform basic activities of daily living [23–28].

By 2050, an increasing incidence of dementias (including Alzheimer's disease) is expected to have tripled from 2010, with a consequent increase in the number of informal caregivers [24].

The informal caregiver is the person who provides more time to monitor and meet the needs of the person with Alzheimer's disease, in order to provide the continuity of a life with dignity, often being performed by a close relative (spouses, children), an unpaid role in most situations [27]. In addition to the challenges of their own daily lives, the informal caregiver is subject to a high risk of exposure to situations of chronic stress, with consequent impact at physical, emotional, social and financial levels, being associated with feelings of isolation, anxiety and depressive symptoms, an increased risk of cardiovascular disease, decreased immunity and increased mortality being described in the literature. For this reason, they are denominated as the secondary victims of this disease [21,25].

The ability of informal caregivers to cope with the recurrence of demands influences the quality of care to the person [28]. Lack of strategies to cope with these demands may have a negative impact on the quality of care provided to the person as well as on the quality of life of the informal caregivers themselves. The literature shows that the quality of life of informal caregivers of people with Alzheimer's disease has been shown to be lower than that of informal caregivers of people without Alzheimer's disease, which may be one of the driving factors for the abandonment of care provision, as well as the increase in work restrictions and decrease in productivity rates [24,26].

4.3. Elderly

According to the latest United Nations report on population prospects, the number of people aged 65 years and overrepresented 9% of the world population in 2019, and is expected to reach 16% by 2050, where the number of people aged 80 years and over will be about three times as high [29]. Of this 16%, about half, will develop some kind of disability or limitation that will undoubtedly require assistance from a responsible person, whereby the informal caregiver assumes a preponderant role in the discharge of needs associated with ageing [30].

The principle of aging as well as the process of aging constitute a positive phenomenon at individual and collective level, proving the progress achieved at economic, social and biomedical levels, constituting, utopically, the favourable culmination of human development, translating into gains inherent to longevity, but bringing alongside it increased responsibilities regarding the response to the needs of the frail person by the degenerative process inherent to aging. It is then possible to affirm that the loss of valences, namely physical and mental, can determine the vulnerability and frailty of the elderly person and compromise the success of this same aging process [31,32].

The increase not only in the longevity index but also in the dependency index verified in the last decades [33] poses new challenges at the social level, necessitating the development of care provision models centred on the elderly person and his/her caregiver, contemplating care of excellence and safety for both parties involved [32]. Thus, physical frailty is defined as a consequence of multiple causes inherent to the aging process and characterized by a decrease in strength and resistance, reduction of physiological function, consequent increase of vulnerability and subsequent development of dependence [9,30]. As previously mentioned, family caregivers are mostly family members, partners, spouses, friends or neighbours who assist in a wide range of care assistance to the frail elderly person, experiencing a substantial physical, financial and psychosocial burden, as well as stress associated with decreased quality of life by the continuous character and longevity of their role as caregivers, often going against the satisfaction of their own needs [24,29,30]. Currently, musculoskeletal symptoms are closely related to the provision of care by informal caregivers, influenced by emotional factors, excessive workloads and poor training, particularly at the ergonomic level [29].

4.4. Institutionalization

Increased longevity inevitably associated with increased incidence of morbidities is one of the predominant factors justifying institutionalization [29].

With the ageing of population and the increasing prevalence of chronic diseases affecting all age groups, the integration of home care services is becoming a necessity for frontline health service organizations worldwide [9].

Since hospitalization is one of the key factors in the increased costs associated with the use of health services related to chronic diseases, it is essential to implement effective and safe alternatives to conventional hospitalization [9]. The overload of emergency services and subsequent hospitalizations are closely related to increased risks for the elderly population, namely functional and cognitive imbalance, as well as loss of independence [9]. Home hospitalization emerges as an alternative to providing care in a hospital environment for people who would be institutionalized for acute episodes of disease [9,10,21].

Home appears as one of the most important contexts for the provision of care, performed not only by health professionals, where the role of nurses stands out, but especially by informal caregivers [32]. However, the overload to which informal caregivers may be subjected during this process, which is not always short or linear, as well as the lack of support, has been shown to be a predictor of early institutionalization [21], highlighting the increased risk of depression, fatigue and burnout, summarizing factors which should be taken into account in the whole process of intervention, follow-up and monitoring, with the need for investment in training, involvement and support, not only for the person being cared for, but also for the informal caregivers [11,25,32,34].

4.5. Informal Caregiver

The loss of independence in performing daily life activities that ageing brings about leads the informal caregiver of the elderly person to change routines, lifestyles [35] and family dynamics [36], with negative consequences on his/her physical and mental health. Thus, the informal caregiver is often forced to abandon life projects, especially when witnessing the degradation of the cognitive capacity of the person receiving care [37]. The uninterrupted character that the role of informal caregiver forces in most situations, with an average of 15h of daily care provision, constitutes in itself a factor of overload and weariness [38].

Women are the most representative group of informal caregivers of older people [36,37], presenting a greater burden due to the accumulation of different social roles [35]; however, there are no differences regarding resilience between genders, greater resilience in caregivers of older people being displayed by children or spouses and those who are already retired [36].

The informal caregivers of the elderly person with Alzheimer's recognize that the information they have in order provide care is, in most situations, insufficient for quality care, with inadequate care planning and lack of tools to deal with changes generated by the disease [39]. Thus, the relationship between the caregiver and the older person with Alzheimer's may generate a dynamic that drives conflicts and tensions, directly affecting the person receiving care, the caregiver and family dynamics [39]. On the other hand, the caregiver of the elderly person recognizes that being a caregiver of his relative generates a strengthening of the affective relationship established [36].

Health care, in turn, should include assessments of physical, cognitive, affective, social, financial, environmental and spiritual components, with the purpose of establishing a tangible therapeutic plan and integrated multidisciplinary follow-up, maintaining functional capacity, social reintegration and maintenance, and promoting a decrease in institutionalization [40].

From this perspective, nurses emerge as the health professionals better positioned to fill in information gaps with the informal caregiver, as well as collaborate in adaptive strategies [35,39] through the analysis of the real needs of informal caregivers and can be seen as "social educators" [36] with consequent improvements in the quality of life of this binomial [38]. The preponderant role of transmission of knowledge and skills to the elderly person and the informal caregiver stands out, with a view to a safe transition and adaptation to the new health condition, giving continuity with the care initiated at hospital level, since health–disease transitions with less positive outcomes are generators of dependence [32]. The transition processes are then seen as complex, demanding and implying a paradigm shift in the provision of care to the vulnerable person, requiring reconfiguration of the nurse's role and multidisciplinary conjugation, encompassing all participants in the process, not forgetting the informal caregiver [32,41].

Nevertheless, it is crucial to take into account that a large majority of informal caregivers of the elderly are themselves elderly and also need care [38]. The overload to which these caregivers are subject when performing their role as informal caregivers, often concomitant with their professions, are in themselves generating conflicts that result in the abandonment of care and inevitable institutionalization [9].

Thus, the paradigm of care focused on the elderly person encompasses biological and psychosocial aspects with the aim of a global and integrative perspective with the purpose of fully satisfying human rights, focusing on self-determination, valuing individual characteristics, expectations and potentialities, and emphasizing the quality of the relationship in the provision of care [32].

The goal of holistic, individualized and quality care provided to the elderly, family and/or informal caregiver contemplates room for a care partner, from the initial moment of diagnosis, involving multidisciplinary care, until evaluation, taking into account this multidisciplinary in the intervention plan, the nurse seen as an asset in providing family members and informal caregivers with better training and information, with a view towards the best and most adapted therapeutic process [42].

4.6. Limitations

The limitations of this research are fundamentally based on the fact that it is the first bibliometric analysis on the topic in question, and the amount of data to be extracted was quite large, leading to an exhaustive treatment.

Some publications may not have been analysed because they were not well catalogued or were not published according to the inclusion criteria. Other types of publication such as conference abstracts or books were not included in this analysis, which may have contributed to this limitation. More recent articles may not be included in the analysis, although they do not have a major impact on the final result.

Another limitation may be related to the fact that only one database was used, excluding SCI-E, SCOPUS, and EBSCO, among others.

5. Conclusions

This bibliometric review regarding the informal caregiver allowed us to conclude that there has been a growing interest in this topic by the scientific community, which has been more pronounced in the last 5 years and is usually associated with health areas, more specifically gerontology and mental illness.

In view of the expected increase in ageing and dependence rates in the coming years, it is expected that there will be a growing need for a transition element capable of responding to the needs of an increasingly elderly and dependent population with a view to maintaining quality of life, with the informal caregiver emerging as a partner in care, and adherence to the therapeutic regimen. It is then vital to understand the evolution of the concept itself, which has been suffering a lexometric changing over time, currently the term "informal caregiver" being the most commonly used and on which research tends to focus.

An evolutionary concept analysis according to Rodgers' framework may point to directions to justify the lexometric changes detected.

Due to the great relevance and growing interest in the topic, this represents a concept that still requires further research, particularly regarding the concept definition and its role in today's society as well as its impact on health–illness transitions or continuity of care. It is also concluded that the issues related to Alzheimer's disease, elderly and institutionalization are closely associated with the concept of informal caregiver/family caregiver, which may be incorporated into future research.

Author Contributions: Conceptualization, B.F., A.D. and L.S.; methodology, B.F., A.D., P.S. and L.S.; validation, L.S., P.S., L.P. and. M.L.; formal analysis, B.F., L.S. and P.S.; investigation, B.F., A.D., P.S. and L.S.; resources, B.F., A.D., P.S. and L.S.; data curation, B.F., A.D., P.S. and L.S.; writing—original draft preparation, B.F., A.D., P.S. and L.S.; writing—review and editing, B.F., L.P., C.F. and L.S.; supervision, L.S., M.L.; project administration, L.S. and M.L.; funding acquisition, L.S. All authors have read and agreed to the published version of the manuscript.

Funding: This research received no external funding.

Institutional Review Board Statement: Not applicable.

Informed Consent Statement: Not applicable.

Data Availability Statement: Not applicable.

Conflicts of Interest: The authors declare no conflict of interest.

References

1. World Health Organization. World Health Statistics 2021. Available online: https://apps.who.int/iris/bitstream/handle/10665/342703/9789240027053-eng.pdf (accessed on 23 October 2021).
2. World Health Organization. World Health Statistics 2020. Available online: https://apps.who.int/iris/bitstream/handle/10665/332070/9789240005105-eng.pdf (accessed on 23 October 2021).
3. Instituto Nacional de Estatística, IP. Estatísticas Demográficas 2019. Available online: https://portal.issn.org/resource/ISSN/0377-2284 (accessed on 23 October 2021).
4. Moreira, M.J.G. *Como Envelhecem os Portugueses: Envelhecimento, Saúde, Idadismo*; Fundação Francisco Manuel dos Santos: Lisboa, Portugal, 2020; ISBN 978-989-900-453-5.
5. Meleis, A.I. *Transitions Theory: Middle Range and Situation Specific Theories in Nursing Research and Practice*, 1st ed.; Springer Publishing Company, LLC: New York, NY, USA, 2010; pp. 12–28, ISBN 978-082-610-535-6.
6. Martins, R.; Mesquita, M. Fraturas da Extremidade Superior do Fémur em Idosos. *Millenium* **2016**, *50*, 239–252. Available online: https://www.ipv.pt/millenium/Millenium50/14.pdf (accessed on 23 October 2021).
7. Menoita, E.C.; Sousa, L.M.; Pão-Alvo, I.; Marques-Vieira, C. *Reabilitar a Pessoa Idosa com AVC: Contributos para um Envelhecer Resiliente*, 1st ed.; Lusociência: Loures, Portugal, 2014; ISBN 978-972-893-078-3.
8. Martins, R.; Santos, C. Capacitação do cuidador informal: O papel dos enfermeiros no processo de gestão da doença. *Gestão Desenvolv.* **2020**, *28*, 117–137. [CrossRef]
9. Casteli, C.P.M.; Mbemba, G.I.C.; Dumont, S.; Dallaire, C.; Juneau, L.; Martin, E.; Laferrière, M.P.; Gagnon, M.P. Indicators of home-based hospitalization model and strategies for its implementation: A systematic review of reviews. *Syst. Rev.* **2020**, *9*, 172. [CrossRef]
10. Huang, Y.L.; McGonagle, M.; Shaw, R.; Eastham, J.; Alsaba, N.; Crilly, J. Models of care for frail older persons who present to the emergency department: A scoping review protocol. *Syst. Rev.* **2020**, *9*, 280. [CrossRef] [PubMed]
11. Montgomery, C.L.; Hopkin, G.; Bagshaw, S.M.; Hessey, E.; Rolfson, D.B. Frailty inclusive care in acute and community-based settings: A systematic review protocol. *Syst. Rev.* **2021**, *10*, 83. [CrossRef] [PubMed]
12. Parmar, J.; Anderson, S.; Duggleby, W.; Holroyd-Leduc, J.; Pollard, C.; Brémault-Phillips, S. Developing person-centred care competencies for the healthcare workforce to support family caregivers: Caregiver centred care. *Health Soc. Care Community* **2021**, *29*, 1327–1338. [CrossRef] [PubMed]
13. Kuluski, K.; Reid, R.J.; Baker, G.R. Applying the principles of adaptive leadership to person-centred care for people with complex care needs: Considerations for care providers, patients, caregivers and organizations. *Health Expect.* **2021**, *24*, 175–181. [CrossRef] [PubMed]

14. Lopes, S.; Costa, M.T.; Fernández-Llimós, F.; Amante, M.J.; Lopes, P.F. A Bibliometria e a Avaliação da Produção Científica: Indicadores e ferramentas. Actas do Congresso Nacional de Bibliotecários, Arquivistas e Documentalistas BAD 2012, 11. Available online: https://www.bad.pt/publicacoes/index.php/congressosbad/article/view/429/pdf (accessed on 23 October 2021).

15. Pritchard, A. Statistical Bibliography or Bibliometrics? *J. Doc.* **1969**, *25*, 348–349. Available online: https://www.researchgate.net/publication/236031787_Statistical_Bibliography_or_Bibliometrics (accessed on 23 October 2021).

16. Donthu, N.; Kumar, S.; Mukherjee, D.; Pandey, N.; Lim, W.M. How to conduct a bibliometric analysis: An overview and guidelines. *J. Bus. Res.* **2021**, *133*, 285–296. [CrossRef]

17. Silva, F.; Silva, J.; Sousa, E.; Costa, A. Gestão de eventos: Um estudo bibliométrico e sociométrico da produção científica internacional. *Rev. Gestão Secr.* **2021**, *12*, 122–146. [CrossRef]

18. Mariani, M.S.; Medo, M.; Zhang, Y. Identification of milestone papers through time-balanced network centrality. *J. Informetr.* **2016**, *10*, 1207–1223. [CrossRef]

19. Yu, L.; Xu, G.; Wang, Y.; Zhang, Y.; Li, A.F. ADPE: Adaptive Dynamic Projected Embedding on Heterogeneous Information Networks. *IEEE Access* **2020**, *8*, 38970–38984. [CrossRef]

20. Chen, C.; Hu, Z.; Liu, S.; Tseng, H. Emerging trends in regenerative medicine: A scientometric analysis inCiteSpace. *Expert Opin. Biol. Ther.* **2012**, *12*, 593–608. [CrossRef]

21. Eom, H.; Fortunato, S. Characterizing and Modeling Citation Dynamics. *PLoS ONE* **2011**, *6*, e24926. [CrossRef] [PubMed]

22. Tofthagen, R.; Fagerstrøm, L. Rodgers' evolutionary concept analysis–a valid method for developing knowledge in nursing science. *Scand. J. Caring Sci.* **2010**, *24*, 21–31. [CrossRef]

23. Novais, T.; Dauphinot, V.; Krolak-Salmon, P.; Mouchoux, C. How to explore the needs of informal caregivers of individuals with cognitive impairment in Alzheimer's disease or related diseases? A systematic review of quantitative and qualitative studies. *BMC Geriatr.* **2017**, *17*, 86. [CrossRef]

24. Sarabia-Cobo, C.; Sarriá, E. Satisfaction with caregiving among informal caregivers of elderly people with dementia based on the salutogenic model of health. *Appl. Nurs. Res.* **2021**, *62*, 151507. [CrossRef] [PubMed]

25. Hazzan, A.A.; Ploeg, J.; Shannon, H.; Raina, P.; Oremus, M. Association between caregiver quality of life and the care provided to persons with Alzheimer's disease: Protocol for a systematic review. *Syst. Rev.* **2013**, *2*, 17. [CrossRef] [PubMed]

26. Cranwell, M.; Gavine, A.; McSwiggan, L.; Kelly, T.B. What happens for informal caregivers during transition to increased levels of care for the person with dementia? A systematic review protocol. *Syst. Rev.* **2018**, *7*, 91. [CrossRef]

27. James, C.; Walshe, C.; Froggatt, K. Protocol for a systematic review on the experience of informal caregivers for people with a moderate to advanced dementia within a domestic home setting. *Syst. Rev.* **2020**, *9*, 270. [CrossRef]

28. Faieta, J.M.; Devos, H.; Vaduvathiriyan, P.; York, M.K.; Erickson, K.I.; Hirsch, M.A.; Downer, B.G.; van Wegen, E.E.H.; Wong, D.C.; Philippou, E.; et al. Exercise interventions for older adults with Alzheimer's disease: A systematic review and meta-analysis protocol. *Syst. Rev.* **2021**, *10*, 6. [CrossRef] [PubMed]

29. Figueiredo, L.C.; Gratão, A.C.M.; Barbosa, G.C.; Monteiro, D.Q.; Pelegrini, L.N.D.C.; Sato, T.O. Musculoskeletal symptoms in formal and informal caregivers of elderly people. *Rev. Bras. Enferm.* **2022**, *75*, 1–7. [CrossRef] [PubMed]

30. Ringer, T.; Hazzan, A.A.; Agarwal, A.; Mutsaers, A.; Papaioannou, A. Relationship between family caregiver burden and physical frailty in older adults without dementia: A systematic review. *Syst. Rev.* **2017**, *6*, 55. [CrossRef] [PubMed]

31. Araújo, O.; Sousa, L.; Vieira, T.; Sequeira, C. Envelhecimento e Comunicação: Desafios para os(as) Enfermeiros(as). In *Competências em Enfermagem, Gerontogeriátrica: Uma Exigência para a Qualidade do Cuidado. Série Monográfica Educação e Investigação em Saúde*; Almeida, M.L., Tavares, J., Ferreira, J.S.S., Eds.; Unidade de Investigação em Ciências da Saúde, Enfermagem (UICISA:E)/Escola Superior de Enfermagem de Coimbra (ESEnfC): Coimbra, Portugal, 2021; pp. 43–64, ISBN 978-989-533-641-8.

32. Sousa, L.; Baixinho, C.L.; Diniz, A.M.; Marques, M. Segurança, Qualidade e Gestão do Risco no Cuidado Gerontogeriátrico. In *Competências em Enfermagem, Gerontogeriátrica: Uma Exigência para a Qualidade do Cuidado. Série Monográfica Educação e Investigação em Saúde*; Almeida, M.L., Tavares, J., Ferreira, J.S.S., Eds.; Unidade de Investigação em Ciências da Saúde, Enfermagem (UICISA:E)/Escola Superior de Enfermagem de Coimbra (ESEnfC): Coimbra, Portugal, 2021; pp. 115–132, ISBN 978-989-533-641-8.

33. Tavares, J.; Almeida, M.L.; Ferreira, J. Padrão de Competências: Porquê? Como? Quais? Para quê? In *Competências em Enfermagem, Gerontogeriátrica: Uma Exigência para a Qualidade do Cuidado. Série Monográfica Educação e Investigação em Saúde*; Almeida, M.L., Tavares, J., Ferreira, J.S.S., Eds.; Unidade de Investigação em Ciências da Saúde, Enfermagem (UICISA:E)/Escola Superior de Enfermagem de Coimbra (ESEnfC): Coimbra, Portugal, 2021; pp. 13–42, ISBN 978-989-533-641-8.

34. Camacho-Conde, J.; Galán-López, J. Depressão e Prejuízo Cognitivo em Adultos Mais Antigos Institucionalizados. *Dement. Geriatr. Cogn. Disord.* **2020**, *49*, 107–120. [CrossRef]

35. Martins, A.; Hanzel, C.; Silva, J. Mudanças de comportamento em idosos com Doença de Alzheimer e sobrecarga para o cuidador. *Esc. Anna Nery-Rev. Enferm.* **2016**, *20*, 352–356. [CrossRef]

36. Mateus, M.; Fernandes, S. Resiliência em cuidadores informais familiares de idosos dependentes. *EDUSER Rev. Educ.* **2019**, *11*, 76–92. [CrossRef]

37. Lacerda, M.; Silva, L.; Oliveira, F.; Coelho, K. O cuidado com o idoso fragilizado e a estratégia saúde da família: Perspetivas do cuidador informal familiar. *Rev. Baiana Enferm.* **2021**, *35*, e43127. [CrossRef]

38. Afonso, R.; Tomáz, T.; Brandão, D.; Ribeiro, Ó. Cuidadores de idosos centenários na região da Beira Interior (Portugal). *Análise Psicológica* **2019**, *37*, 147–160. [CrossRef]

39. Oliveira, J.; Ferreira, A.; Fonseca, A.; Paes, G. Desafios de cuidadores familiares de idosos com doença de Alzheimer inseridos em um grupo de apoio. *Rev. Enferm. UFPE Online* **2016**, *10*, 539–544. [CrossRef]
40. Martins, M.M.; Faria, A.; Ribeiro, O. *Gestão no Cuidado Gerontogeriátrica In Competências em Enfermagem, Gerontogeriátrica: Uma Exigência para a Qualidade do Cuidado. Série Monográfica Educação e Investigação em Saúde*; Almeida, M.L., Tavares, J., Ferreira, J.S.S., Eds.; Unidade de Investigação em Ciências da Saúde, Enfermagem (UICISA:E)/Escola Superior de Enfermagem de Coimbra (ESEnfC): Coimbra, Portugal, 2021; pp. 199–215, ISBN 978-989-533-641-8.
41. Sousa, S.; Ferreira, D.; Gonçalves, L.; Polaro, S.; Fernandes, D. Sobrecarga do cuidador familiar da pessoa idosa com Alzheimer. *Rev. Enferm. Bras.* **2020**, *19*, 246–252. [CrossRef]
42. Cordeiro, R.; Reis do Arco, H.; Carvalho, J.C. Trabalho Interdisciplinar no Cuidado à Pessoa Idosa, Família e/ou Cuidador Informal. In *Competências em Enfermagem, Gerontogeriátrica: Uma Exigência para a Qualidade do Cuidado. Série Monográfica Educação e Investigação em Saúde*; Almeida, M.L., Tavares, J., Ferreira, J.S.S., Eds.; Unidade de Investigação em Ciências da Saúde, Enfermagem (UICISA:E)/Escola Superior de Enfermagem de Coimbra (ESEnfC): Coimbra, Portugal, 2021; pp. 133–140, ISBN 978-989-533-641-8.

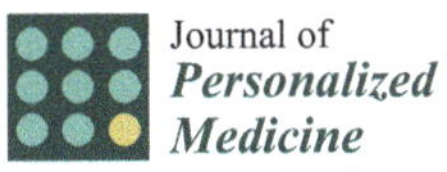

Journal of
Personalized Medicine

Article

Effects of Therapeutic and Aerobic Exercise Programs on Pain, Neuromuscular Activation, and Bite Force in Patients with Temporomandibular Disorders

Paula Manuela Mendes Moleirinho-Alves [1,2,3,*], Pedro Miguel Teixeira Cravas Cebola [2,3],
Paulo Duarte Guia dos Santos [1], José Pedro Correia [1], Catarina Godinho [2],
Raul Alexandre Nunes da Silva Oliveira [1] and Pedro Luís Cemacelha Pezarat-Correia [1]

[1] CIPER Neuromuscular Research Lab, Faculty of Human Kinetics, University of Lisbon,
    1499-002 Cruz Quebrada, Portugal; l2013123@fmh.ulisboa.pt (P.D.G.d.S.); jpcorreia.ft@gmail.com (J.P.C.);
    roliveira@fmh.ulisboa.pt (R.A.N.d.S.O.); ppezarat@fmh.ulisboa.pt (P.L.C.P.-C.)
[2] Grupo de Patologia Médica, Nutrição e Exercício Clínico (PaMNEC) do Centro de Investigação
    Interdisciplinar Egas Moniz (CiiEM), 2829-511 Monte de Caparica, Portugal;
    cebola_ped@hotmail.com (P.M.T.C.C.); cgcgodinho@gmail.com (C.G.)
[3] Sleep and Temporomandibular Disorder Department, Cuf Tejo Hospital, 130-352 Lisboa, Portugal
*   Correspondence: pmoleirinhoa@gmail.com; Tel.: +351-96645791

Citation: Moleirinho-Alves, P.M.M.;
Cebola, P.M.T.C.; dos Santos, P.D.G.;
Correia, J.P.; Godinho, C.; Oliveira,
R.A.N.d.S.; Pezarat-Correia, P.L.C.
Effects of Therapeutic and Aerobic
Exercise Programs on Pain,
Neuromuscular Activation, and Bite
Force in Patients with
Temporomandibular Disorders. *J.
Pers. Med.* **2021**, *11*, 1170. https://
doi.org/10.3390/jpm11111170

Academic Editor: José Carmelo
Adsuar Sala

Received: 9 September 2021
Accepted: 8 November 2021
Published: 10 November 2021

Abstract: Pain in masticatory muscles is one of the most frequent symptoms in patients with temporomandibular disorders (TMD) and can lead to changes in the patterns of neuromuscular activity
of masticatory muscles and decrease in bite force. This study assesses the effects of three eight-week
exercise programs on pain intensity, neuromuscular activation, and bite force of masticatory muscles
in patients with TMD. Forty-five patients were divided into three groups: a therapeutic exercise
program (G1), a therapeutic and aerobic exercise program (G2), and an aerobic exercise program
(G3). The masticatory muscles' pain was evaluated using the numeric pain rating scale (NPRS),
surface electromyographic (sEMG) activity of the masseter was recorded during maximum voluntary
contraction and at rest, and bite force was evaluated using a dynamometer. These parameters were
evaluated twice at baseline (A01/A02), at the end of the eight-week intervention period (A1), and
8–12 weeks after the end of the intervention (A2). After intervention, G2 showed the best results,
with a significantly decrease in masticatory muscles' pain and increase in bite force. These results
suggest that interventions to reduce pain in patients with TMD should be multimodal.

Keywords: temporomandibular disorders; physiotherapy; surface electromyography; aerobic exercise;
therapeutic exercise

1. Introduction

Temporomandibular disorder (TMD) is the second most common cause of mouth and
face pain, only surpassed by odontogenic pain, and presents a high potential to evolve
into persistent/chronic pain [1,2]. It is estimated that the worldwide prevalence is between
5% and 12% of the adult population and that women are affected at least twice as much
as men [3]. Regarding TMD subgroups, myofascial pain disorders have been found in
45.3% of patients, and women constitute the majority of patients in all TMD subgroups,
especially in muscle-related TMD [4]. The most frequent symptoms of TMD muscle-related
dysfunction are pain, changes in mouth opening, and jaw movements [1]. However, pain
is the main issue and the most common reason for seeking medical care [5], which is why a
large number of studies have aimed to evaluate the effectiveness of various pain-related
intervention measures [6]. Pain in the masticatory muscles in individuals with TMD can
lead to changes in neuromuscular activation patterns, which may be more evident in
maximum voluntary contraction (MVC) [7], with some studies indicating a decrease in bite
force (BF) in these patients [8].

Several studies carried out using different approaches in TMD have obtained contradictory results [9–12]. Physiotherapy plays a prominent role in the treatment of TMD [13] and has several intervention strategies, including therapeutic exercises [14,15]; however, although several studies have evaluated the effects of therapeutic exercise on pain control [13–15], the significant methodological heterogeneity among studies makes it difficult to reach a consensus. Exercise is an important component of pain management strategies for most patients and is also vital for their general health and well-being [15]. Several studies report that exercise reduces the sensitivity to painful stimuli in healthy individuals [15–19], which is termed exercise-induced analgesia or hypoalgesia [20–22]. High-intensity aerobic exercise has been known to produce a large hypoalgesic effect in healthy individuals [23]; other studies carried out in subjects with chronic pain, including fibromyalgia, undergoing aerobic exercise have also shown that intense exercise can decrease pain [24,25]. However, there is a lack of studies investigating the role of aerobic exercise in patients with TMD. Therefore, the present study aims to assess the effects of three eight-week exercise intervention programs on pain, neuromuscular activity, and bite force of masticatory muscles in patients with muscle-related TMD.

2. Materials and Methods

2.1. Study Design

In the present longitudinal study, a non-probabilistic convenience sampling method was used.

2.2. Sampling and Recruitment

Participants were recruited between July 2019 and February 2020 at Egas Moniz University Clinic and Egas Moniz Dental Clinic by two dentists and a physiotherapist, all three being specialists in TMD with over five years' experience in the field. The inclusion criteria were 18–50 years of age, a diagnosis of local myalgia and myofascial pain (for bilateral masseter and temporalis muscles) according to Diagnostic Criteria for Temporomandibular Disorders (DC-TMD) [26], and signing the free and informed consent form. Patients with any musculoskeletal, psychiatric, cardiovascular, pulmonary, autoimmune, active malignant neoplastic, metabolic, and/or neurological disease; with any other medical consideration that prevented the performance of aerobic exercises of moderate intensity; a history of face trauma; using orthodontic and/or occlusal bite appliances; with pregnancy, alcoholism or drug addiction, drug intake that can affect neuromuscular system, or who had used painkillers and or anti-inflammatory drugs in the 48 h prior to data collection were excluded.

The sample size was calculated using GPower 3.0 version 3.0.10 (Heinrich-Heine-Universität, Dusseldorf, Germany), and a total of 45 subjects were recruited according to the highest value obtained in the different statistical methodologies used and considering an alpha of 5% and a power of 80%.

2.3. Ethics and Procedures

The study protocol was approved by the Ethical Committee of Egas Moniz University Institute on 13 February 2019 (ID N° 675/2019). All individuals gave their informed consent in accordance with the Helsinki Declaration and understood that they were free to withdraw from the study at any time.

Patients were distributed among the three exercise groups. Those who did not agree to perform aerobic exercise were allocated to experimental group 1 (G1), and the remaining patients were randomly allocated to the other two groups (G2 and G3), using a computer program (randomized.com). G1 carried out a protocol of specific therapeutic exercises for the masticatory muscles, G2 carried out the same therapeutic exercise protocol directed at the masticatory muscles associated with aerobic exercise, and G3 carried out the same aerobic exercise program as G2. At the first moment of assessment (A01), pain intensity and sEMG data at the resting position (RP) and maximum voluntary contraction (MVC) were collected. Two weeks later, a new evaluation (A02) was carried out without any intervention between these two moments. Then, the G1, G2, and G3 exercise programs were started. Eight weeks after the start of the intervention protocols, a new evaluation moment (A1) was carried out, which took place 48 h after the end of the exercise programs. Eight to twelve weeks after the end of the intervention, the patients returned to the clinic for the last evaluation moment (A2) (Figure 1). All evaluation data were collected by an independent researcher who was blinded to the group allocation.

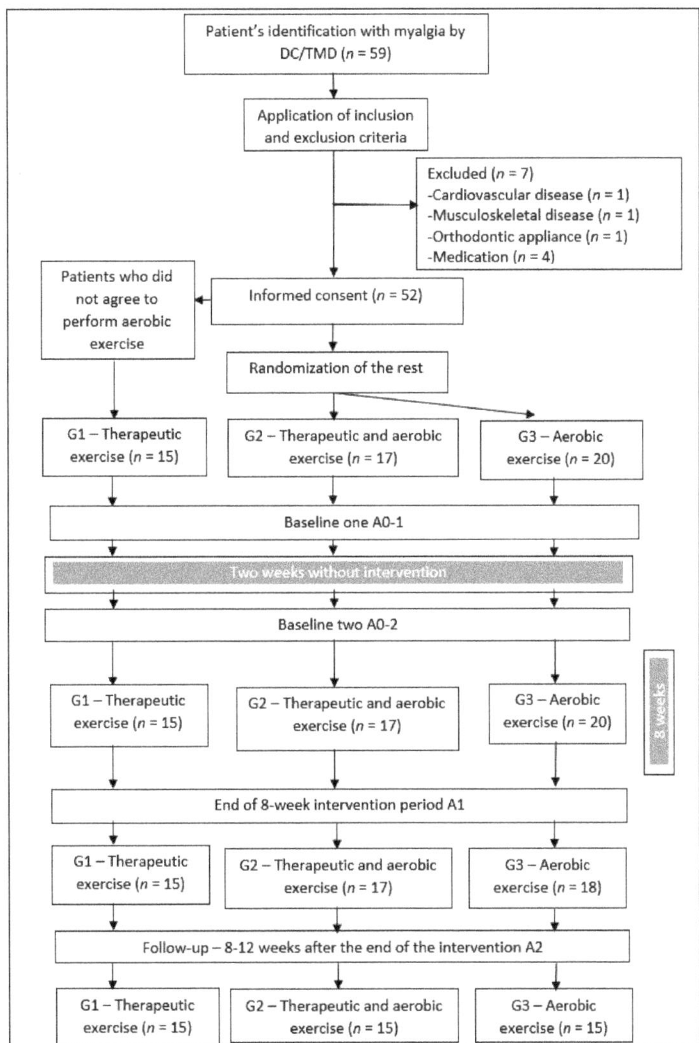

Figure 1. Study design flow chart.

Patients in the G1 group participated in a weekly exercise session for a period of 8 weeks. The physiotherapy session was the same for all participants, the techniques were always applied in the same sequence, and they were always performed by the same physiotherapist for 30 min. Each session consisted of the following techniques: compression, transverse, and longitudinal massage of the masseter muscle, bilaterally; longitudinal massage of the temporal muscle, bilaterally; compression of the medial pterygoid muscle, bilaterally; passive stretching of the masseter and medial pterygoid, bilaterally; isotonic strengthening exercises through resisted mouth opening and closing and resisted left and right deviation (10 repetitions of each exercise); and coordination exercises through mouth opening and closing exercises and laterals (10 repetitions of each exercise) [27–30].

Patients in the G2 group participated in a weekly physiotherapy session for a period of 8 weeks. The physical therapy session was the same as described for G1. The G2 group exercise program also included two weekly cycle ergometer training sessions, which were always supervised by the same physiotherapist and lasted for 30 min. The participants cycled the first 5 min (warm-up period) with an intensity of 50% of the heart rate reserve (HRR), the next 24 min with an intensity of 70% of the HRR, and the last minute at 50% of the HRR for active recovery. The speed and/or resistance of the cycle ergometer were adjusted throughout the training period in order to keep the exercise intensity within the predefined value. HRR was determined according to the Karvonen formula [31], and resting heart rate (HR) was assessed on three consecutive days, after five minutes of rest in a chair with the arms supported. The average value was calculated and used as the resting HR.

Patients in the G3 group underwent only two weekly cycle ergometer training sessions for eight weeks, which were always supervised by the same physiotherapist and lasted for 30 min. The protocol performed was the same as that defined for G2.

2.4. Data Collection

Pain intensity was evaluated using an analog algometer (Baseline® 11LBS model, 5 kg, with 1 cm [2] of stainless steel contact surface, Fabrication Enterprises Inc., White Plains, NY, USA), with the patients comfortably positioned in the supine position and fully relaxed. The evaluator placed the end of the contact surface of the algometer perpendicularly and exerted a gradual pressure on the three portions of the masseter (upper, middle, and lower) and temporal (anterior, middle, and posterior) muscles bilaterally, according to the physical examination indications of the DC-TMD [26]. Changes in pain intensity were evaluated by applying a constant pressure (1 Kg) [26] using the NPRS. The subjects were instructed to classify the pain intensity at the maximum pressure exerted. Pain was measured three times at each of the points mentioned above, with an interval of 10 s between each measure at the same point and 30 s between different points. For each point, the average of the three measurements was calculated to determine the NPRS. The minimum clinically important difference considered was two points [32].

sEMG procedures and data acquisition were performed by a physiotherapist with previous experience in sEMG. All procedures and sEMG data were collected with patients in a calm and quiet environment with a constant room temperature, seated comfortably in a chair without head support, hands resting on their legs and aligned with their shoulders, hips, and knees at 90° of flexion, and instructed to look ahead and avoid facial and orbicular expressions. Before the start of data collection, sEMG data acquisition procedures were prepared. AMBU® BlueSensor N electrodes (AMBU, Ballerup, Denmark), which were bipolar (pre-gelled Ag-AgCl, 10 mm diameter disc), were positioned parallel to the muscle fibers and fixed on the skin in the masseter muscle (superficial portion), bilaterally. To determine electrode placement, an isometric contraction of the masseter in maximum intercuspation was requested, in order to guarantee the same position of the temporomandibular joint was maintained in all subsequent procedures. The electrodes were placed in the muscle belly, with the upper electrode at the intersection between the tragus-labial commissure and the exocanthion–gonion lines [33], and were positioned 20 mm apart according to SENIAM recommendations [34]. Skin preparation was performed by gentle sanding and cleaning with cotton wool soaked in a 70% alcoholic solution. A bracelet ground electrode was placed over the wrist styloid apophyses. For the collection of sEMG data, an eight-channel system with active electrodes connected to a bioPLUX research 2010 system (PLUX, Lisbon, Portugal) was used, with a common mode rejection ratio of 110 dB, input impedance > 100 MΩ, and gain of 1000. The data were recorded with a sampling frequency of 1000 Hz. Prior to processing, the raw sEMG signals were inspected by an experienced researcher to assess their quality. Afterwards, the signals were digitally filtered (10–490 Hz), rectified, and smoothed using a 4th-order 5-Hz Butterworth low-pass filter. The normalization of the resting sEMG value was performed using the MVC sEMG value as a reference. To quantify sEMG intensity, the average EMG signal amplitude was determined during the defined time periods. All sEMG signal processing was performed through routines developed with Matlab software (The Mathworks Inc., Natick, MA, USA). The recording of sEMG activity in the RP was performed by maintaining the masticatory muscles at rest for one minute. The 10 s between 40 and 50 s were selected to assess muscle activity at rest. sEMG during MVC was assessed by maintaining a maximum contraction for three seconds and was controlled using a bite force dynamometer (model IDDK, Kratos Equipamentos Industriais Ltd.a, Cotia, São Paulo, Brazil), which was placed between the first and second premolars. The defined procedure was performed bilaterally and repeated three times on each side. Both used software programs, sEMG, and Matlab, were configured to store all generated data files in a solid state disk encrypted with Bitlocker, accessible only to the principal investigator of this study. All collected data were properly anonymized.

2.5. Data Analysis

Categorical variables were analyzed using Pearson's Chi-Square Test to confirm equality between groups at the time A01. For continuous variables, a non-parametric Kruskal–Wallis Test was performed to confirm equality between groups at time A01. A two-way mixed ANOVA was used to assess the behavior of the variables at the various assessment times (random factor) and for the three intervention groups (fixed factor). A 95% confidence interval was determined for all tests, and a 5% significance level was used. The Statistical Package for the Social Sciences (SPSS®) version 26 (IBM Corp., Armonk, NY, USA) was used for all statistical analyses. Cohen's d effect size was also calculated: effect sizes up to 0.2 were considered irrelevant, those between 0.2 and 0.5 were considered small, those between 0.5 and 0.8 were considered moderate, and values above 0.8 were considered large.

3. Results

The sample consisted of 52 patients, out of which 45 (86.5%) completed the four evaluation moments (15 in each of the three experimental groups). Of the 52 initial patients, there were seven dropouts (two who did not attend the third evaluation moment (A-1) and five who did not attend the last evaluation moment (A-2)), which represented a value of 13.5% that confirmed a good adherence to the study. The statistical analysis performed only included the 45 participants who completed the four evaluation moments. Each group was composed of 13 females and 2 males (H = 1.61, p = 0.45), ranging from 18 to 35 years of age. The mean age and standard deviation was 26.9 ± 5.5 years for G1, 26 ± 4.4 years for G2, and 24.9 ± 3.4 years for G3. In G1 and G2, myofascial pain was the most common diagnostic subgroup (86.7%), while myalgia (86.7%) was the most common in G3. The distribution of diagnostic subgroups was significantly different between the exercise groups (χ^2 = 22.88, p < 0.001).

4. Pain Intensity

Both the left and right masseter and temporalis muscles' NPRS did not present significant differences (H = 2.1, p = 0.36; H = 0.30, p = 0.86 for the left and right masseter, respectively; H = 0.54, p = 0.77; H = 0.18, p = 0.91 for the left and right temporalis, respectively) between groups at either A01 or A02. After the intervention programs (A1), NPRS improved significantly more in G2 and G1 than in G3. The effect size of this difference was large for the masseter muscle in the three groups; however, the G2 group stood out for this indicator, with d = 4.0 on the right and 5.4 on the left masseter, respectively; in the other groups, there were effect sizes of 2.1 and 2.8 in G1 (right and left sides, respectively) and of 1.0 and 1.3 in G3 (right and left sides, respectively). Regarding the temporal muscle, there was a large effect on G1, with values of 1.2 and 1.8 (right and left sides, respectively) and on G2, with 2.3 and 3.3 (right and left sides, respectively), while G2 showed moderate effect sizes of $d = 0.4$ and 0.5 in the right and left sides, respectively. Between A1 and A2, there was a marginal increase in the mean of the NPRS in all groups, which was neither significant nor had a notable effect size (Figure 2A–D).

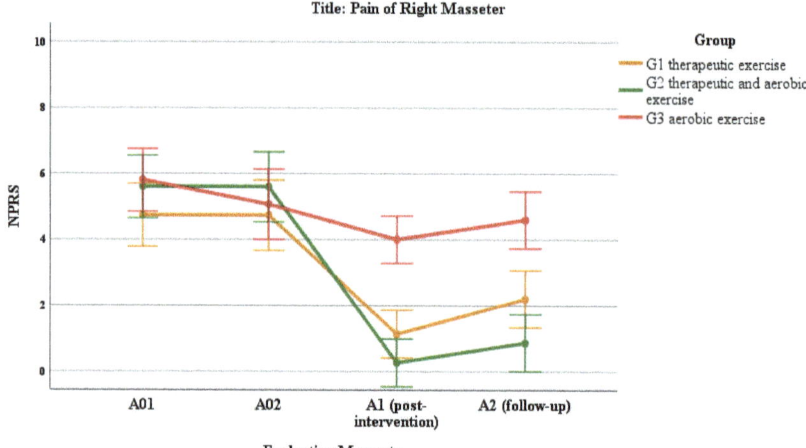

Subtitle: G1 – experimental group that carried out a therapeutic exercise program; G2 – experimental group that associated a therapeutic exercise program with aerobic exercise; G3 – experimental group that carried out an aerobic exercise program; A01 - evaluation baseline one; A02 – evaluation baseline two; A1 – evaluation post-intervention; A2 – follow-up; NPRS – 11-item numerical pain scale.

(A)

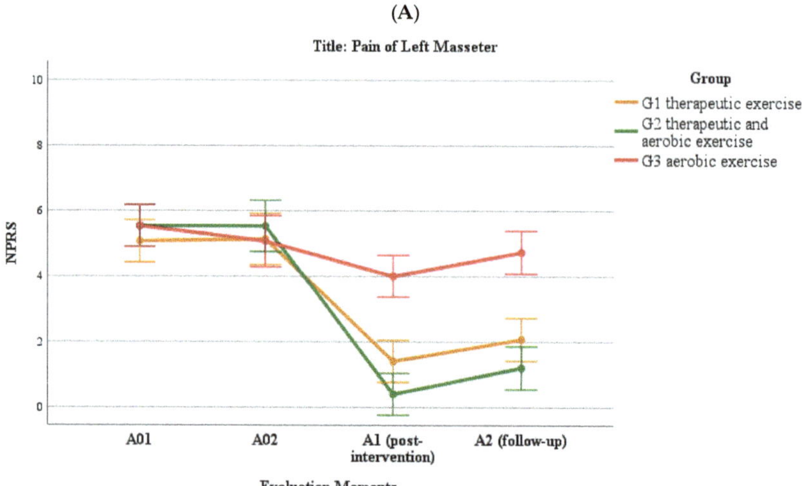

Subtitle: G1 – experimental group that carried out a therapeutic exercise program; G2 – experimental group that associated a therapeutic exercise program with aerobic exercise; G3 – experimental group that carried out an aerobic exercise program; A01 - evaluation baseline one; A02 – evaluation baseline two; A1 – evaluation post-intervention; A2 – follow-up; NPRS – 11-item numerical pain scale.

(B)

Figure 2. *Cont.*

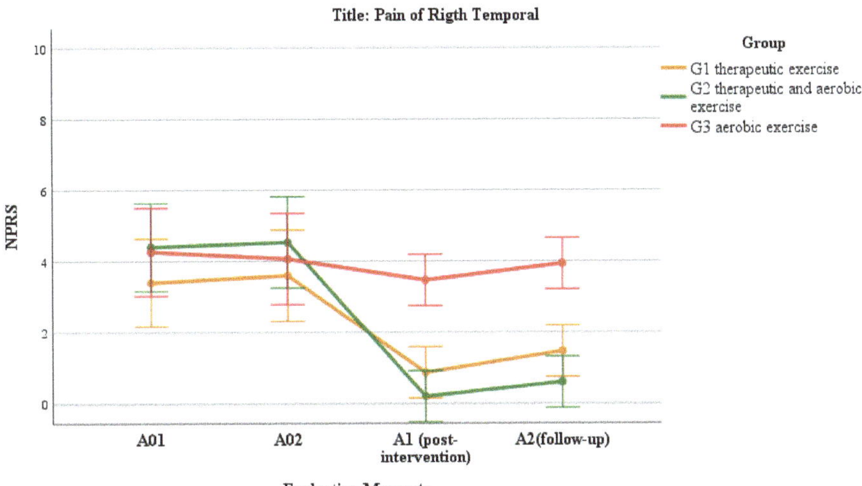

Subtitle: G1 – experimental group that carried out a therapeutic exercise program; G2 – experimental group that associated a therapeutic exercise program with aerobic exercise; G3 – experimental group that carried out an aerobic exercise program; A01 - evaluation baseline one; A02 – evaluation baseline two; A1 – evaluation post-intervention; A2 – follow-up; NPRS – 11-item numerical pain scale.

(C)

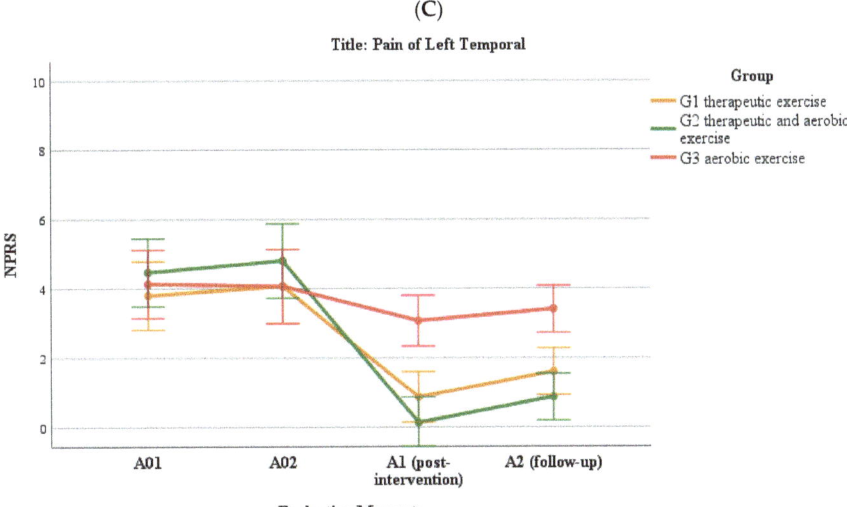

Subtitle: G1 – experimental group that carried out a therapeutic exercise program; G2 – experimental group that associated a therapeutic exercise program with aerobic exercise; G3 – experimental group that carried out an aerobic exercise program; A01 - evaluation baseline one; A02 – evaluation baseline two; A1 – evaluation post-intervention; A2 – follow-up; NPRS – 11-item numerical pain scale.

(D)

Figure 2. (**A**) Changes in the NPRS of the right masseter muscle at the different time points. (**B**) Changes in the NPRS of the left masseter muscle at the different time points. (**C**) Changes in the NPRS of the right temporal muscle at the different time points. (**D**) Changes in the NPRS of the left temporal muscle at the different time points.

5. Neuromuscular Activity—sEMG

The average amplitude of the normalized sEMG signal was calculated for masseter muscle of both sides (left and right). In resting position, the average sEMG was calculated for a time window of 10 s (between 40 and 50 s) and in the MVC for a time window of 0.250 s around the maximum peak.

There were no significant differences between groups in the mean sEMG of the masseter muscle during MVC (H = 4.98, p = 0.19; H = 0.18, p = 0.91 for the left and right sides, respectively) or RP (H = 0.71, p = 0.54; H = 1.25, p = 0.92 for the left and right sides, respectively) on either side at A01 or A02. There were also no significant differences in MVC and RP sEMG between groups at A1, A2, or between these two time points (Table 1).

Table 1. Changes in sEMG during MVC and RP in each group at the different time points.

sEMG of MVC and RP		G1 (Mean)	Lower Bound	Upper Bound	G2 (Mean)	Lower Bound	Upper Bound	G3 (Mean)	Lower Bound	Upper Bound
			95% Confidence Interval			95% Confidence Interval			95% Confidence Interval	
A01	sEMG Right MVC	93.3	91.672	95.005	92.5	90.858	94.192	92.4	90.736	94.069
	sEMG Left MVC	90.8	89.246	92.265	91.4	89.924	92.943	91.2	89.663	92.682
	Right RP	6.1	4.031	8.044	5.0	2.950	6.963	5.4	3.355	7.367
	Left RP	7.2	4.920	9.560	5.5	3.154	7.794	6.2	3.881	8.521
A02	sEMG Right MVC	90.8	88.938	92.583	91.9	90.068	93.713	90.8	88.978	92.623
	sEMG Left MVC	90.5	88.844	92.161	90.6	88.901	92.218	89.5	87.834	91.151
	Right RP	6.0	3.892	8.144	5.1	3.015	7.267	5.6	3.478	7.730
	Left RP	7.3	4.967	9.553	5.6	3.352	7.938	6.3	3.971	8.557
A1	sEMG Right MVC	92.0	90.353	93.732	92.3	90.570	93.949	92.3	90.653	94.032
	sEMG Left MVC	90.8	88.986	92.668	91.8	89.977	93.658	90.5	88.666	92.347
	Right RP	4.4	2.740	6.115	3.2	1.469	4.844	4.6	2.900	6.276
	Left RP	4.6	2.821	6.385	3.6	1.788	5.352	5.3	3.481	7.045
A2	sEMG Right MVC	92.3	90.584	93.916	92.1	90.445	93.778	91.9	90.221	93.553
	sEMG Left MVC	90.9	89.056	92.667	91.3	89.474	93.084	91.7	89.921	93.531
	Right RP	4.6	2.800	6.431	3.5	1.660	5.292	5.1	3.315	6.947
	Left RP	4.7	2.979	6.560	3.7	1.902	5.484	5.8	4.068	7.650

Abbreviations: G1—experimental group that carried out a therapeutic exercise program; G2—experimental group that associated a therapeutic exercise program with aerobic exercise; G3—experimental group that carried out an aerobic exercise program; A01—evaluation baseline one; A02—evaluation baseline two; A1—evaluation post-intervention; A2—follow-up; sEMG—electromyography activity; MVC—maximal voluntary contraction (%); RP—rest position.

6. Bite Force

There were no differences in BF (H = 1.25, p = 0.54; H = 2.31, p = 0.31 for the left and right sides, respectively) between groups either on the right or the left sides at both A01 and A02. From baseline to A1, BF significantly increased in G1 and G2, while G3 showed no significant differences. There was a large effect size in G1 on the right (d = 1.5) and left (d = 1.7) sides and on the left side in G2 (d = 0.8), while a moderate effect size was seen in the G2 group on the right side (d = 0.7), and a small effect size was seen in G3 both on the right and on the left sides (d = 0.3). There were no significant changes from A1 to A2 on either side in any of the groups (Figure 3A,B).

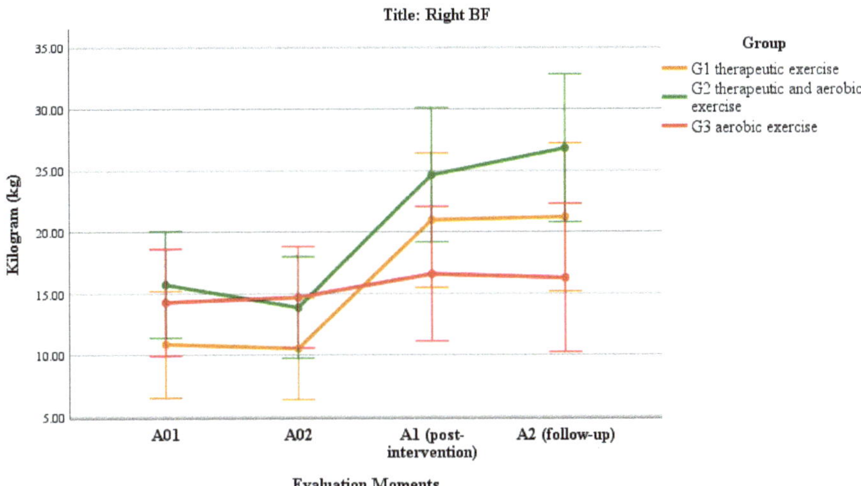

Subtitle: G1 – experimental group that carried out a therapeutic exercise program; G2 – experimental group that associated a therapeutic exercise program with aerobic exercise; G3 – experimental group that carried out an aerobic exercise program; A01 - evaluation baseline one; A02 – evaluation baseline two; A1 – evaluation post-intervention; A2 – follow-up; BF - bite force (kg).

(**A**)

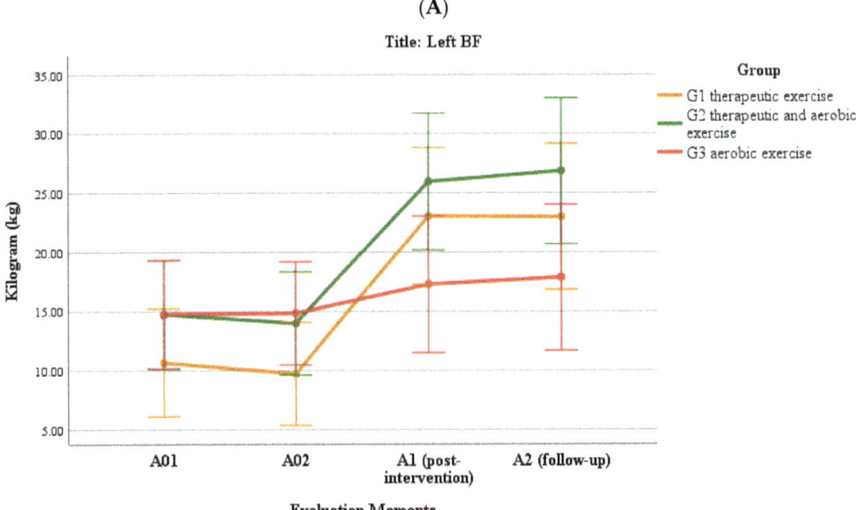

Subtitle: G1 – experimental group that carried out a therapeutic exercise program; G2 – experimental group that associated a therapeutic exercise program with aerobic exercise; G3 – experimental group that carried out an aerobic exercise program; A01 - evaluation baseline one; A02 – evaluation baseline two; A1 – evaluation post-intervention; A2 – follow-up; BF – bite force (kg).

(**B**)

Figure 3. (**A**) Changes in right BF at the different time points. (**B**) Changes in left BF at the different time points.

7. Discussion

To our knowledge, this is the first study to analyze the effects of a combination of therapeutic and aerobic exercise on participants with TMD. A treatment regimen of aerobic exercise combined with therapeutic exercise over an 8-week period significantly decreased pain and increased BF. However, changes in sEMG activity were not significant. The study hypothesis was therefore partially confirmed.

8. Pain Intensity

Pain decreased in all groups after the intervention programs were carried out, with a greater effect size for the G2 group, followed by G1. Changes in pain were evaluated by applying a constant pressure (1 Kg), using the numerical pain scale (NPRS). The minimum clinically important difference considered was two points [32].

In G1 and G2, the intervention programs led to a clinically important reduction in NPRS, with this reduction being greater in G2. In G3, there was no clinically significant reduction in NPRS after performing the aerobic exercise program.

NPRS was higher for the masseter muscle (right and left) than for the temporal muscle (right and left) in all groups. This difference between muscles may result from the average of the initially reported NPRS, which was always higher for the masseter muscle, since when analyzing the mean NPRS values after the eight-week intervention period, the reported final NPRS values were similar for both muscles (masseter and temporal) bilaterally.

The results obtained in G1 are in line with those observed by Kalamir et al. [35], who found that a therapeutic exercise program led to a reduction in pain in the masticatory muscles. The different type of intervention (which included intra-oral myofascial therapy, condylar distraction, isometric contractions, and mobilization of the temporal and medial pterygoid) and duration (two weekly sessions for five weeks) relative to our study does not allow for further comparisons.

In G3, the results obtained in the masseter and temporal muscle were in line with those identified by Naugle et al. [16], in which the authors concluded that aerobic exercise led to a wide range of hypoalgesic effects (between 0.04 and 1.47). However, it is necessary to interpret these data carefully, since the cited study was carried out in healthy individuals.

Studies of aerobic exercise in patients with chronic pain, including fibromyalgia, have found a decrease in pain with a subset of physical activity [24,25]. Since patients with TMD show central sensitization [36,37], the aerobic exercise seem to promote similar results and should be included in TMD intervention. Thus, the results obtained by G3, in relation to the masseter (large effect size) and the temporal (moderate effect size) muscle, may result from the majority of the participants in this group having myalgia (presence of local pain on palpation) and as such having less change in pain processing than patients with health conditions that lead to major changes in central pain processing, such as those involving the presence of myofascial pain (radiating pain on palpation within the limits of the assessed muscle). Patients with myofascial pain can present an increase in the size of receptor fields, a greater susceptibility to painful stimuli, and a lower threshold of neuronal depolarization. These differences may be due to the different subtypes of TMD, with some patients presenting only peripheral involvement and others presenting both peripheral and central involvement [38].

The group with better results (greater effect sizes) was the one that associated therapeutic exercises with aerobic exercises (G2), which suggests that the simultaneous use of both types of intervention improves outcomes. However, it is important to note that the effects seen in G1 showed a pattern of effects similar to those observed in G2, but smaller. The larger effect sizes seen in G2 may result from the association between the effect of therapeutic exercise and the decrease in sensitivity to painful stimuli as a result of the activation of opioid and non-opioid systems resulting from aerobic exercise. Exercise induces the release of endogenous opioids in peripheral, spinal, and/or central sites, which leads to pain modulation [39] and can also contribute to the release of neurotransmitters (serotonin and norepinephrine) according to the defined exercise parameters [40], which can produce analgesia when activating cannabinoid receptors [22]. Additionally, the increase in blood pressure and heart rate during exercise [41], as well as the activation of descending pathways [42], may have contributed to hypoalgesia. Considering the multidimensional experience of pain and the complexity of the processes involved in the mechanisms of analgesia, the most likely explanation is that there may be an interaction between different systems, in different patients, and at different times depending on the set of factors that in each situation are contributing to the presence of pain.

The effects obtained immediately after the completion of the intervention programs were maintained during the final follow-up in all groups.

9. Bite Force and Neuromuscular Activation of Masticatory Muscles

The sEMG activity during MVC did not change significantly in any of the groups after the intervention programs. Previous studies that carried out intervention strategies to decrease pain in masticatory muscles also did not find changes in the masseter sEMG activity after the decrease in pain intensity [43,44]. However, comparisons are difficult to make, since in those studies the normalization of MVC occurred through the interposition of folded articulating paper between the teeth, and the authors did not use a dynamometer to control the BF, as was done in the present study.

A study of experimentally induced masseter pain found that the increase in pain led to a decrease in sEMG activity, not only during the period when the pain was present, but also after its disappearance [45]. The fact that most of the patients in our study reported pain in the masticatory muscles for more than six months may have contributed to the lack of variation in sEMG activity, since it may already be the result of an anticipatory and protective response developed by the central nervous system (CNS). In the final follow-up, there were also no changes in sEMG activity in any of the groups. Thus, in our study, there was no change in the sEMG activity of patients after the intervention programs were performed, despite the decrease in pain intensity seen in all groups.

BF increased in all groups after the completion of the intervention programs, with greater effect sizes in G1 and G2, while the increase was much lower in G3.

The results are in line with those observed by other authors, who found that the decrease in masticatory muscle pain intensity led to an increase in BF [46]. Another set of studies evaluating the BF of patients with TMD in comparison with healthy subjects found that the masticatory MVC was reduced in the group of participants with TMD [8,47]. Cho and Lee [7] obtained similar results, since they found that the presence of pain led to a decrease in BF, although it is necessary to emphasize that in these studies, pain was experimentally induced. There remains no consensus on the relationship between pain in the masticatory muscles and BF, since other authors have not identified this correlation [33,48]. In the present study, the group with better results (as demonstrated by the greater effect size) was G1, followed by G2. There seems to be a relationship between the decrease in pain in the masticatory muscles and the increase in BF, since in G1 and G2, where there was a greater decrease in pain intensity, a greater increase in BF was also observed.

The different results observed for relationship between BF and pain in different studies [7,33,35] may be due to the patients presenting different levels of pain intensity, anxiety, fear, pain catastrophizing, and different psychological characteristics [49]. The sensory system, one of the components of the neuromuscular system, is multidimensional and includes several inter-individual factors, with contributions from sensory-discriminatory, cognitive-evaluative and motivational-affective components, where factors such as the pain location, intensity, and characteristics can lead to supraspinal and suprabulbar modulation, thus modifying the effects of pain on motor activity [48,50].

Several hypotheses can be theorized to explain the increase in BF without a corresponding increasing in sEMG activity during MVC. Given the complexity of the neuromuscular system, the increased BF without increasing MVC sEMG may result from the development of different combinations of muscle activation strategies, which may show intra- and inter-individual variability. For example, a better synchronization between muscles can be a strategy to coordinate muscle activity and lead to increased force production without changes in the activation intensity in each muscle [51]. The increase in strength may also have resulted from an increase in synergistic muscle activity regardless of activation neural activity of agonists [52]. Finally, there may have been a decrease in antagonist co-activation, since it is counterproductive to the production of maximum force because it generates a force opposite to the desired movement [53]. This decreased co-activation of antagonistic muscles would be expected through reciprocal inhibition [54]. On the other hand, sEMG activity depends on the ability of the CNS to direct a central drive to the motoneuron pool, which may be influenced by the pain intensity, levels of anxiety, individual psychological characteristics, fear of movement, and pain catastrophizing [49], which contributes to increasing the complexity of the mechanisms involved. It is plausible to state that the complexity and multidimensionality inherent to the neuromuscular system can lead to different neuromuscular recruitment strategies for the performance of a given task, which are composed by complex and individualized reactions that can lead to an increase in BF without being accompanied by an increase in the sEMG activity during the MVC.

Regarding sEMG in the PR, despite the decreasing trend seen in the three groups after the exercise interventions, there were no significant differences. Studies that have compared the sEMG activity at rest between patients with TMD and healthy individuals have shown contradictory findings, with some authors identifying greater activity in individuals with TMD [55] and others not reporting significant differences [56]. The effects obtained immediately after completing the intervention program were maintained at the final follow-up.

We recommend that physiotherapists carry out multimodal training programs that include therapeutic exercise associated with aerobic exercise to reduce the pain intensity of the masseter and temporal muscles and increase BF in patients with TMD.

This study has some limitations. First, we used a small, convenience-based sample, which means that the findings may not be generalizable to other populations. The sample also included only subjects between 18 and 35 years, which does not allow extrapolation of results to other age groups. The non-acceptance by several patients of joining groups G2 and G3, which included the performance of the aerobic exercise program, may have contributed to some heterogeneity between groups at baseline regarding the type of TMD (in group G3, the majority of patients presented myalgia-type TMD, while in the other groups, the dominant was myofascial-type TMD), but the statistical analysis did not show differences at baseline between the G1 and G2/G3 groups (the differences are between G3 and G1/G2), so the allocation to the groups was considered to have not interfered with the results obtained. Despite the strict compliance with the electrode placement protocol, it is impossible to guarantee that we were able to exactly reproduce the electrode placement in the different evaluations of each subject. In a similar way, despite our efforts to reproduce the dynamometer placement protocol between the premolars in the different evaluations, we cannot be sure that there was no variability in this placement, which might have influenced the BF produced.

Future studies should recruit a larger sample and randomize patients across the three groups so that the results can be extrapolated to other populations. An intervention program which includes aerobic exercises of moderate intensity to facilitate the participants' adherence and carry out an intervention program with a shorter duration (six weeks) should also be considered to check whether similar results would be obtained in a shorter period of time of intervention.

10. Conclusions

The therapeutic exercise program associated with aerobic exercise showed the greatest effects on pain intensity (decrease) and BF (increase), although there were no significant differences in the group that performed therapeutic exercise alone. Interventions in patients with TMD experiencing pain must have a multimodal component, and aerobic exercise was shown to be an important component. There were no changes in the sEMG activity during MVC and at rest after carrying out any of the three exercise programs. All effects obtained after carrying out the exercise programs were maintained at follow-up.

Author Contributions: P.M.M.M.-A. was involved in conceptualization, methodology, software, validation, formal analysis, investigation, resources, data curation, writing—original draft preparation, and writing—review and editing; P.M.T.C.C. was involved in investigation, writing—original draft preparation, and writing—review and editing; P.D.G.d.S. was involved in software, formal analysis, and data curation; J.P.C. was involved in writing—original draft preparation and writing—review and editing; C.G. was involved in writing—original draft preparation and writing—review and editing; R.A.N.d.S.O. was involved in conceptualization, methodology, software, validation, formal analysis, investigation, resources, data curation, writing—original draft preparation, and writing—review and editing; P.M.T.C.C. was involved in investigation, writing—original draft preparation, and writing—review and editing; and P.L.C.P.-C. was involved in conceptualization, methodology, software, validation, formal analysis, investigation, resources, data curation, writing—original draft preparation, and writing—review and editing. All authors have read and agreed to the published version of the manuscript.

Funding: This research did not receive any specific grant from funding agencies in the public, commercial, or not-for-profit sectors.

Institutional Review Board Statement: The study was conducted according to the guidelines of the Declaration of Helsinki, and approved by the Institutional Review Board (or Ethics Committee) of Egas Moniz Higher Institute of Health Science on 13 February 2019 (ID N° 675/2019).

Informed Consent Statement: Informed consent was obtained from all subjects involved in the study.

Data Availability Statement: The data presented in this study are available on request from the first author.

Acknowledgments: This work is financed by national funds through the FCT—Foundation for Science and Technology, I.P., under the project UIDB/04585/2020. The researchers would like to thank the Centro de Investigação Interdisciplinar Egas Moniz (CiiEM) for the support provided for the publication of this article. We thank the informatic engineer Luis Alves and the statistics professor Isabel Flores. We also thank all participants in the study.

Conflicts of Interest: The authors declare no potential conflict of interest.

Ethical Approval: Before conducting the study, a research protocol was analyzed and approved by the Ethical Committee of Egas Moniz University Institute on 13 February 2019 (ID N° 675/2019).

References

1. Dworkin, S.F.; Massoth, D.L. Temporomandibular disorders and chronic pain: Disease or illness? *J. Prosthet. Dent.* **1994**, *72*, 29–38. [CrossRef]
2. Lipton, J.A.; Ship, J.A.; Larach-Robinson, D. Estimated prevalence and distribution of reported orofacial pain in the United States. *J. Am. Dent. Assoc.* **1993**, *124*, 115–121. [CrossRef] [PubMed]
3. National Institute of Dental and Craniofacial Research. Facial Pain, July 2018. Available online: https://www.nidcr.nih.gov/research/data-statistics/facial-pain (accessed on 12 December 2020).
4. Blanco-Hungria, A.; Blanco-Aguilera, A.; Blanco-Aguilera, E.; Serrano-del-Rosal, R.; Biedma-Velázquez, L.; Rodríguez-Torronteras, A.; Segura-Saint-Gerons, R. Prevalence of the different Axis I clinical subtypes in a sample of patients with orofacial pain and temporomandibular disorders in the Andalusian Healthcare Service. *Med. Oral Patol. Oral Cir. Bucal* **2016**, *21*, 169–177. [CrossRef]
5. Oral, K.; Küçük, B.B.; Ebeoğlu, B.; Dinçer, S. Etiology of temporomandibular disorder pain. *J. Turk. Soc. Algol.* **2009**, *21*, 89–94.
6. Fricton, J.R.; Ouyang, W.; Nixdorf, D.R.; Schiffman, E.L.; Velly, A.M.; Look, J.O. Critical appraisal of methods used in randomized controlled trials of treatments for temporomandibular disorders. *J. Orofac. Pain* **2010**, *24*, 139–151.
7. Cho, G.; Lee, Y. Analysis of Masticatory Muscle Activity Based on Presence of Temporomandibular Joint Disorders. *Med. Sci. Monit.* **2020**, *26*, e921337. [CrossRef]
8. Todic, J.; Martinovic, B.; Pavlovic, J.; Tabakovic, S.; Staletovic, M. Assessment of the impact of temporomandibular disorders on maximum bite force. *Biomed. Pap.* **2019**, *163*, 274–278. [CrossRef]
9. Pficer, K.J.; Dodic, S.; Lazic, V.; Trajkovic, G.; Milic, N.; Milicic, B. Occlusal stabilization splint for patients with temporomandibular disorders: Meta-analysis of short and long term effects. *PLoS ONE* **2017**, *12*, e0171296. [CrossRef]
10. Xu, G.Z.; Jia, J.; Jin, L.; Li, J.H.; Wang, Z.Y.; Cao, D.Y. Low-Level Laser Therapy for Temporomandibular Disorders: A Systematic Review with Meta-Analysis. *Pain Res. Manag.* **2018**, *2018*, 4230583. [CrossRef]
11. Al-Moraissi, E.A.; Alradom, J.; Aladashi, O.; Goddard, G.; Christidis, N. Needling therapies in the management of myofascial pain of the masticatory muscles: A network meta-analysis of randomised clinical trials. *J. Oral Rehabil.* **2020**, *47*, 910–922. [CrossRef]

12. Al-Moraissi, E.A.; Conti, P.C.R.; Alyahya, A.; Alkebsi, K.; Elsharkawy, A.; Christidis, N. The hierarchy of different treatments for myogenous temporomandibular disorders: A systematic review and network meta-analysis of randomized clinical trials. *Oral Maxillofac. Surg.* **2021**, 1–15. [CrossRef]

13. Armijo-Olivo, S.; Pitance, L.; Singh, V.; Neto, F.; Thie, N.; Michelotti, A. Effectiveness of manual therapy and therapeutic exercise for temporomandibular disorders: Systematic review and meta-analysis. *Phys. Ther.* **2016**, *96*, 9–25. [CrossRef] [PubMed]

14. Dickerson, S.M.; Weaver, J.M.; Boyson, A.N.; Thacker, J.A.; Junak, A.A.; Ritzline, P.D.; Donaldson, M.B. The effectiveness of exercise therapy for temporomandibular dysfunction: A systematic review and meta-analysis. *Clin. Rehabil.* **2017**, *31*, 1039–1048. [CrossRef] [PubMed]

15. Paço, M.; Peleteiro, B.; Duarte, J.; Pinho, T. The effectiveness of physiotherapy in the management of temporomandibular disorders: A systematic review and meta-analysis. *J. Oral Facial Pain Headache* **2016**, *30*, 210–220. [CrossRef]

16. Naugle, K.M.; Fillingim, R.B.; Riley, J.L., III. A meta-analytic review of the hypoalgesic effects of exercise. *J. Pain* **2012**, *13*, 1139–1150. [CrossRef]

17. Koltyn, K.F.; Garvin, A.W.; Gardiner, R.L.; Nelson, T.F. Perception of pain following aerobic exercise. *Med. Sci. Sports Exerc.* **1996**, *28*, 1418–1421. [CrossRef]

18. Meeus, M.; Roussel, N.A.; Truijen, S.; Nijs, J. Reduced pressure pain thresholds in response to exercise in Chronic Fatigue Syndrome but not in Chronic Low Back Pain: An experimental study. *J. Rehabil. Med.* **2010**, *42*, 884–890. [CrossRef]

19. Vierck Jr, C.J.; Staud, R.; Price, D.D.; Cannon, R.L.; Mauderli, A.P.; Martin, A.D. The effect of maximal exercise on temporal summation of second pain (windup) in patients with Fibromyalgia Syndrome. *J. Pain* **2001**, *2*, 334–344. [CrossRef] [PubMed]

20. Koltyn, K.F. Analgesia following exercise: A review. *Sports Med.* **2000**, *29*, 85–98. [CrossRef] [PubMed]

21. Koltyn, K.F. Exercise-induced hypoalgesia and intensity of exercise. *Sports Med.* **2002**, *32*, 477–487. [CrossRef]

22. Koltyn, K.F.; Brellenthin, A.G.; Cook, D.B.; Sehgal, N.; Hillard, C. Mechanisms of Exercise-Induced Hypoalgesia. *J. Pain* **2014**, *15*, 1294–1304. [CrossRef]

23. Naugle, K.M.; Naugle, K.E.; Fillingim, R.B.; Samuels, B.; Riley, J.L., 3rd. Intensity Thresholds for Aerobic Exercise-Induced Hypoalgesia. *Med. Sci. Sports Exerc.* **2014**, *46*, 817–825. [CrossRef]

24. Bidone, J.; Busch, A.J.; Schachter, C.L.; Overend, T.J.; Kim, S.Y.; Góes, S.M.; Boden, C.B.; Foulds, H.J. Aerobic exercise training for adults with fibromyalgia. *Cochrane Database Syst. Rev.* **2017**, *21*, CD012700. [CrossRef]

25. Polaski, A.M.; Phelps, A.L.; Kostek, M.C.; Szucs, K.A.; Kolber, B.J. Exercise-induced hypoalgesia: A meta-analysis of exercise dosing for the treatment of chronic pain. *PLoS ONE* **2019**, *14*, e0210418. [CrossRef]

26. Schiffman, E.; Ohrbach, R.; Truelove, E.; Look, J.; Anderson, G.; Goulet, J.; List, T.; Svensson, P.; Gonzalez, Y.; Lobbezoo, F.; et al. Diagnostic criteria for temporomandibular disorders (DC/TMD) for clinical and research applications: Recommendations of the International RDC/TMD Consortium Network and Orofacial Pain Special Interest Group. *J. Oral Facial Pain Headache* **2014**, *28*, 6–27. [CrossRef]

27. Gay, C.W.; Alappattu, M.J.; Coronado, R.A.; Horn, M.E.; Bishop, M.D. Effect of a single session of muscle-biased therapy on pain sensitivity: A systematic review and meta-analysis of randomized controlled trials. *J. Pain Res.* **2013**, *6*, 7–22. [CrossRef]

28. Okeson, J. *Management of Temporomandibular Disorders and Occlusion*, 8th ed.; Elsevier: Maryland Heights, MO, USA, 2019.

29. Simons, D.G. Understanding effective treatments of myofascial trigger points. *J. Bodyw. Mov. Ther.* **2002**, *6*, 81–88. [CrossRef]

30. Shimada, A.; Ishigaki, S.; Matsuka, Y.; Komiyama, O.; Torisu, T.; Oono, Y.; Sato, H.; Naganawa, T.; Mine, A.; Yamazaki, Y.; et al. Effects of exercise therapy on painful temporomandibular disorders. *J. Oral Rehabil.* **2019**, *46*, 475–481. [CrossRef]

31. Karvonen, M.; Kentala, E.; Mustala, O. The Effects of Training on Heart Rate: A Longitudinal Study. *Ann. Med. Exp. Biol. Fenn.* **1957**, *35*, 307–315.

32. Farrar, J.T.; Young Jr, J.P.; LaMoreaux, L.W.; Werth, J.L.; Poole, M.R. Clinical importance of changes in chronic pain intensity measured on an 11-point numerical pain rating scale. *Pain* **2001**, *94*, 149–158. [CrossRef]

33. Tartaglia, G.M.; Lodetti, G.; Paiva, G.; De Felicio, C.M.; Sforza, C. Surface electromyographic assessment of patients with long lasting temporomandibular joint disorder pain. *J. Electromyogr. Kinesiol.* **2011**, *21*, 659–664. [CrossRef]

34. Hermens, H.J.; Freriks, B.; Disselhorst-Klug, C.; Rau, G. Development of recommendations for sEMG sensors and sensor placement procedures. *J. Electromyogr. Kinesiol.* **2000**, *10*, 361–374. [CrossRef]

35. Kalamir, A.; Pollard, H.; Vitiello, A.; Bonello, R. Intra-oral myofascial therapy for chronic myogenous temporomandibular disorders: A randomized, controlled pilot study. *J. Man. Manip. Ther.* **2010**, *18*, 139–146. [CrossRef]

36. Chichorro, J.G.; Porreca, F.; Sessle, B. Mechanisms of craniofacial pain. *Cephalalgia* **2017**, *37*, 613–626. [CrossRef]

37. Svensson, P.; Kumar, A. Assessment of risk factors for oro-facial pain and recent developments in classification: Implications for management. *J. Oral Rehabil.* **2016**, *43*, 977–989. [CrossRef]

38. Pfau, D.; Rolke, R.; Nickel, R.; Treede, R.; Daublaender, M. Somatosensory profiles in subgroups of patients with myogenic temporomandibular disorders and Fibromyalgia Syndrome. *Pain* **2009**, *147*, 72–83. [CrossRef]

39. Thorén, P.; Floras, J.; Hoffmann, P.; Seals, D.R. Endorphins and exercise: Physiological mechanisms and clinical implications. *Med. Sci. Sports Exerc.* **1990**, *22*, 417–428.

40. Dietrich, A.; McDaniel, W.F. Endocannabinoids and exercise. *Br. J. Sports Med.* **2004**, *38*, 536–541. [CrossRef] [PubMed]

41. Koltyn, K.; Trine, M.; Stegner, A.; Tobar, D.A. Effect of Isometric Exercise on Pain Perception and Blood Pressure in Men and Women. *Med. Sci. Sports Exerc.* **2001**, *33*, 282–290. [CrossRef]

42. Villemure, C.; Bushnell, M. Cognitive modulation of pain: How do attention and emotion influence pain processing? *Pain* **2002**, *95*, 195–199. [CrossRef]

43. Herpich, C.; Leal-Junior, E.; Gomes, C.; Gloria, I.; Amaral, A.; Amaral, M.; Politti, F.; Biasotto-Gonzalez, D. Immediate and short-term effects of phototherapy on pain, muscle activity, and joint mobility in women with temporomandibular disorder: A randomized, double-blind, placebo-controlled, clinical trial. *Disabil. Rehabil.* **2017**, *40*, 2318–2324. [CrossRef] [PubMed]

44. Rodrigues, D.; Siriani, A.; Bérzin, F. Effect of conventional TENS on pain and electromyographic activity of masticatory muscles in TMD patients. *Braz. Oral Res.* **2004**, *18*, 290–295. [CrossRef] [PubMed]

45. Shimada, A.; Hara, S.; Svensson, P. Effect of experimental jaw muscle pain on EMG activity and bite force distribution at different level of clenching. *J. Oral Rehabil.* **2013**, *40*, 826–833. [CrossRef] [PubMed]

46. Goiato, M.C.; Zuim, P.R.J.; Moreno, A.; Dos Santos, D.M.; da Silva, E.V.F.; de Caxias, F.P.; Turcio, K.H.L. Does pain in the masseter and anterior temporal muscles influence maximal bite force? *Arch. Oral Biol.* **2017**, *83*, 1–6. [CrossRef]

47. Testa, M.; Geri, T.; Pitance, L.; Lentz, P.; Gizzi, L.; Erlenwein, J.; Petkze, F.; Falla, D. Alterations in jaw clenching force control in people with myogenic temporomandibular disorders. *J. Electromyogr. Kinesiol.* **2018**, *43*, 111–117. [CrossRef]

48. Peck, C.; Murray, G.; Gerzina, T. How does pain affect jaw muscle activity? The Integrated Pain Adaptation Model. *Aust. Dent. J.* **2008**, *53*, 201–207. [CrossRef]

49. Maulina, T.; Amhamed, M.; Whittle, T.; Gal, J.; Akhter, R.; Murray, G.M. The Effects of Experimental Temporalis Muscle Pain on Jaw Muscle Electromyographic Activity During Jaw Movements and Relationships with Some Psychological Variables. *J. Oral Facial Pain Headache* **2018**, *32*, 29–39. [CrossRef]

50. Ferreira, P.; Sandoval, I.; Whittle, T.; Mojaver, Y.N.; Murray, G.M. Reorganization of masseter and temporalis muscles single motor unit activity during experimental masseter muscle pain. *J. Oral Facial Pain Headache* **2020**, *34*, 40–52. [CrossRef]

51. Mellor, R.; Hodges, P. Motor unit synchronization between medial and lateral vasti muscles. *Clin. Neurophysiol.* **2005**, *116*, 1585–1595. [CrossRef]

52. Cormie, P.; McGuigan, M.R.; Newton, R.U. Developing Maximal Neuromuscular Power. *Sports Med.* **2011**, *41*, 17–38. [CrossRef]

53. Aagaard, P.; Simonsen, E.B.; Andersen, J.L.; Magnusson, S.P.; Bojsen-Møller, F.; Dyhre-Poulsen, P. Antagonist muscle coactivation during isokinetic knee extension. *Scand. J. Med. Sci. Sports* **2000**, *10*, 58–67. [CrossRef]

54. Milner, T.E.; Cloutier, C.; Leger, A.B.; Franklin, D.W. Inability to activate muscles maximally during cocontraction and the effect of joint stiffness. *Exp. Brain Res.* **1995**, *107*, 293–305. [CrossRef]

55. Lauriti, L.; Motta, L.J.; Godoy, C.H.L.; Biasotto-Gonzalez, D.A.; Politti, F.; Mesquita-Ferrari, R.A.; Fernandes, K.P.S.; Bussadori, S.K. Influence of temporomandibular disorder on temporal and masseter muscles and occlusal contacts in adolescents: An electromyographic study. *BMC Musculoskelet. Disord.* **2014**, *15*, 123. [CrossRef] [PubMed]

56. Barros, B.; Biasotto-Gonzalez, D.; Bussadori, S.K.; Gomes, C.; Politti, F. Is there a difference in the electromyographic activity of the masticatory muscles between individuals with temporomandibular disorder and healthy controls? A systematic review with meta-analysis. *J. Oral Rehabil.* **2020**, *47*, 672–682. [CrossRef] [PubMed]

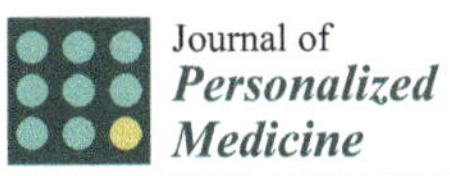

Journal of
Personalized Medicine

MDPI

Article

The Effects of Different Types of Dual Tasking on Balance in Healthy Older Adults

Graça Monteiro de Barros [1,2], Filipe Melo [3], Josefa Domingos [4], Raul Oliveira [5], Luís Silva [6], Júlio Belo Fernandes [4] and Catarina Godinho [4,*]

1   Fisio-Lógica Centro de Fisioterapia, Lda, 1350-275 Lisboa, Portugal; gracamantua@gmail.com
2   Escola Superior de Saúde Atlântica, 2730-036 Barcarena, Portugal
3   Laboratório de Comportamento Motor, Faculdade de Motricidade Humana, Universidade de Lisboa, 1495-688 Cruz Quebrada, Portugal; fmelo@fmh.ulisboa.pt
4   Grupo de Patologia Médica, Nutrição e Exercício Clínico (PaMNEC) do Centro de Investigação Interdisciplinar Egas Moniz (CiiEM), Escola Superior de Saúde Egas Moniz, Caparica, 2829-511 Almada, Portugal; domingosjosefa@gmail.com (J.D.); juliobelo01@gmail.com (J.B.F.)
5   Neuromuscular Research Lab, CIPER, Faculdade de Motricidade Humana, Universidade de Lisboa, 1495-688 Cruz Quebrada, Portugal; roliveira@fmh.ulisboa.pt
6   Physics Department, LIBPhys-UNL, Nova School of Science and Technology, Universidade Nova de Lisboa, Caparica, 2829-516 Almada, Portugal; lmd.silva@fct.unl.pt
*   Correspondence: cgcgodinho@gmail.com; Tel.: +351-910077492

Abstract: Numerous of our daily activities are performed within multitask or dual task conditions. These conditions involve the interaction of perceptual and motor processes involved in postural control. Age-related changes may negatively impact cognition and balance control. Studies identifying changes related to dual-task actions in older people are need. This study aimed to determine the effects of different types of dual-tasking on the balance control of healthy older adults. The sample included 36 community-living older adults, performing two tests—a sway test and a timed up-and-go test—in three conditions: (a) single motor task; (b) dual motor task; and (c) dual motor task with cognitive demands. Cognitive processes (dual-task and cognition) affected static balance, increasing amplitude ($p < 0.001$) and frequency ($p < 0.001$) of the center of mass displacements. Dynamic balance revealed significant differences between the single motor condition and the other two conditions during gait phases ($p < 0.001$). The effect of dual-tasking in older adults suggests that cognitive processes are a main cause of increased variability in balance and gait when under an automatic control. During sit-to-stand, turning, and turn-to-sit movements under dual-tasking, the perceptive information becomes the most important focus of attention, while any cognitive task becomes secondary.

Keywords: dual-tasking; cognitive function; postural control; older adults

Citation: de Barros, G.M.; Melo, F.; Domingos, J.; Oliveira, R.; Silva, L.; Fernandes, J.B.; Godinho, C. The Effects of Different Types of Dual Tasking on Balance in Healthy Older Adults. *J. Pers. Med.* **2021**, *11*, 933. https://doi.org/10.3390/jpm11090933

Academic Editor: Rajendra D Badgaiyan

Received: 4 August 2021
Accepted: 16 September 2021
Published: 18 September 2021

Publisher's Note: MDPI stays neutral with regard to jurisdictional claims in published maps and institutional affiliations.

1. Introduction

Daily life is occupied by dual-tasking behaviors, such as walking while talking with someone or while taking a picture on the phone. Effective daily functioning requires people to share their attention resources between the cognitive and the postural requirements necessary to complete the tasks [1]. This ability to perform concurrent performances is known as dual-tasking. A decreased capacity to perform dual-tasking may reduce the person's ability to participate in their life roles [2]. Due to the aging process and prevalence of chronic diseases, older adults show some levels of decline when performing postural tasks while dual-tasking [3]. Upholding and improving older adults' ability to perform under dual-task situations is an imperative goal for extending their functionality.

The literature reports several factors that are considered to influence the person's ability to divide their attention resources between the two tasks, namely external factors, such as the tasks' complexity, and intrinsic factors, such as physical status, executive function, and task prioritization [4,5].

Activities such as driving or walking are considered automatic motor sequences, largely operating independently from more cognitively intensive processes such as communication. When combined into a dual-task activity, the interaction of the perceptual-motor and cognitive neurophysiologic processes may have an influence upon the postural control that has a primary support function [6,7]. The turning characteristics during ambulating are a major contributor to motor disability, falls, and reduced quality of life in older people, largely because the necessary (intrinsic) dynamic balance control decreases with age [8].

Previous research indicates that postural control and gait in older adults lose some level of automaticity, defined as the capacity to be independently executed with minimum attentional costs, and indicated by alterations of motor patterns during dual-task activities [9,10]. The degree to which postural control and gait change during the simultaneous performance of other tasks is considered related to the level of difficulty of the concurrent task [3].

Questions remain regarding the overall amount of influence of different dual-task combinations (motor–motor versus motor–cognition) on postural control and gait. Although different aspects of the influence that dual-task activities have on postural control and gait have been observed in healthy older adults [11,12], the factors that contribute to postural control and gait changes, in response to "dual-tasking" among this population have not been fully clarified. It is hypothesized that in a homogeneous sample of healthy older adults with no perturbation in mobility and cognitive function, postural control and gait will remain under greater automatic control and thus, dual-task decrement, although present, will remain at a reduced level.

It is of great relevance to develop a normative evaluation of the postural control during static and dynamic equilibrium conditions [13]. This evaluation should include the performance of single and dual-tasks in order to determine which parameters may be altered with aging.

Postural and gait analysis obtained during the execution of different motor tasks will allow for the understanding of the interaction between motor and cognitive capacity, as well as the effects upon healthy aging subjects [14].

The objective of this study was to evaluate the effects of dual-task activities on balance control in healthy older individuals, namely, by exploring its influence on the temporal and space parameters of static activities such as postural sway in addition to dynamic tasks (standing and sitting on a chair and walking in conjunction to rotational movements) while performing a balance control task such as carrying a tray with a full glass of water.

2. Materials and Methods

2.1. Study Design

This investigation was based on an observational cross-sectional study with a single moment evaluation.

2.2. Sampling and Recruitment

Healthy older adults were recruited from the community by advertisements on social media and at seniors' centers by phone or in person. The sampling method selection was non-probabilistic by convenience.

Subjects were included if they were seniors—aged 65 years and over, independent in their daily activities, and presenting independent walking.

Subjects were excluded if they presented vestibular disorders, neurological diseases, lack of cognitive skills according to the results of Mini Mental Score (MMS) < 20, musculoskeletal impairments that could affect gait, and inability to stand and walk unassisted.

2.3. Ethics and Procedures

This study follows the principles of the Declaration of Helsinki. All participants provided written informed consent and the study was approved by the Ethics Council of the Faculty of Human Kinetics (ID: CEFMH N°4/2016 in 15 February 2016).

2.4. Data Collection

Subjects were asked to perform two different tests randomly—the instrumented sway test (ISWAY) and the instrumented timed up-and-go test (ITUG)—during three task conditions that were applied randomly: (a) single motor task; (b) dual motor task (single motor task carrying a tray with a full glass of water); and (c) dual motor task with cognitive demands (the same as the dual motor task including counting back from 100, three by three). During the ISWAY test, subjects had to maintain a stable standing position.

Balance and gait were measured using four Opal inertial sensors and automated algorithms from Mobility Lab, by APDM (APDM Inc., Portland, OR, USA). Sensors were placed on both ankles, the chest, and the posterior trunk at the level of L5 (Center of Mass—CM), with elastic Velcro bands sufficiently stable to avoid any undesirable dress movement (Figure 1).

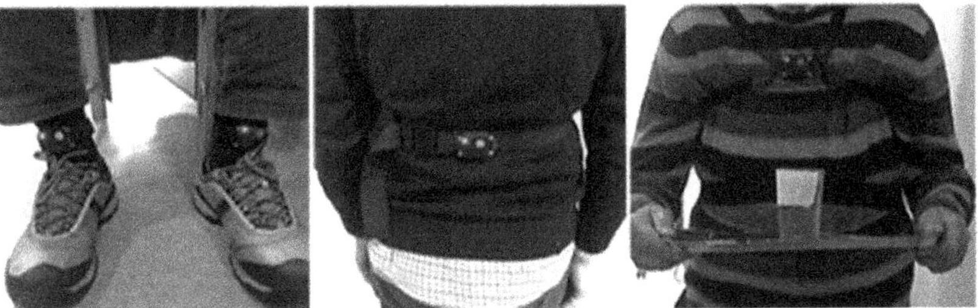

Figure 1. Placement of the Opal sensors and tray with a glass of water.

Inertial sensor data was collected and wirelessly streamed to a laptop for automatic generation of gait and balance metrics provided in specific reports by the Mobility Lab software. In the ISWAY test, subjects were asked to stand quietly for 30 s. In the ITUG test, subjects had to stand up from a chair without using their arms, walk 7 m, turn around to walk back to the chair, and sit down. Subjects repeated the ITUG test three times, once for each test condition (single motor task, dual motor task and, dual motor task with cognitive demands). Before the tests, each subject was submitted to a familiarization trial.

2.5. Data Analysis

The APDM automated analysis algorithm identified the standing position of the ISWAY test as well as the sit-to-stand, gait, turning and turn-to-sit components/phases of the ITUG test, providing a total of 52 spatial-temporal metrics [15]. From this automatic analysis, we monitored the following measures: Postural Sway (ISWAY test)—Forward/Backward and Right/Left amplitude (cm), Frequency (Hz), and Ellipse Sway area (m^2/s^4); ITUG: Sit-to-Stand—Time duration (s), Peak velocity (^{0}/s), and Trunk range of movement (RoM) (^{0}); Gait—Duration (s), Stride length (% of height), Cadence (steps/min), Stride velocity (% of height/s), Double support time (% of total gait cycle duration), Swing phase (% of total gait cycle duration), and Stance phase (% of total gait cycle duration); Turning—Duration (s), Number of steps (n°), Turn Peak velocity (^{0}/s), and Step duration during turning (s); Turn-to-Sit—Duration (s), Turn Peak velocity (^{0}/s), and Trunk range of movement (RoM) (^{0}).

Data results were subjected to analysis to identify the presence of any outliers. The assumption of normality was verified by Kolmogorov–Smirnov test. Kurtosis and skewness of the distributions were also analyzed. A repeated measures ANOVA was used for comparisons among the three conditions—(1) single motor task, (2) dual motor task, and (3) dual motor task with cognitive demands.

Sphericity was verified by Mauchly's test, and when this assumption could not be accepted, this parameter was corrected through the Greenhouse–Geisser Epsilon. Significant differences in ANOVA led to multiple comparisons with Bonferroni adjustment. Friedman's test was applied when the normality assumption was not verified, and in case of significant differences, Dunn's multiple comparisons were applied. The level of significance was set at 0.05. Data analysis included kinematic parameters during the two different tests (ISWAY and ITUG) during the three different conditions (single motor task, dual motor task, and dual motor task with cognitive demands).

3. Results

3.1. ISWAY Test

Thirty-six healthy older adults (9 men and 27 women, 73 $\pm$ 5.7 years) were recruited from the community. All participants consistently altered their static balance and gait pattern in response to additional dual-task load, although specific kinematic changes varied according to task conditions. Postural control in standing position, measured via the ISWAY, was only affected during the dual motor task with cognitive demands, due to the increased cognitive complexity when compared with the other two conditions (single task and dual motor task). There were no differences in kinematic data between the other two motor tasks (single and dual motor tasks). Specifically, instrumental assessments related to the ISWAY test showed an increase in the postural sway parameters of the center of mass (CM) movement in terms of forward–backward (χ^2 (2) = 19.385; $p < 0.001$; $N = 26$), and right–left ($F_{(2,50)}$ = 18.956; $p < 0.001$) displacement amplitude, forward–backward (χ^2 (2) = 20.846; $p < 0.001$; $N = 26$) and right–left (χ^2 (2) = 22.020; $p < 0.001$; $N = 26$) displacement frequency, and ellipse sway area ($F_{(1.488, 37.194)}$ = 27.361; $p < 0.001$). Figure 2 shows significant differences in pairwise comparisons for ISWAY test parameters and the respective boxplots.

3.2. ITUG Test

The dynamic balance analyzed during the ITUG test revealed highly significant differences ($p < 0.001$) between the single motor condition and the other two dual task conditions (dual motor task and dual motor task with cognitive demands) in the kinematic data of the ITUG test different phases.

3.2.1. Sit-to-Stand Phase

With respect to time duration, there were no significant differences among the different test conditions, but there were highly significant ($p < 0.001$) differences in peak velocity (χ^2 (2) = 46.545; $N = 33$) and trunk range of movement (RoM) ($F_{(2,64)}$ = 41,861; $p < 0.001$) between the single motor task and the other two tasks (dual motor task and dual motor task with cognitive demands) although there were no statistical significant differences between the two dual-task activities.

Figure 3 shows significant differences in pairwise comparisons for sit-to-stand parameters and the respective boxplots.

3.2.2. Gait Phase

Significant differences in time duration were observed among all three conditions ($F_{(1.681, 58.831)}$ = 61,377; $p < 0.001$). Since there were significant differences between all conditions, showing that the gait duration increases as the level of complexity of the task also increases.

Stride length revealed significant differences among all conditions ($F_{(2, 70)}$ = 39.375; $p < 0.001$), again with the reduction in stride length relative to the level of complexity of the task.

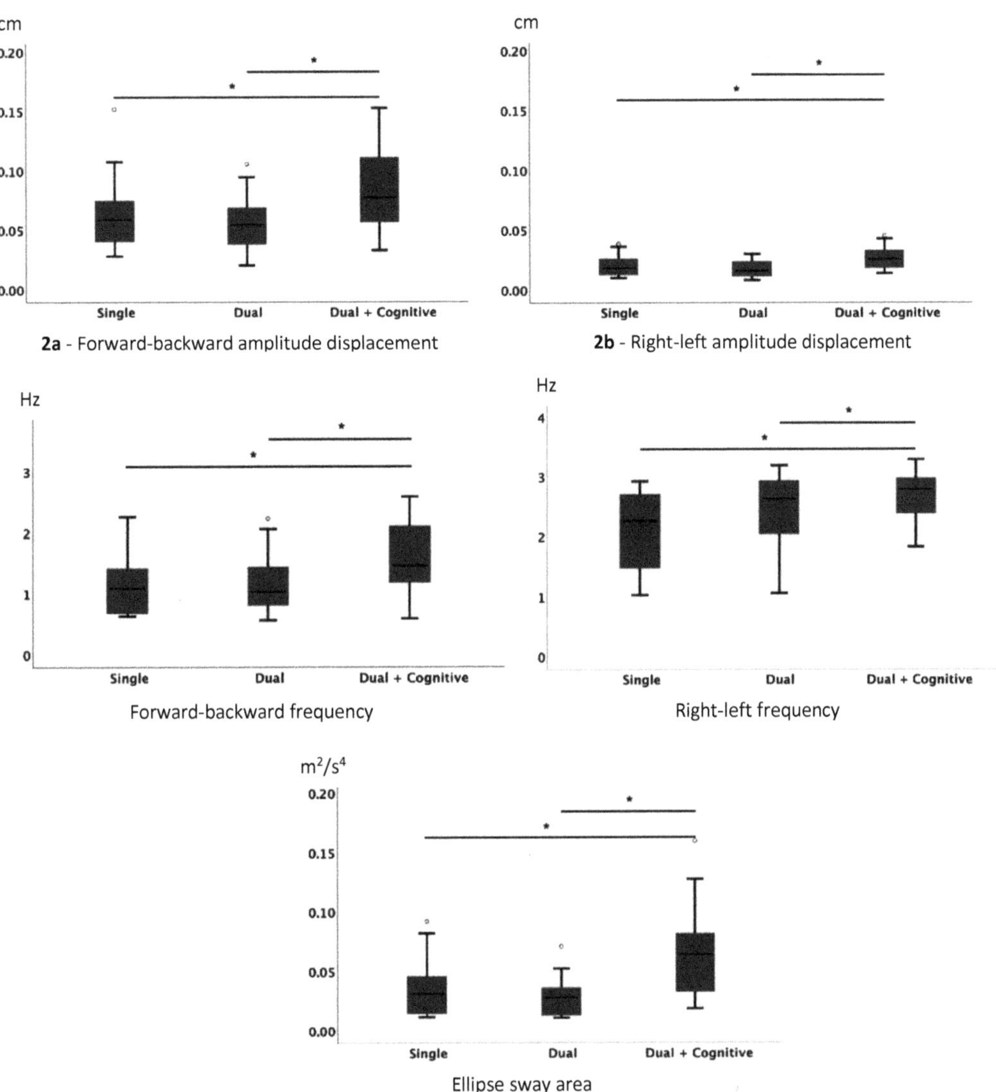

Figure 2. Balance parameters for the three conditions: single task, dual task, and dual and cognitive task during the ISWAY test. * Significant differences for pairwise comparisons.

The cadence parameter demonstrated significant differences between the dual motor task with cognitive demands condition and the other two conditions (single motor task and dual motor task) ($F_{(1.408, 49.281)}$ = 41.767; <0.001). There were no significant differences between the other two conditions.

Stride velocity showed significant differences among all task conditions ($F_{(1.590, 55.665)}$ = 54.459; $p < 0.001$), with a reduction of the results related to the level of complexity of the task.

Double support time revealed significant differences between the single motor task and the dual motor task with cognitive demands condition (χ^2 (2) = 44.169; $p < 0.001$; $N = 36$). No significant differences were observed between the other two conditions.

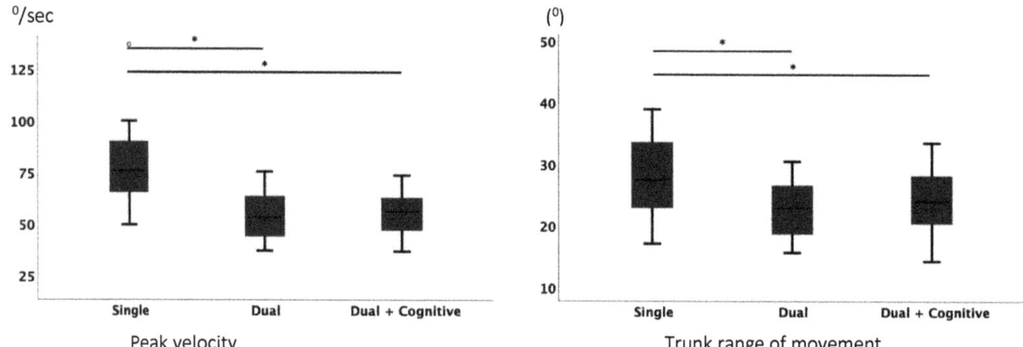

Peak velocity   Trunk range of movement

Figure 3. Sit-to-stand parameters for the three conditions: single task, dual task, and dual and cognitive task during the ITUG test. * Significant differences for pairwise comparisons.

Similarly, assessment of swing phase only demonstrated significant differences between the single motor task and the dual motor task with cognitive demands condition ($F_{(1.672,\ 58.529)}$ = 48.018; $p < 0.001$), showing a marked reduction in swing time. No significant differences were found between the other two conditions.

Stance phase showed significant differences between the single motor task and the dual motor task compared to the dual motor task with cognitive demands condition (χ^2 (2) = 43.504; $p < 0.001$; N = 36). No significant differences were observed between the other two conditions.

Figure 4 shows significant differences in pairwise comparisons for gait parameters and the respective boxplots.

3.2.3. Turning Phase

Turning duration showed significant differences between all the conditions ($F_{(2,64)}$ = 87.413; $p < 0.001$), with an increase in time corresponding to the level of complexity of the task. For all other turning-related assessments, there was a consistent pattern of statistically significant changes when comparing the single motor task to the dual motor task activity but no statistically significant changes when comparing the dual motor task with the dual motor task with cognitive demands conditions.

The number of steps revealed significant differences between the different conditions (χ^2 (2) = 42.365; $p < 0.001$; N = 32), with the single motor task condition presenting smaller values in relation to the other two dual motor task conditions. No statistically significant differences in the number of steps were identified during the two dual motor task conditions themselves (Figure 5).

Similarly, highly significant differences in peak velocity were identified comparing the single motor task to both other dual motor task conditions ($F_{(1.349,\ 41834)}$ = 72.817; $p < 0.001$). There were no statistically significant differences observed between the two dual motor task conditions.

Figure 5 shows significant differences in pairwise comparisons for turning parameters and the respective boxplots.

3.2.4. Turn-to-Sit Phase

Turn-to-sit duration revealed also significant differences only between the single motor task and the two dual motor tasks conditions (χ^2 (2) = 33.515; $p < 0.001$; N = 33), with no statistically significant differences between the two dual motor task conditions (Figure 6).

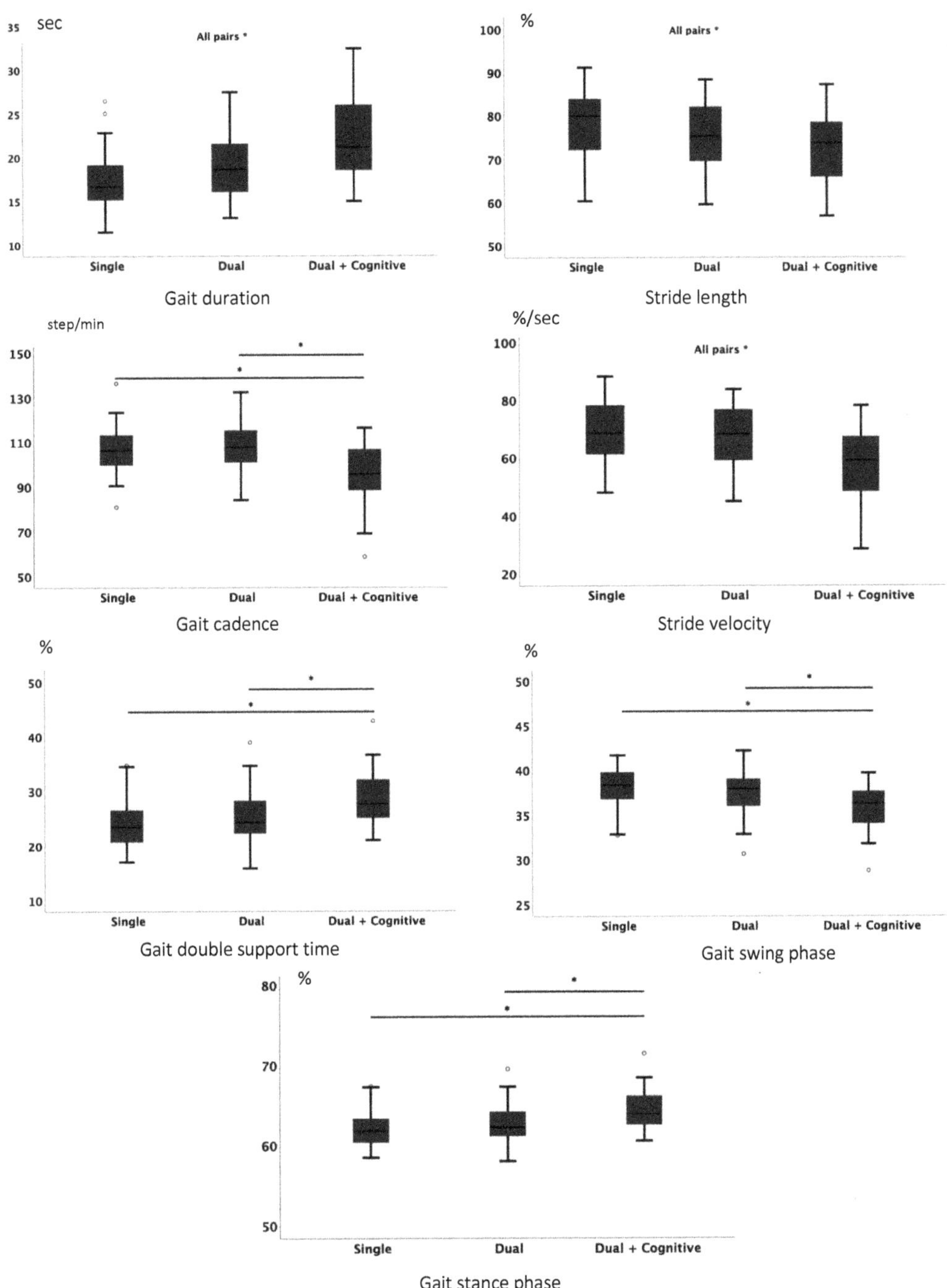

Figure 4. Gait parameters for the three conditions: single task, dual task, and dual and cognitive task during the ITUG test. * Significant differences for pairwise comparisons.

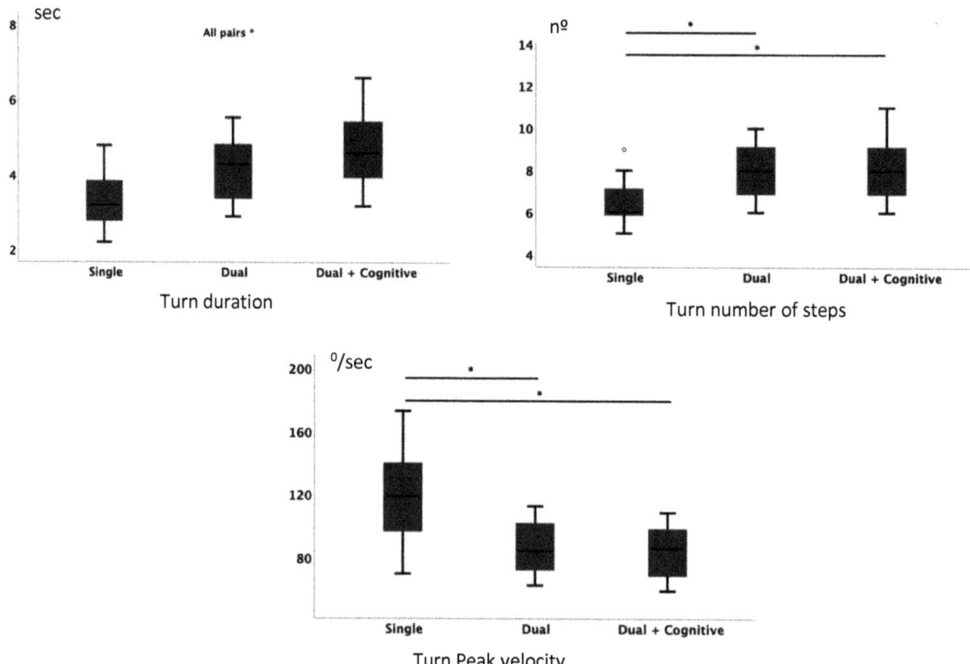

Figure 5. Turning parameters for the three conditions: single task, dual task, and dual and cognitive task during the ITUG test. * Significant differences for pairwise comparisons.

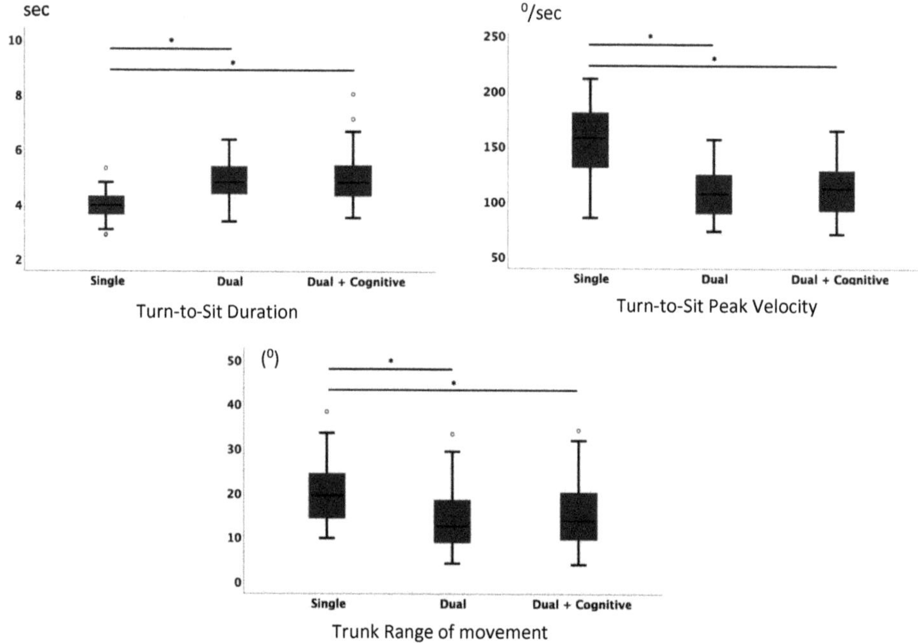

Figure 6. Turn-to-sit parameters for the three conditions: single task, dual task, and dual and cognitive task during the ITUG test. * Significant differences for pairwise comparisons.

Turn peak velocity revealed significant differences between the single motor task condition and both other dual motor task conditions, ($F_{(2,64)}$ = 64.977, $p < 0.001$ and $F_{(1.696, 54.267)}$ = 49.739, $p < 0.001$, respectively). There were no significant differences between either of the dual motor task conditions.

Trunk range of movement revealed significant differences between the different conditions ($F_{(1.696, 54.267)}$ = 49.739; $p < 0.001$) with the single motor task condition being responsible for these differences, showing a smaller trunk amplitude related to the other two conditions which did not show significant differences.

Figure 6 shows significant differences in pairwise comparisons for turn-to-sit parameters and the respective boxplots.

4. Discussion

The process of ageing is associated with functional decline that affects the speed of the executive function processes, which are the main neurocognitive processes for the proper development of daily life activities [16]. Simple actions including walking while talking require people to divide attention between the two tasks. When cognitive functions deteriorate and processing two actions becomes difficult, older people are placed at risk, and independence is compromised [17]. Healthy adults have the ability to develop dual-task activities; however, as a result of the ageing process and/or stages of neurological disorders, the ability to perform multiple tasks can be affected [1,7]. Consequently, preserving and improving a person's walking ability during other daily life activities is a crucial aim for extending functionality.

This study revealed that a change in walking performance was observed with the increasing path complexity and under dual-task conditions. Recent studies also showed that performing two tasks or dividing one's attention between tasks can result in the decrease of walking performance not only in healthy adults [9] but also in people with neurological pathologies [7,18].

Consistently, dual motor tasks with cognitive demands resulted in the most instances of statistically significant differences between the two types of dual-task activity identified while monitoring static balance and gait. The demands of a single motor task highlighted statistically significant differences when monitoring more complex movements like sit-to-stand, turning, and turn-to-sit, as well as during tasks involved in changes in movement direction or height control. These types of actions are associated with girdle dissociative control, which, in our sample of healthy older adults, is constrained by a counter-control strategy based on a pelvic and scapular girdle blockage.

Regarding the different conditions and tasks involved, we may consider that standing and walking are motor actions that can be performed under an automatic control, mediated by subcortical structures, releasing our attention to concurrent tasks needing greater engagement like in cognitive operations.

Previous studies have also shown how older adults under dual task testing contexts show a reduced gait velocity, cadence, and stride time variability [11,12]. Our study is in line with previous research showing that gait performance change deteriorates, and instability increases when a cognitive load is augmented. These results have clinical impact, since low performance in dual-task activities is associated with an increased risk for dementia [19,20], falls, and functional decline [21,22]. Furthermore, in older adults low gait speed is a significant clinical parameter associated with functional decline, falls, morbidity, and survival [23,24]. Significant improvements in the standard walking speed are related with increased subsistence in community dwelling [24].

Turning requires dynamic balance control, which often deteriorates with age. Our results suggest that cognitive processes are highly involved in the increased variability identified during tasks where movement is under an automatic control (like in standing or walking) in our sample composed of healthy older adults. However, during more complex activities such as sit-to-stand, turning and turn-to-sit, where the efficiency and control of the secondary motor task (carrying a tray with a full glass of water) implies a need for additional attention, the primary focus appears to be upon the perceptive information and any cognitive task becomes secondary. Nevertheless, motor actions that require the manipulation and control of sliding objects, or changes in body movement direction or heights, may involve a greater need for attention in order to control and accomplish the intended task. When evaluating the performances of the balance tests, also measuring the accuracy of the given additional task may produce more objective data.

Overall, the study results revealed that there was an adaptation in the motor control of the different tasks, and this should be contemplated in active aging programs of physical activity in order to maintain the effectiveness of the different perceptual-motor processes. The promoting training incorporating neuroplasticity principles, must be considered so that the performance capacity to perform dual tasks can be improved [25]. Using frequent and varied repetitions of different specific exercises is necessary for improving or maintaining performance [26,27].

5. Conclusions

The results from this study show that dual-tasking influences balance behavior in healthy older adults. By increasing the task complexity with an additional cognitive task, we change balance control. Healthy older adults are prone to focus on the challenging dual motor task or dual motor task with cognitive demands and sacrifice balance performance to some extent.

Further investigations should test the effects of dual task training protocols in older adults' balance and walking speed. The application of dual task training appears to be promising to improve the use of these parameters. Furthermore, longitudinal studies that assess the detraining effects are also needed. Therefore, we recommend that this assessment should be carried out in future studies and highlight the need to compare older populations with healthy young and adult subjects.

Author Contributions: Conceptualization; Formal analysis; Investigation; Methodology; Writing and Reviewing, G.M.d.B.; Conceptualization; Formal analysis; Investigation; Methodology; Writing and Reviewing; writing—original draft preparation; Project administration, F.M.; Conceptualization; Data curation; Formal analysis; Investigation; Methodology; Writing—Reviewing and Editing, J.D.; Formal analysis; Investigation; Methodology; Writing and Reviewing, R.O.; Methodology; Formal analysis; Writing and Reviewing, L.S.; Methodology; Writing—Reviewing and Editing, J.B.F.; Conceptualization; Formal analysis; Project administration; Writing—Reviewing and Editing, C.G. All authors have read and agreed to the published version of the manuscript.

Funding: This research did not receive any specific grant from funding agencies in the public, commercial, or not-for-profit sectors.

Institutional Review Board Statement: The study was conducted according to the guidelines of the Declaration of Helsinki, and approved by the Institutional Review Board and Ethics Committee of Faculty of Human Kinetics (ID: CEFMH N°4/2016 in 15 February 2016).

Informed Consent Statement: Informed consent was obtained from all subjects involved in the study.

Data Availability Statement: The data presented in this study are available on request from the first author.

Acknowledgments: This work is financed by national funds through the FCT—Foundation for Science and Technology, I.P., under the project UIDB/04585/2020. The researchers would like to thank the Centro de Investigação Interdisciplinar Egas Moniz (CiiEM) for the support provided for the publication of this article.

Conflicts of Interest: The authors declare that they have no conflict of interests.

References

1. Raichlen, D.A.; Bharadwaj, P.K.; Nguyen, L.A.; Franchetti, M.K.; Zigman, E.K.; Solorio, A.R.; Alexander, G.E. Effects of simultaneous cognitive and aerobic exercise training on dual-task walking performance in healthy older adults: Results from a pilot randomized controlled trial. *BMC Geriatr.* **2020**, *20*, 83. [CrossRef]
2. Agmon, M.; Kodesh, E.; Kizony, R. The effect of different types of walking on dual-task performance and task prioritization among community-dwelling older adults. *Sci. World J.* **2014**, *2014*, 259547. [CrossRef]
3. Ruffieux, J.; Keller, M.; Lauber, B.; Taube, W. Changes in Standing and Walking Performance under Dual-Task Conditions across the Lifespan. *Sports Med.* **2015**, *45*, 1739–1758. [CrossRef]
4. Liu-Ambrose, T.; Katarynych, L.A.; Ashe, M.C.; Nagamatsu, L.S.; Hsu, C.L. Dual-task gait performance among community-dwelling senior women: The role of balance confidence and executive functions. *J. Gerontol. Series A Biol. Sci. Med. Sci.* **2009**, *64*, 975–982. [CrossRef] [PubMed]
5. Muci, B.; Keser, I.; Meric, A.; Karatas, G.K. What are the factors affecting dual-task gait performance in people after stroke? *Physiother. Theory Pract.* **2020**, *16*, 1–8. [CrossRef] [PubMed]
6. Ghai, S.; Ghai, I.; Effenberg, A.O. Effects of dual tasks and dual-task training on postural stability: A systematic review and meta-analysis. *Clin. Interv. Aging* **2017**, *12*, 557–577. [CrossRef] [PubMed]
7. Hunter, S.W.; Omana, H.; Madou, E.; Wittich, W.; Hill, K.D.; Johnson, A.M.; Divine, A.; Holmes, J.D. Effect of dual-tasking on walking and cognitive demands in adults with Alzheimer's dementia experienced in using a 4-wheeled walker. *Gait Posture* **2020**, *77*, 164–170. [CrossRef]
8. Mancini, M.; Schlueter, H.; El-Gohary, M.; Mattek, N.; Duncan, C.; Kaye, J.; Horak, F.B. Continuous Monitoring of Turning Mobility and Its Association to Falls and Cognitive Function: A Pilot Study. *J. Gerontol.* **2016**, *71*, 1102–1108. [CrossRef]
9. Fraser, S.A.; Dupuy, O.; Pouliot, P.; Lesage, F.; Bherer, L. Comparable Cerebral Oxygenation Patterns in Younger and Older Adults during Dual-Task Walking with Increasing Load. *Front. Aging Neurosci.* **2016**, *8*, 240. [CrossRef]
10. Richer, N.; Lajoie, Y. Automaticity of Postural Control while Dual-tasking Revealed in Young and Older Adults. *Exp. Aging Res.* **2020**, *46*, 1–21. [CrossRef]
11. Hillel, I.; Gazit, E.; Nieuwboer, A.; Avanzino, L.; Rochester, L.; Cereatti, A.; Croce, U.D.; Rikkert, M.O.; Bloem, B.R.; Pelosin, E.; et al. Is every-day walking in older adults more analogous to dual-task walking or to usual walking? Elucidating the gaps between gait performance in the lab and during 24/7 monitoring. *Eur. Rev. Aging Phys. Act.* **2019**, *16*, 6. [CrossRef] [PubMed]
12. Smith, E.; Cusack, T.; Blake, C. The effect of a dual task on gait speed in community dwelling older adults: A systematic review and meta-analysis. *Gait Posture* **2016**, *44*, 250–258. [CrossRef] [PubMed]
13. Hemmati, L.; Rojhani-Shirazi, Z.; Malek-Hoseini, H.; Mobaraki, I. Evaluation of Static and Dynamic Balance Tests in Single and Dual Task Conditions in Participants with Nonspecific Chronic Low Back Pain. *J. Chiropr. Med.* **2017**, *16*, 189–194. [CrossRef] [PubMed]
14. Mancini, M.; King, L.; Salarian, A.; Holmstrom, L.; McNames, J.; Horak, F.B. Mobility Lab to Assess Balance and Gait with Synchronized Body-worn Sensors. *J. Bioeng. Biomed. Sci.* **2011**, *7* (Suppl. S1). [CrossRef]
15. Salarian, A.; Horak, F.B.; Zampieri, C.; Carlson-Kuhta, P.; Nutt, J.G.; Aminian, K. iTUG, a sensitive and reliable measure of mobility. *IEEE Trans. Neural Syst. Rehabil. Eng.* **2010**, *18*, 303–310. [CrossRef]
16. Falbo, S.; Condello, G.; Capranica, L.; Forte, R.; Pesce, C. Effects of Physical-Cognitive Dual Task Training on Executive Function and Gait Performance in Older Adults: A Randomized Controlled Trial. *BioMed Res. Int.* **2016**, *2016*, 5812092. [CrossRef]
17. Azadian, E.; Torbati, H.R.; Kakhki, A.R.; Farahpour, N. The effect of dual task and executive training on pattern of gait in older adults with balance impairment: A Randomized controlled trial. *Arch. Gerontol. Geriatr.* **2016**, *62*, 83–89. [CrossRef]
18. Ries, J.D. Rehabilitation for Individuals with Dementia: Facilitating Success. *Curr. Geriatr. Rep.* **2018**, *7*, 59–70. [CrossRef]
19. Åhman, H.B.; Cedervall, Y.; Kilander, L.; Giedraitis, V.; Berglund, L.; McKee, K.J.; Rosendahl, E.; Ingelsson, M.; Åberg, A.C. Dual-task tests discriminate between dementia, mild cognitive impairment, subjective cognitive impairment, and healthy controls—A cross-sectional cohort study. *BMC Geriatr.* **2020**, *20*, 258. [CrossRef]
20. Montero-Odasso, M.M.; Sarquis-Adamson, Y.; Speechley, M.; Borrie, M.J.; Hachinski, V.C.; Wells, J.; Riccio, P.M.; Schapira, M.; Sejdic, E.; Camicioli, R.M.; et al. Association of Dual-Task Gait With Incident Dementia in Mild Cognitive Impairment: Results From the Gait and Brain Study. *JAMA Neurol.* **2017**, *74*, 857–865. [CrossRef] [PubMed]
21. Li, F.; Harmer, P. Prevalence of Falls, Physical Performance, and Dual-Task Cost While Walking in Older Adults at High Risk of Falling with and Without Cognitive Impairment. *Clin. Interv. Aging* **2020**, *15*, 945–952. [CrossRef]
22. Tomas-Carus, P.; Biehl-Printes, C.; Pereira, C.; Veiga, G.; Costa, A.; Collado-Mateo, D. Dual task performance and history of falls in community-dwelling older adults. *Exp. Gerontol.* **2019**, *120*, 35–39. [CrossRef] [PubMed]
23. Jung, H.W.; Jang, I.Y.; Lee, C.K.; Yu, S.S.; Hwang, J.K.; Jeon, C.; Lee, Y.S.; Lee, E. Usual gait speed is associated with frailty status, institutionalization, and mortality in community-dwelling rural older adults: A longitudinal analysis of the Aging Study of Pyeongchang Rural Area. *Clin. Interv. Aging* **2018**, *13*, 1079–1089. [CrossRef] [PubMed]
24. Studenski, S.; Perera, S.; Patel, K.; Rosano, C.; Faulkner, K.; Inzitari, M.; Brach, J.; Chandler, J.; Cawthon, P.; Connor, E.B.; et al. Gait speed and survival in older adults. *JAMA* **2011**, *305*, 50–58. [CrossRef] [PubMed]
25. Yuan, P.; Koppelmans, V.; Reuter-Lorenz, P.A.; De Dios, Y.E.; Gadd, N.E.; Wood, S.J.; Riascos, R.; Kofman, I.S.; Bloomberg, J.J.; Mulavara, A.P.; et al. Increased Brain Activation for Dual Tasking with 70-Days Head-Down Bed Rest. *Front. Syst. Neurosci.* **2016**, *10*, 71. [CrossRef] [PubMed]

26. Patel, V.; Craig, J.; Schumacher, M.; Burns, M.K.; Florescu, I.; Vinjamuri, R. Synergy Repetition Training versus Task Repetition Training in Acquiring New Skill. *Front. Bioeng. Biotechnol.* **2017**, *5*, 9. [CrossRef]
27. Ranganathan, R.; Lee, M.H.; Newell, K.M. Repetition without Repetition: Challenges in Understanding Behavioral Flexibility in Motor Skill. *Front. Psychol.* **2020**, *11*, 2018. [CrossRef]

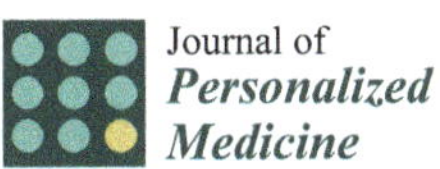

Journal of
Personalized Medicine

MDPI

Study Protocol

Addressing Ageism—Be Active in Aging: Study Protocol

Júlio Belo Fernandes [1,2,*], Catarina Ramos [1,3,4], Josefa Domingos [2], Cidália Castro [1,5], Aida Simões [1,5], Catarina Bernardes [1,2], Jorge Fonseca [1,2,6], Luís Proença [3,5], Miguel Grunho [2,7], Paula Moleirinho-Alves [2,8], Sérgio Simões [1,2], Diogo Sousa-Catita [2], Diana Alves Vareta [9] and Catarina Godinho [1,2]

[1] Escola Superior de Saúde Egas Moniz, 2829-511 Almada, Portugal; cramos@egasmoniz.edu.pt (C.R.); ccastro@egasmoniz.edu.pt (C.C.); aidasimoes@gmail.com (A.S.); cbernardes@egasmoniz.edu.pt (C.B.); jorgedafonseca@hotmail.com (J.F.); sergio_23@netcabo.pt (S.S.); cgcgodinho@gmail.com (C.G.)

[2] Grupo de Patologia Médica, Nutrição e Exercício Clínico (PaMNEC), Centro de Investigação Interdisciplinar Egas Moniz (CiiEM), 2829-511 Almada, Portugal; domingosjosefa@gmail.com (J.D.); miguelgrunho@gmail.com (M.G.); pmoleirinhoa@gmail.com (P.M.-A.); diogo.rsc2@gmail.com (D.S.-C.)

[3] Instituto Universitário Egas Moniz, 2829-511 Almada, Portugal; lproenca@egasmoniz.edu.pt

[4] LabPSI, Centro de Investigação Interdisciplinar Egas Moniz (CiiEM), 2829-511 Almada, Portugal

[5] Centro de Investigação Interdisciplinar Egas Moniz (CiiEM), 2829-511 Almada, Portugal

[6] Department of Gastroenterology, Hospital Garcia de Orta EPE (HGO), 2805-267 Almada, Portugal

[7] Department of Neurology, Hospital Garcia de Orta, 2805-267 Almada, Portugal

[8] Sleep and Temporomandibular Disorder Department, Cuf Tejo Hospital, 1350-352 Lisboa, Portugal

[9] Department of Nursing, Centro Hospitalar de Setúbal, 2900-182 Setúbal, Portugal; diana_vareta@hotmail.com

* Correspondence: juliobelo01@gmail.com

Citation: Fernandes, J.B.; Ramos, C.; Domingos, J.; Castro, C.; Simões, A.; Bernardes, C.; Fonseca, J.; Proença, L.; Grunho, M.; Moleirinho-Alves, P.; et al. Addressing Ageism—Be Active in Aging: Study Protocol. *J. Pers. Med.* **2022**, *12*, 354. https://doi.org/10.3390/jpm12030354

Academic Editor: Amelia Filippelli

Received: 20 December 2021
Accepted: 24 February 2022
Published: 25 February 2022

Publisher's Note: MDPI stays neutral with regard to jurisdictional claims in published maps and institutional affiliations.

Abstract: Ageism refers to stereotyping (how we think), prejudice (how we feel), and discrimination (how we act) against people based on their age. It is a serious public health issue that can negatively impact older people's health and quality of life. The present protocol has several goals: (1) adapt the Ambivalent Ageism Scale for the general Portuguese population and healthcare professionals; (2) assess the factorial invariance of the questionnaire between general population vs. healthcare professionals; (3) evaluate the level of ageism and its predictors in the general population and evaluate the level of ageism and its predictors in healthcare professionals; (4) compare the levels of ageism between groups and the invariance between groups regarding the explanatory model of predictors of ageism. This quantitative, cross-sectional, descriptive, observational study will be developed in partnership with several Healthcare Professional Boards/Associations, National Geriatrics and Gerontology Associations, and the Universities of the Third Age Network Association. The web-based survey will be conducted on a convenience sample recruited via various social media and institutional channels. The survey consists of three questionnaires: (1) Demographic data; (2) Ambivalent Ageism Scale; (3) Palmore-Neri and Cachioni questionnaire. The methodology of this study will include translation, pilot testing, semantic adjustment, exploratory and confirmatory factor analysis, and multigroup analysis of the Ambivalent Ageism Scale. Data will be treated using International Business Machines Corporation (IBM®) Statistical Package for the Social Sciences (SPSS) software and Analysis of Moment Structures (AMOS). Descriptive analysis will be conducted to assess the level of ageism in the study sample. The ageism levels between the two groups will be compared using the t-student test, and two Structural Equation Modeling will be developed to evaluate the predictors of ageism. Assessing ageism is necessary to allow healthcare professionals and policymakers to design and implement strategies to solve or reduce this issue. Findings from this study will generate knowledge relevant to healthcare and medical courses along with anti-ageism education for the Portuguese population.

Keywords: ageism; stereotyping; prejudice; discrimination; older adults; assessment; aging

1. Introduction

The demographic aging of the population is one of humanity's greatest triumphs and challenges. By 2050 the number of people aged 60 or older is expected to rise from 962 million in 2017 to 2.1 billion in 2050 and 3.1 billion in 2100 [1].

In the European Union, Portugal has the fourth-highest percentage age of older people [2]. In 2000, the Portuguese population aging index was 98.8%, having almost doubled in 2018, to 157.7%, increasing the dependency index from 24% to 33.6% [3].

Aging becomes a problem when society is not prepared for its own aging, presenting negative attitudes towards this stage of life [4].

Ageism, a term first coined by Robert Butler, refers to stereotyping (thoughts), prejudice (feelings), and discrimination (actions or behavior) against people by their age [5], has been identified as a serious threat to active aging and a major public health issue [6]. Despite being described in the bibliography since the late 60s, it took more than 30 years for ageism to be addressed within human rights instruments like the Madrid International Plan of Action on Ageing [7]. It is a multidimensional concept that includes different dimensions (cognitive, affective, and behavioral) operating at a micro-level (singular person), meso-level (social networks), and macro-level (cultural or institutional) and can occur consciously (explicitly) or unconsciously (implicitly) [4].

Ageism can have different targets, as it can be directed towards others or oneself [8]. In addition, ageism can also affect people of different ages, but children, adolescents, and older adults feel it more frequently. In our study, we intend to obtain data about the age-based attitudes and discrimination affecting older adults, and therefore the term "ageism" used here is applied for this context.

Definitions of ageism refer to older people, aging, and the aging process as being seen in an undesirable fashion. Ageist attitudes are of great complexity as they fit the paternalistic stereotype. Older adults are seen as warm but incompetent, ending in hostile and benevolent forms of prejudice [9,10]. Because most people consider the manifestation of protective behaviors and attitudes towards older adults positive, it is more challenging to address the benevolent forms of ageism [9,10].

Numerous studies have verified that ageism negatively impacts older people in several distinct dimensions such as memory and cognitive performance [11,12], health and wellbeing [13], social isolation and loneliness [14], job performance [15], decreased quality of life [13], and even their will-to-live [16]. These findings suggest that negative stereotypes, prejudice, or discrimination against people by their age can become internalized to such an extent that conscious or unconscious influence the person's cognitive and/or physical capacity.

While negative representations of older adults may lead to exclusion, hostile attitudes and behaviors [8,9], and social exclusion [17], favorable depictions often provoke well-intended benevolent behaviors, like providing unneeded support [18,19].

It is common to find ageism in many sectors of society, including those providing health and social care. Considering healthcare systems, older adults represent a significant group of users, and their care has a crucial impact on the overall financial costs [20]. However, these systems are designed considering the care needs of a younger population, aiming to achieve a quick turnover and not prioritizing the complexity of older adults' health and social concerns. Several studies involving healthcare professionals support that ageism contributes to worse received care for older adults with poorer health outcomes [21,22]. Conversely, healthcare professionals who have positive perceptions of older adults are more prone to assess and manage their healthcare concerns and social needs [23]. Additionally, if we consider that health professionals broadly foster a paradigm shift towards active aging, it becomes essential to assess the presence of ageism in this population as ageism may be reflected in their clinical practice. Health professionals must take the lead in promoting active aging and ensuring that their care practices enable and empower older adults to remain as autonomous and independent as possible for as long as possible [24].

Therefore, it is crucial to assess the presence of ageism and its predictors in the population, with a special focus on healthcare professionals.

The research will have two phases. Phase 1 aims to evaluate ageism in Portuguese healthcare professionals and identify its predictors. In Phase 2, we will expand the study to a representative sample of the Portuguese population.

We chose the Ambivalent Ageism Scale to evaluate ageism because it is a useful tool for researchers to measure attitudes toward older adults, allowing us to assess different elements of ageist attitudes and benevolent and hostile ageism [9].

1.1. Research Questions

(a)   What is the level of ageism in Portuguese healthcare professionals?
(b)   What are the predictors of ageism in Portuguese healthcare professionals?
(c)   What is the level of ageism in the Portuguese population?
(d)   What are the predictors of ageism in the Portuguese population?

1.2. Objective

Given the research questions mentioned above, the study goals are: (a) adapt the Ambivalent Ageism Scale for the general Portuguese population and for healthcare professionals; (b) assess the factorial invariance of the questionnaire between both groups (general population vs. healthcare professionals); (c) evaluate the level of ageism and its predictors in the general population; (d) evaluate the level of ageism and its predictors in healthcare professionals; (e) compare the levels of ageism between groups and the invariance between groups regarding the explanatory model of predictors of ageism.

2. Methods

2.1. Design

A quantitative, cross-sectional, descriptive, observational study conducted based on a web-based survey.

2.2. Time Period

January 2022–June 2024 (Gantt Chart Figure 1).

	1	2	3	4	5	6	7	8	9	10	11	12	13	14	15	16	17	18
Planning	■	■																
Questionnaire		■	■	■	■													
Standardization		■	■	■	■													
Translation					■	■	■	■	■									
Survey										■	■	■	■					
Data analysis														■	■	■	■	
Reporting																■	■	■

Figure 1. Project schedule.

2.3. Population and Recruitment

We will use a convenience sampling to recruit participants via various social media and institutional channels.

2.3.1. Phase 1

The study population consists of healthcare professionals (i.e., nurses, physiologists, physiotherapists, psychologists, speech therapists, occupational therapists, and doctors).

2.3.2. Phase 2

The study population consists of Portuguese citizens.

2.4. Inclusion Criteria

2.4.1. Phase 1

- Portuguese health care professional's (i.e., Portuguese nurses, physiologists, physiotherapists, psychologists, speech therapists, occupational therapists, doctors);
- Willingness to participate in the study.

2.4.2. Phase 2

- Portuguese population;
- People aged 18 years and above;
- Willingness to participate;
- Ability to understand, provide informed consent and comply with all the proceedings.

2.5. Exclusion Criteria

Target population under the age of 18, and an unwillingness/inability to understand, provide informed consent, or comply with all the proceedings.

2.6. Sample Size Calculation

The total sample consists of 168 participants, which will be divided into 2 groups (84 healthcare professionals and 84 participants from general population from Portugal). The sample size was obtained based on a power calculation (5% level of significance) indicating that a total sample size of 140 will have 95% power, for a small effect size (0.25). Therefore, sample size was increased to 168 participants to accommodate a 20% of exclusions.

2.7. Partner Institutions

In Phase 1, the study will be conducted in collaboration with the Board of Nurses, Board of Physiotherapists, Board of Psychologists, Board of Medicine, and the Portuguese Association of Exercise Physiologists.

These partners will use their database to forward an email (with a link to access the survey), inviting their members/associates to participate in the study. At the same time, we will create a campaign to publicize the study on different social media channels to maximize the number of respondents.

In phase 2 the study will be conducted in collaboration with the National Association of Social Gerontology, the Portuguese Society of Geriatrics and Gerontology, and the Universities of the Third Age Network Association. In addition, we will start a campaign to publicize the study on different social media channels to maximize the number of respondents.

2.8. Data Collection

Data collection will be carried out through the application of the web-based survey using Qualtrics. Participants will answer the survey. At the end of all the questionnaires, participants can see the contact details of the researchers for any questions or comments, as well as links to other organizations that provide information or intervention in the area of ageism. The survey's first page will clarify the objectives and procedures of the study and the guarantee to ensure the confidentiality and anonymity of the data. Before completing the survey, informed consent will be obtained from all study participants.

2.9. The Survey

Part 1—Demographic data: Multiple choice and quick answer questions are presented to allow the sociodemographic characterization of the sample. Participants will report information such as gender, age, nationality, education, professional status, frequency, and quality of intergenerational contact.

Part 2—Ambivalent Ageism Scale: To assess the presence of benevolent and hostile ageism, we will use the Ambivalent Ageism Scale developed by Cary, Chasteen, and Remedios [9]. Participants will report their agreement on a 7-point Likert-type scale with 13 statements regarding older adults. Nine of those items allow assessing the presence of benevolent ageism, and the remaining four items the presence of hostile ageism (e.g., "It is helpful to repeat things to old people because they rarely understand the first time.", "It is good to tell old people that they are too old to do certain things; otherwise they might get their feelings hurt when they eventually fail." or "Old people are a drain on the health care system and the economy.").

Part 3—Palmore-Neri and Cachioni questionnaire: To assess the level of knowledge concerning aging, we will use the Palmore-Neri and Cachioni questionnaire [25]. The questionnaire is an adaptation of the Palmore Aging Quiz, consisting of 25 items covering general knowledge about aging and questions about older adults' physical, psychological, and social dimensions.

Ageism and level of knowledge are constructs that can be influenced by social desirability. Therefore, to control for social desirability bias, we will include a short text before the presentation of the questionnaires (based on the text from Goetzke, Nitzko, and Spiller [26]). In addition, we will also apply the Balanced Inventory of Desirable Responding (BIDR) short scale (Winkler, Kroh, & Spiess [27]; adapted to English by Goetzke, Nitzko, and Spiller [26]), as a complementary measure to control for social desirability bias.

2.10. Ambivalent Ageism Scale Translation and Cultural Validation

The Ambivalent Ageism Scale will be translated in accordance with World Health Organization best practice guidelines [28].

The translation process will be performed through different stages, namely: forward translation, an expert panel, back-translation, pre-testing, and cognitive interviewing. Our team has already gained permission by email correspondence to use and translate the Ambivalent Ageism Scale. Translation and cultural validation will take place between May 2022 and September 2022.

2.10.1. Stage I—Forward Translation

The translation of the questionnaire from the original English version into the Portuguese language will be accomplished by two independent bilingual translators. One translator will be an expert on Ageism, providing a translation that more closely resembles the original instrument. The other will be a naïve translator, who is unaware of the questionnaire's aim, producing another translation so that subtle variances in the original questionnaire might be perceived. Any divergences in the translation will be debated and resolved between the two translators or, if needed, a third unbiased translator fluent in both languages. With the forward translation, we aim to translate the questionnaire and determine its conceptual equivalence in Portuguese, reflecting the nuances of the target language.

2.10.2. Stage II—Back-Translation

The back-translation will be performed independently from the forward translation to ensure the accuracy of the translation. This stage will be done independently by two further translators fluent in both Portuguese and English. Following the best practice recommendation, these two translators will not have previous exposure to the original questionnaire. As in the previous stage, any divergences in the translation will be debated and resolved between the two translators or, if needed, a third unbiased translator. In this stage, we aim to reveal any misunderstandings or unclear wording in the initial translation.

2.10.3. Stage III—Questionnaire Pilot Test and Semantic Adjustment

The translated version will be applied to a small (34, 20%, from the total sample), randomly selected sample of men and women to discuss the items' understanding and arrive at the final translation of the Portuguese version of the questionnaires Ambivalent Ageism Scale. The Ambivalent Ageism Scale will be pilot tested through a think-aloud protocol [29] as per the best practice recommendation. Participants will be asked to fill out the questionnaire while verbalizing their thought processes. This process enables researchers to gather information on how participants understood the questionnaire and its instructions and allows the verification of the questionnaire comprehensibility for Portuguese speakers.

Subsequently, researchers will apply the instruments to the general and healthcare samples within the scope of the investigation protocol.

2.11. Data Analysis

Data will be treated using Statistical Package for the Social Sciences (SPSS) software (International Business Machines Corporation (IBM) SPSS Statistics®, v.27.0, IBM® Corp, Armonk, NY, USA) and Analysis of Moment Structures (AMOS®) (v.27.0, SPSS Inc., Chicago, IL, USA). To assess the construct validity of the Ambivalent Ageism Scale, exploratory factor analyses (EFA) will be performed. The principal components method will be used for the extraction of common factors and the Varimax rotation for the factor rotation [30]. Confirmatory factor analyses will be performed using Structural Equation Modeling (SEM) with Maximum Likelihood as estimator. Confirmatory factor analyses models will be evaluated with chi-square, and an alpha level of 0.05 will be used to determine statistical significance. Model fit will be assessed using the comparative fit index (CFI), the goodness of fit index (GFI), and the root mean square error of approximation (RMSEA). Values above 0.90 on the CFI and the GFI and below 0.05 on the root mean square error of approximation are indicators of good model fit [31]. Model invariance between groups (general population and healthcare professionals samples) regarding baseline model and resulting models will be calculated using $\Delta\text{CFI}(\leq 0.01)$ [31]. After the final version of the Ambivalent Ageism Scale is obtained, a descriptive analysis (i.e., mean, standard deviation, minimum, maximum) of ageism will be conducted to assess the level of ageism in both groups. The ageism levels between the two groups will be compared using the t-student test. In order to evaluate the predictors of ageism, two versions of Structural Equation Modeling will be developed, one for the general population sample and the other for the healthcare professionals sample, with ageism as the dependent variable and with the following variables as independent variables: level of knowledge concerning aging, gender, age, nationality, education, professional status, frequency, and quality of intergenerational contact. The same criteria mentioned above will be used to evaluate the model fit. The invariance between the Structural Equation Modeling models of ageism predictors of the general population and the healthcare professionals will be assessed through a multigroup analysis. The same criteria for assessing model invariance mentioned above will be applied.

2.12. Ethics and Procedures

This research will be conducted in accordance with the Helsinki Declaration (as revised in 2013) and will seek approval from the Egas Moniz Ethics Committee.

All the participants must complete an informed consent question embedded on the first page of the questionnaire. It will state that participation is entirely voluntary. Participants are also free to not reply to some questions, change or review their responses, or voluntarily quit at any time. Consent will be obtained before proceeding to the next page if participants answer "YES" to the form's first question, agreeing to participate in the study. Participants who answer "NO" to the informed consent question will be directed to the end of the survey. Data will be conducted in compliance with ethical principles guaranteeing the participants' anonymity. Therefore, no individual answers to the questionnaire will be accessible.

2.13. Confidentiality and Data Retention

In this study, all data collected from participants will be strictly anonymous and confidential. Researchers are not interested in individual responses. Only the project managers will have access to all data. Essential documents will be archived in a way that ensures that they are readily available, upon request, to the competent authorities. All paper copies will be stored in a locked file. Data collected from the survey will be coded and stored on a password-protected and backed-up computer drive. For five years, all data will remain locked in a file cabinet at Egas Moniz University. The project managers will destroy all data when this retention period is complete.

3. Discussion

This study represents a starting point to change the narrative around age and aging among the Portuguese population. Up to now, there has been no significant study that addresses ageism in Portugal. Ageism can harm members of society individually and collectively, with negative consequences for their health and wellbeing, being responsible for a heavy economic burden on society. For example, in the United States of America, age stereotypes led to excess annual costs of US$63 billion for the eight most expensive health conditions [32]. Ageist behaviors can be combatted. However, collective action is needed to increase awareness and address this issue for this to happen. Increasing peoples' awareness of ageist behaviors is essential to decreasing ageism as a persistent social phenomenon.

There are several scales designed to measure hostile ageism, potentially making it difficult for clinicians to decide which to choose for better practices. Notably, the Ambivalent Ageism Scale is the first dedicated to measuring both hostile and benevolent ageism since hostile and benevolent ageist attitudes exist and do not predict the same outcomes [9]. This scale had good test-retest reliability ($r = 0.80$) and good internal consistency ($\alpha = 0.91$). The internal consistency of the benevolent subscale was $\alpha = 0.89$, for the hostile ageism subscale $\alpha = 0.84$ [9]. Besides being a useful tool for researchers to assess hostile and benevolent ageism, respondents do not perceive their participation in the survey as difficult or time-consuming when compared to the Ambivalent Ageism Scale (consisting of report agreement with 13 statements) [9].

The data collected in this study may play a central role in raising awareness of ageism among the Portuguese population, with a particular focus on healthcare professionals. After its completion, it is expected that the team of researchers will work with key partners to develop content related to ageism and share this content on various social media platforms to raise awareness of this problem.

Assessing ageism is the first step that allows healthcare professionals and policymakers to develop and implement strategies (e.g., education strategies) to solve this issue. Previous studies investigated strategies to combat ageism. For example, research developed in Canada addressed the effect of educational programs on nursing students' knowledge and ageist behaviors. Researchers concluded that education had a positive impact on the way students view older adults [33].

Other studies also show that increased aging knowledge was significantly correlated with reduced ageist behaviors [34–36]. Therefore, raising awareness about ageism followed by increasing knowledge about aging should be the strategy to minimize the burden of this public health problem. Furthermore, knowledge and skills can be transmitted by developing educational activities enhancing understanding and empathy regarding aging.

In addition, previous studies have shown that a high level of encounters in the right setting decreases ageism, so multidisciplinary intervention to promote intergenerational contact should be promoted [37–39]. There is a clear need to increase aging knowledge combined with open, natural, and mutual relationships that will enable the reduction of negative attitudes towards aging.

This study protocol presents our aims, methodological approach, and plan to operationalize the research. The findings are expected to have direct relevance to several healthcare and medical courses across Portugal, along with anti-ageism education for the general public.

It is necessary to develop the capacity to challenge, rather than perpetuate, stereotypes, prejudice, and discrimination against people by their age. Therefore, this study is of vital importance.

This study has the advantage of contributing to a more complete representation of ageism among the Portuguese population. Nevertheless, we emphasize that the study has limitations. The first is the possibility that participants might deny or minimize their ageist behaviors if they recognize them as incorrect or socially undesirable. Alternatively, if participants perceive it to be socially desirable, they might overstate the frequency of their behavior, increasing the frequency of the positive items. Second, by relying upon recruiting participants via various social media, we may not generalize the survey result to the population as a whole as there is the possibility of under-or over-representation.

Author Contributions: Conceptualization, J.B.F., C.R., J.D., C.C., A.S., D.A.V. and C.G.; methodology, J.B.F., C.R., J.D., C.C., A.S., C.B., J.F., L.P., M.G., P.M.-A., S.S., D.S.-C., D.A.V. and C.G.; writing—original draft preparation, J.B.F., C.R., J.D., C.C., A.S., C.B., J.F., L.P., M.G., P.M.-A., S.S., D.S.-C., D.A.V. and C.G.; writing—review and editing, J.B.F., C.R., J.D., C.C., A.S., C.B., J.F., L.P., M.G., P.M.-A., S.S., D.S.-C., D.A.V. and C.G.; supervision, J.B.F. and C.G.; project administration, J.B.F. and C.G. All authors have read and agreed to the published version of the manuscript.

Funding: This research received no external funding.

Institutional Review Board Statement: Not applicable.

Informed Consent Statement: Not applicable.

Data Availability Statement: Not applicable.

Acknowledgments: This publication is financed by national funds through the FCT—Foundation for Science and Technology, I.P., under the project UIDB/04585/2020. The researchers would like to thank the Centro de Investigação Interdisciplinar Egas Moniz (CiiEM) for the support provided for the publication of this article.

Conflicts of Interest: The authors declare no conflict of interest.

References

1. United Nations Department of Economic and Social Affairs. *The 2017 Revision, Key Findings and Advance Tables*; United Nations: New York, NY, USA, 2017.
2. Eurostat. *Aging Europe: Looking at the Lives of Older People in the EU*; Publications Office of the European Union: Luxembourg, 2019.
3. Instituto Nacional de Estatística (National Institute of Statistics). Available online: https://www.pordata.pt/Portugal/Indicadores+de+envelhecimento-526 (accessed on 4 December 2021).
4. World Health Organization. *Global Report on Ageism*; World Health Organization: Geneva, Switzerland, 2021.
5. Butler, R.N. Age-ism: Another form of bigotry. *Gerontologist* **1969**, *9*, 243–246. [CrossRef] [PubMed]
6. Officer, A.; de la Fuente-Núñez, V. A global campaign to combat ageism. *Bull. World Health Organ.* **2018**, *96*, 95–296. [CrossRef] [PubMed]
7. United Nations. *Political declaration and Madrid Plan of Action on Aging*; United Nations: New York, NY, USA, 2002.
8. Ayalon, L.; Tesch-Römer, C. Taking a closer look at ageism: Self- and other-directed ageist attitudes and discrimination. *Eur. J. Ageing* **2017**, *14*, 1–4. [CrossRef] [PubMed]
9. Cary, L.A.; Chasteen, A.L.; Remedios, J. The Ambivalent Ageism Scale: Developing and Validating a Scale to Measure Benevolent and Hostile Ageism. *Gerontologist* **2017**, *57*, e27–e36. [CrossRef]
10. Sublett, J.F.; Vale, M.T.; Bisconti, T.L. Expanding Benevolent Ageism: Replicating Attitudes of Overaccommodation to Older Men. *Exp. Aging Res.* **2021**, 1–14. [CrossRef]
11. Chan, S.; Au, A.; Lai, S. The detrimental impacts of negative age stereotypes on the episodic memory of older adults: Does social participation moderate the effects? *BMC Geriatr.* **2020**, *20*, 452. [CrossRef]
12. Molden, J.; Maxfield, M. The impact of aging stereotypes on dementia worry. *Eur. J. Ageing* **2016**, *14*, 29–37. [CrossRef]
13. Chang, E.S.; Kannoth, S.; Levy, S.; Wang, S.Y.; Lee, J.E.; Levy, B.R. Global reach of ageism on older persons' health: A systematic review. *PLoS ONE* **2020**, *15*, e0220857. [CrossRef]
14. Silva, M.F.; Silva, D.; Bacurau, A.; Francisco, P.; Assumpção, D.; Neri, A.L.; Borim, F. Ageism against older adults in the context of the COVID-19 pandemic: An integrative review. *Rev. Saude Publica* **2021**, *55*, 4. [CrossRef]

15. Clendon, J.; Walker, L. Nurses aged over 50 and their perceptions of flexible working. *J. Nurs. Manag.* **2016**, *24*, 336–346. [CrossRef]
16. Marques, S.; Lima, M.L.; Abrams, D.; Swift, H. Will to live in older people's medical decisions: Immediate and delayed effects of aging stereotypes. *J. Appl. Soc. Psychol.* **2014**, *44*, 399–408. [CrossRef]
17. Fernandes, J.B.; Fernandes, S.B.; Almeida, A.S.; Vareta, D.A.; Miller, C.A. Older Adults' Perceived Barriers to Participation in a Falls Prevention Strategy. *J. Pers. Med.* **2021**, *11*, 450. [CrossRef] [PubMed]
18. Swift, H.J.; Chasteen, A.L. Ageism in the time of COVID-19. *Group Process Intergr. Relat.* **2021**, *24*, 246–252. [CrossRef]
19. Vale, M.T.; Bisconti, T.L.; Sublett, J.F. Benevolent ageism: Attitudes of overaccommodative behavior toward older women. *J. Soc. Psychol.* **2020**, *160*, 548–558. [CrossRef] [PubMed]
20. Kalseth, J.; Halvorsen, T. Health and care service utilisation and cost over the life-span: A descriptive analysis of population data. *BMC Health Serv. Res.* **2020**, *20*, 435. [CrossRef]
21. Inouye, S.K. Creating an anti-ageist healthcare system to improve care for our current and future selves. *Nat. Aging* **2021**, *1*, 150–152. [CrossRef]
22. Meisner, B.A. Physicians' attitudes toward aging, the aged, and the provision of geriatric care: A systematic narrative review. *Crit. Public Health* **2012**, *22*, 61–72. [CrossRef]
23. Giles, H.; Ryan, E.B.; Anas, A.P. Perceptions of intergenerational communication by young, middle-aged, and older Canadians. *Can. J. Behav. Sci.* **2008**, *40*, 21–30. [CrossRef]
24. World Health Organization. *Global Strategy and Action Plan on Ageing and Health*; World Health Organization: Geneva, Switzerland, 2017.
25. Neri, A.L.; Cachioni, M.; Resende, M.C. Atitudes em relação à velhice. In *Tratado de Geriatria e Gerontologia*; Freitas, E.V., Py, L., Néri, A.L., Cançado, F.A.X., Gorzoni, M.L., Rocha, S.M., Eds.; Guanabara Koogan: Rio de Janeiro, Brazil, 2002; pp. 972–998.
26. Goetzke, B.; Nitzko, S.; Spiller, A. Consumption of organic and functional food. A matter of well-being and health? *Appetite* **2014**, *1*, 96–105. [CrossRef]
27. Winkler, N.; Kroh, M.; Spiess, M. *Entwicklung Einer Deutschen Kurzskala zur Zweidimensionalen Messung von Sozialer Erwünschtheit [Development of a German Short Scale for Two-Dimensional Measurement of Social Desirability]*; DIW Discussion Papers; Deutsches Institut für Wirtschaftsforschung (DIW): Berlin, Germany, 2006.
28. World Health Organization: Process of Translation and Adaptation of Instruments. Available online: http://www.who.int/substance_abuse/research_tools/translation/en/ (accessed on 5 November 2021).
29. Jääskeliänien, R. Think-aloud protocol. In *Handbook of Translation Studies*; Gambier, Y., van Doorslaer, L., Eds.; John Benjamins Publishing: Amsterdam, The Netherlands, 2010; pp. 371–383.
30. Marôco, J. *Análise Estatística com o SPSS Statistics*, 5th ed.; Report Number: Pêro Pinheiro, Portugal, 2011.
31. Byrne, B.M. *Structural Equation Modeling with AMOS: Basic Concepts Applications, and Programming*, 2nd ed.; N Routledge: New York, NY, USA, 2010.
32. Levy, B.R.; Slade, M.D.; Chang, E.S.; Kannoth, S.; Wang, S.Y. Ageism Amplifies Cost and Prevalence of Health Conditions. *Gerontologist* **2020**, *60*, 174–181. [CrossRef]
33. Potter, G.; Clarke, T.; Hackett, S.; Little, M. Nursing students and geriatric care: The influence of specific knowledge on evolving values, attitudes, and actions. *Nurse Educ. Pract.* **2013**, *13*, 449–453. [CrossRef] [PubMed]
34. Cherry, K.E.; Erwin, M.J.; Allen, P.D. Aging knowledge and self-reported ageism. *Innov. Aging* **2019**, *3*, S81. [CrossRef]
35. Cooney, C.; Minahan, J.; Siedlecki, K.L. Do Feelings and Knowledge About Aging Predict Ageism? *J. Appl. Gerontol.* **2021**, *40*, 28–37. [CrossRef]
36. Donizzetti, A.R. Ageism in an Aging Society: The Role of Knowledge, Anxiety about Aging, and Stereotypes in Young People and Adults. *J. Environ. Res. Public Health* **2019**, *16*, 1329. [CrossRef]
37. Verhage, M.; Schuurman, B.; Lindenberg, J. How young adults view older people: Exploring the pathways of constructing a group image after participation in an intergenerational programme. *J. Aging Stud.* **2021**, *56*, 100912. [CrossRef] [PubMed]
38. Ermer, A.E.; York, K.; Mauro, K. Addressing ageism using intergenerational performing arts interventions. *Gerontol. Geriatr. Educ.* **2021**, *42*, 308–315. [CrossRef]
39. Burnes, D.; Sheppard, C.; Henderson, C.R.; Wassel, M.; Cope, R.; Barber, C.; Pillemer, K. Interventions to Reduce Ageism Against Older Adults: A Systematic Review and Meta-Analysis. *Am. J. Public Health* **2019**, *109*, e1–e9. [CrossRef]

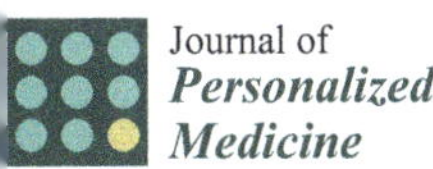

Journal of *Personalized Medicine*

Article

Rehabilitation Nurse's Perspective on Transitional Care: An Online Focus Group

Rita Pedrosa [1,*], Óscar Ferreira [1] and Cristina Lavareda Baixinho [1,2]

1   Nursing School of Lisbon, Nursing Research, Innovation and Development Centre of Lisbon (CIDNUR), 1600-090 Lisbon, Portugal; oferrera@esel.pt (Ó.F.); crbaixinho@esel.pt (C.L.B.)
2   Center for Innovative Care and Health Technology (ciTechCare), Polytechnic of Leiria, 2410-541 Leiria, Portugal
*   Correspondence: anaritapedrosa@esel.pt

Abstract: The increasing incidence of chronic and dependence leads to the need for hospitalization and adaptation in the process of returning home, as well as transition between care levels to ensure continuity of care. The World Health Organization has been warning about this problem since 2016, and consider reorganizing the care model as one of the solutions. The present study aimed to analyse the nurses' perspective on transitional care for dependent people with rehabilitation care needs after hospital discharge. Methods: A focus *group* was developed with the participation of Rehabilitation Nurses from the hospital and community context, and content analysis was defined a *posteriori*. Results: From the content analysis emerged four related categories: promotion of continuity of care, nurse of advanced practice as a care manager, capacitation of the person and caregiver, and promotion of the care coordination. Conclusions: The present study allowed the strategies identification that minimize fragmentation risk of care and promote the person participation in transitional care. Ensuring transitional care is imperative to increase the quality of care, the satisfaction of professionals, clients, and the development of a system of sustainable health.

Keywords: advanced nursing practice; rehabilitation nursing; transitional care; hospital discharge; continuity of care

Citation: Pedrosa, R.; Ferreira, Ó.; Baixinho, C.L. Rehabilitation Nurse's Perspective on Transitional Care: An Online Focus Group. *J. Pers. Med.* **2022**, *12*, 582. https://doi.org/10.3390/jpm12040582

Academic Editors: Fábio G. Teixeira, Catarina Godinho, Júlio Belo Fernandes and José Carmelo Adsuar Sala

Received: 8 February 2022
Accepted: 3 April 2022
Published: 5 April 2022

Publisher's Note: MDPI stays neutral with regard to jurisdictional claims in published maps and institutional affiliations.

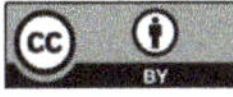

1. Introduction

The population aging associated with the increased prevalence of chronic diseases is a current problem and to which health systems seek to adapt responses through the development of strategies that provide better health outcomes and reduce the costs associated with the sector.

According to the World Health Organization (WHO), health systems have the responsibility to improve the population health and protect them from the financial costs associated with the disease situation, as well as to treat them with dignity. This would be made possible through increasing the capacity and quality of care delivery, ensuring coverage for the whole population, and ensuring that these services remain accessible to all [1].

Continuity and coordination of care are broad, interconnected concepts that can even overlap, and that contribute significantly to the way people experience their experiences in the health sector [1–3]. According to the WHO, there are eight priority practices that should be implemented at different levels of the health system and care, which ensure their continuity: (1) continuity (in the relationship) with primary health care professionals; (2) shared care and decision-making; (3) case management for people with complex needs; (4) services defined or with a single access point; (5) transitional or intermediate care; (6) integral service along the entire process; (7) technology to support continuity and coordination; (8) building the working capacity [1].

Transitional care refers to the care provision during the transition from hospital to home, from home to hospital and from illness or injury to recovery and independence—they can, in fact, involve the person's reintegration into their employment and broader social role, or support the transition to palliative and end-of-life care. This holistic and biopsychosocial approach to transitional care should be culturally sensitive and involve the family, caregivers, employer and local community [1].

Countries with a health system based on Primary Health Care have a population with better health outcomes, lower rates of potentially avoidable hospitalizations, have lower socio-economic inequalities in reported health status and unmet needs. These outcomes are particularly relevant when interpreted in the face of an ageing population, and the consequent profile of the elderly (mostly users of primary health care and with frequent transition between levels of care): the integration and continuity of care are central and should provide the person, depending on their individual situation, access to the type and intensity of care they actually need, in the proper time and place [4,5].

The articulation between care levels requires a multi and interdisciplinary team that ensures quality and safety, avoiding the decline of functionality in the post-discharge period and unnecessary rehospitalisations due to foreseeable risks and complications. Ensuring a safe transition from the hospital to the community is, for this reason, an appropriate strategy to be followed by the different health services, by the potential in promoting autonomy and independence for self-care [6–8]. Nevertheless, transition between care levels often cannot be planned, which leads to consequences in the preparation of patients and caretakers and contributes to hospital readmissions. The reasons for readmission vary, but one of the most important components are assessment of community resources and whether they can fit patients' needs [7–9]. A French study estimated that, for patients 75 years old or older, hospital readmission rate within 30 days after discharge was 14%, and according to the researchers one quarter of these events was preventable [7].

There are few studies on transitional care to support care continuity in the rehabilitation context and they have not systematized professionals' interventions, which impacts the development of health policies oriented toward transitional rehabilitation care [9].

The present study aimed to analyse the nurses' perspective on transitional care for dependent people with rehabilitation care needs after hospital discharge.

2. Materials and Methods

2.1. Study Design

This was a qualitative, descriptive and exploratory study to answer the following research question: "How rehabilitation nurses see the needs and organization of transitional care?" The study protocol consisted of five phases: planning, preparation, moderation, data analysis, and dissemination of results [10,11].

The *focus group* (FG) is a research method that aims to collect qualitative data from a group of people (between 4 and 12 participants) through their interaction and discussion on a topic presented by the researcher. The implementation of this method of data collection allows a greater intervention of participants on topics defined in a script, which can be carried out at different moments of the research process [10,11].

2.2. Participants

In the present study, the participants were defined as the following inclusion criteria: rehabilitation nurses, with clinical experience in rehabilitation care of dependent older persons' with need of rehabilitation nursing care and with experience in transitional care programmes.

Given the nature of transitional care that starts at the hospital and continues after returning home, the option was to have 50% of participants with clinical practice in hospital and 50% with clinical practice in home care, integrated into primary health care. In accordance with the literature review that assume that transitional care and the management of the transition from hospital to home can happen in three stages: before the person leaves the hospital, at hospital discharge, or within 48 h to 30 days after discharge [1–3,7,9].

The number of participants was established a priori according to the ideal number of participants defined by the same authors, for online FG [10].

2.3. Data Collection

The literature review was crucial for structuring the interview script, which was organized around the follow stimulus questions: What are the transitional care needs presented by dependent older persons and their caregivers? What difficulties do they experience in ensuring continuity of care between hospital and community? How do you think transitional care can be planned to ensure continuity of rehabilitation care?

In the e-mail sent to nurses and at the beginning of the focus group, participants were informed about the aim of the study, the estimated duration (90 min), avoiding early dropouts at the start of the group discussions [11], and also about the presence and identification of the moderator and co-moderator.

The role of the moderator was to support the group in exploring the topic, and introducing new insights that may arise [11]. The stimulus questions and the work of the moderator were previously reviewed by the team to ensure the necessary moderation skills, group dynamics, and control of possible critical elements to ensure a successful FG. The choice of a co-moderator was in line with the recommendations of the authors, and was designed to increase the rigor of the process. His primary goal was to help the moderator manage the recording equipment, be aware of the conditions and logistics of the physical setting, respond to unexpected interruptions, and take notes on the group discussion [11].

Data collection was carried out online in February 2021, through the Zoom® platform, with an approximate duration of 90 min. It was moderated by two impartial and experienced researchers.

2.4. Data Analysis

The recording was watched twice before being transcribed by one of the researchers present in the FGs so they could "visualize" what had occurred in the group.

After transcription, content analysis was performed according to Bardin [12], supported by webQDA software®.

It was conducted through the construction of categories of analysis a posteriori valuing and interpreting the information shared by the participants. Coding was carried out by the researcher who transcribed the recordings of the FGs, and then validated by the research team. Representativeness, comprehensiveness, homogeneity, and relevance were ensured when the categories were defined. A code was assigned to each participant (P1, 2, 3 ...).

The research phases were rigorously conducted and validated by the entire team so that the results accurately represented the participants' experiences. After coding the findings, they were returned to the participants for their validation, ensuring the credibility of the study.

Confirmability was guaranteed by the communication that took place during the coding process, by the literature, among the team, and by an expert who evaluated the codes that emerged from the findings.

Transferability was demonstrated by the depth of the analysis, the methodological description, and presentation of the results, which increase the likelihood of the findings being significant in other similar contexts.

2.5. Ethical Considerations

Ethical approval was obtained from the Ethics Committee of the hospital Vila Franca de Xira—Portugal (Protocol number—HVFX2020).

Anonymity and confidentiality were ensured and the data were encoded, without identification of the source. During the development of the research work, there was no provision for damage to the study participants or costs arising from their participation.

3. Results

Through the defined criteria, the study was developed through the participation of six rehabilitation nurses, aged between 40 and 53 years (representing an average age of 46.5 years), being mostly female (83.3%). All participants had a professional experience of more than 10 years, three of the participants performed functions in the hospital unit, and three in Community Care units integrated in the geographical area covered by the hospital unit.

From the content analysis emerged four categories and sixteen subcategories (presented in Table 1), being: promotion of continuity of care (with 93 units of registration), nurse of advanced practice as care manager (with 41 units of registration), capacitation of the person and caregiver (with 34 units of registration), and promotion of the coordination of care (with 96 units) (Table 1).

Table 1. Corpus of the content analysis from the focus group, Lisbon, 2021.

Category	Subcategory	Registration Units
Promoting continuity of care	Continuity of care	38
	Access difficulties	13
	Difficulties in articulation	31
	Health–disease transition	2
	Transition to the role of caregiver	9
	Subtotal:	93
Advanced practice nurse as care manager	Gains with structured project—Person	22
	Gains with structured design—Family	4
	Gains with structured design—Professionals	15
	Subtotal:	41
Training of the person and caregiver	Information	6
	Rehabilitation nurse intervention—Person	16
	Rehabilitation nurse intervention—Family	11
	Rehabilitation nurse intervention—Home	1
	Subtotal:	34
Promoting care coordination	Gains with transitional care	5
	Needs felt by professionals	59
	Difficulties experienced by professionals	30
	Rehabilitation nurse intervention—Team	2
	Subtotal:	96
	TOTAL:	264

3.1. Promoting Continuity of Care

The promotion of continuity of care should include actions aimed, overall, at improving the health care provided and satisfaction of the person/family, minimizing the fragmentation of care, avoiding readmissions and consequently contributing to a more sustainable health system. In this context, rehabilitation nurses feel that all people would benefit from rehabilitation care, including dependents with reduced recovery potential and who would benefit from passive mobilizations for their comfort and safety. The participants recognize that the rehabilitation nurse will permanently be an added value in the continuity of care process, namely in the continuity of information.

> " . . . *even in a completely dependent person who has come to the Emergency by extreme weight loss, by poor general condition, by the appearance [of] pressure zones, he may even be very dependent on his Barthel scale, but maybe if it is in a situation like the one I am describing, it makes perfect sense to be a rehabilitation nurse to go to the house*" (P5);

> "*A user with multiple goings to the Emergency Service, with an identified caregiver, is necessary a person with quality, sufficient qualification to intervene in the process of management of those care that is being implemented, because if the person is going several*

times to the Emergency Service, there is a plan that has to be stipulated and corrected what is being done wrong. In my opinion it is a Rehabilitation Nurse who has human, technical capacity, whatever it is to define and to see what is badly stratified there at that moment, in the patient itself" (P6);

"It would have to be the assessment that is made at the patient's admission, the evaluation made at the time of discharge, the gains acquired during hospitalization, or not, and the plan, what was the plan that was instituted that patient, the identification, who was the caregiver identified and who was made the teachings, or not, could have been only the user" (P5).

The intervention of the rehabilitation nurse, for the participants, is simultaneously relevant in facilitating the transition process of health disease and, simultaneously, in the transition to the role of caregiver. If, on the one hand, there is a need to readapt the person to the health event and his/her disability, on the other hand, the family often sees moments of tension and anxiety associated with the moment of transition:

" … having to start a life over with the problem you have at that moment, don't you? And with the difficulties they will encounter" (P3);

"What I believe is that, usually these are older people who have a partner, or a partner, also the same age and that instead of coming an old man or the old woman, comes a child or daughter-in-law, because only they can move, and it is about those who do the teachings, they are the ones who are really targeted in care, obviously a user when he returns to the home, who is there is the husband or wife who is the same age" (P4).

Nevertheless, they reveal the existence of difficulty in accessing care (UR = 13) during the transition, associated with difficulty in articulation (UR = 31).

" … we had no information about what had happened, whether or not they had been in the hospital, and what the diagnosis was, and how quickly we had to make a home visit" (P1);

"And you have no information, in hospital terms, that that user is already followed by us, that caregiver has been followed by us for a long time." (P1);

" … he comes to a place and we start from scratch, we start asking the same questions and teaching the same things, and in a way maybe different. It doesn't make any sense, does it?" (P5).

The participants recognize difficulty in access and articulation, arguing that the rehabilitation nurse should take the lead in the organizational process of continuity care even if it lacks homogeneity of procedures. Through the focus group, it was possible to interpret the understanding about the health–disease transition process, the need to adapt to the present; however, the participants did not contemplate the integration of their desires and objectives in the rehabilitation process.

3.2. Advanced Practice Nurse as Care Manager

The category of advanced practice nurse as care manager (UR = 41) emerged from the subcategories related to the gains associated with the implementation of structured projects. Advanced nursing, and specifically advanced practice nurses, have been increasingly explored topics in research, namely in the contribution of these professionals with a characteristic profile, specialized knowledge, complex decision-making skills, skills and competencies for practice, whose characteristics must adapt to the context in which it is inserted.

Rehabilitation Nurses recognize gains associated with the person under going for care:

"From the safe transition, when we go, most of them already come in a much better process in terms of autonomy." (P1);

"And this transition is seen, and is mirrored in gains in the health of users, of patients who go to the emergency department, particularly those chronic users in which they

had a certain number of already high emergency episodes, and that the community is absorbing them after our referral and are doing an excellent job with them." (P6);

At the same time, gains associated with the family are identified by the participants:

"It is an added value too, just to complement a little, families verbalize" (P2);

" ... caregiver's anxiety" (P1);

" ... even for family members themselves, it holds family members accountable and you help us in a completely different way from what you have done until then" (P6).

They also recognize gains associated with professionals:

" ... also when we enter their house ... gives another chega, another lens, so to speak, because it remains a conductive wire" (P2);

" ... success is of articulation between all and has resulted very well" (P1).

From the content analysis of this category, it is possible to conclude that rehabilitation nurses share a vision about their advanced and specialized practice, namely their contribution to improving the quality and access to care, resulting in benefits for the person in care, the family, and the professionals involved.

As already mentioned above, despite the recognition of professionals regarding the integration and coordination of care, the bibliographic sample analyzed in the integrative review of the literature demonstrates that the experience of the person himself translates into a non-inclusive role both in decision-making and in hospital discharge planning, associating the experience of the family that mentions distancing from professionals during hospitalization with consequent lower confidence in the rehabilitation process.

3.3. Training of the Person and Caregiver

In a similar perspective, the category of training of the person and caregiver emerges (UR = 34). In this context, and according to the specific competencies of rehabilitation nurses, it is extremely important to have early intervention by the rehabilitation nurse in the preparation of discharge, with the training of the dependent person promoting their functional readaptation and also intervening with their caregiver.

In the first instance, rehabilitation nurses approach the transmission of information to the person and caregiver, emphasizing the same importance of the training and learning process and its transversal language, both in the hospital context and in a home context:

"Despite believing that all the teachings that are done inhospital are certainly very well accomplished, but our reality when we arrive on the first day to the family, they do not know anything and are completely lost" (P3);

"In fact when the colleagues in the community come and approach this person, they already know what we have done and can have a thread here to continue working on that person and have positive results" (P6).

With regard to the intervention of the rehabilitation nurse in the person in the community after hospital discharge, this begins after referral still in the hospital context (via email or telephone) in order to continue the care plan already established, reinforcing some information that is considered fundamental.

"Whenever a user comes ... and that in the discharge letter or in the email is already referred to rehabilitation nurse, we try to always be [the Rehabilitation Nurse] to make the first evaluation" (P3);

" ... dependence on self-care, dependence on mobilization, the risk of pressure ulcer, the risk of fall, the need for respiratory rehabilitation, are all criteria that we all have to speak the same language, we hospital for community and vice versa, right? And vice versa, if this happens, if it already comes with this identification and with this reference, the identification of these needs of the person." (P5).

With regard to the family, which assumes the informal caregiver role, it emerges as a partner in rehabilitation nursing care in the home context, also lacking interventions by the rehabilitation nurse.

> *" … it is up to the Rehabilitation Nurse to evaluate the situation and then, from there, to be able to establish a plan together with the caregiver in a way that brings benefits to this patient"* (P6);

> *"After this identification of the caregiver, it will have to be taught, instructed and trained in the needs that have been identified to optimize the potential of that person, both the person and the caregiver"* (P5);

It is also stressed by one of the participants the possible need for intervention in the housing context so that transitional care can be guaranteed, namely:

> *"The evaluation of architectural barriers, here already by the colleague who is in the community, can also be something that is important for this continuity for the community"* (P5).

The susceptibility and vulnerabilities of the person and family in a transitional situation are a life-cycle phenomena influenced by several factors and variables, and that can ensure adherence to the rehabilitation program. The rehabilitation nurse assumes a fundamental role in the training of the person and caregiver, in an individualized and objective intervention, mobilizing instruments that allow identifying results and translating health gains.

3.4. Promoting Care Coordination

The category that presents the greatest expressiveness in content analysis is the Promotion of care coordination, with 96 registration units.

Care coordination should involve integrating interventions between care levels, in line with tools aimed at optimising care planning, including the transmission of information and monitoring of information and the current care plan.

Through content analysis, it is possible to observe that rehabilitation nurses value the optimization of care delivery in order to maximize the quality of care provided, believing that the moments of recourse to health services can still be experienced in a more pleasant way, reducing the rehospitalizations and minimizing the tension currently experienced.

The gains from transitional care are therefore clear for rehabilitation nurses:

> *" … by creating the basic conditions, fighting hard for this, we would be able to ensure that the safe transition had a key role in patient care. To any of them."* (P6);

> *"If this were the case, we would certainly avoid many readmissions"* (P4).

Nevertheless, the participants express their intention to intervene with the teams to ensure the coordination of care and knowledge of the reality of the care of each context, thus assuming a leadership role.

> *" … we should all get a view of what this is about, and you what's [d]here, it's more of an approximation. We had already talked here a few years ago about regular meetings, formal meetings."* (P4);

On the other hand, rehabilitation nurses identify difficulties and needs in the implementation of their rehabilitation programs. It is reported by several participants that there is an increasing identification of people with oncological, palliative, or mental pathology who need the intervention of the rehabilitation nurse, and that it is difficult to respond to these requests concomitantly by the asymmetry of available resources.

> *"In n functions, ready … Wherever it is, it has n functions, and it goes there a arrive, here and there, to try to safeguard everything, but it is not enough."* (P4);

> *"And we have no possibility of allocating resources, we have no means to deal with solicitudes"* (P2);

"Nothing, nothing, on the contrary, we have to adjust when they should be themselves [computer applications] responding to our needs." (P4).

They also state that it is not possible for them to provide exclusively specialized care in rehabilitation, accumulating interventions that could be developed by general care nurses, but there is, on the part of the context, the need to monetize home visits.

"In the ideal world there were enough nurses to be able to mobilize. So, they would have to have very defined functions within multidisciplinary teams and work with the social worker, with nutritionist, with the psychologist, with the ... I don't know, with the physiatra, to make a reference to the Network [National Care Network]" (P5).

Although the benefits of transitional care and the evidence of the role of leader of these professionals in the projects are clear to the participants, they are referred to as an opportunity to improve the development of guidelines for referencing the person to the community, communication between professionals (method and language) and peer training, ensuring, for example, the identification of the need for visit by the rehabilitation nurse, or even in the continuity of teaching and training programs with the person and family.

Compared to the results obtained through the analysis of the bibliographic sample, health professionals, despite recognizing the success of transitional care dependent on the reintegration of care fragments, did not identify their opportunities for improvement explicitly, highlighting exclusively the barriers to integration and coordination of care (e.g., the lack of time available from the team for this investment).

4. Discussion

The results obtained allow us to affirm that, although there is a transition between levels of care, transitional rehabilitation care does not always exist. This results in an increased risk of fragmented care and the absence of continuity of care increases the risk of adverse events and complications in the period after discharge, contributing to hospital readmissions, loss of quality of life and increased co-morbidity. It is clear, for this reason, the need for transitional care that provides a positive impact in promoting independence for self-care and functionality to avoid complications after hospital discharge, which is corroborated by the results of the focus group [13].

Published studies state that, in the process of transition of care, the person identifies as fundamental the recovery of their autonomy, learning about self-care, the relationship with caregivers and professionals and the involvement in the transition of care (and their planning). From the experience of this transition emerge six indicative themes, namely: the need of the person himself to become independent, to learn about self-care, the relationship of support with caregivers, the relationship with professionals, the search for information, and the discussion and negotiation of the transitional care plan [14].

The rehabilitation nurses included in the focus group recognize that knowing the reality of the care of each context would be a facilitating aspect for the preparation of the return to home.

Despite being one of the priority practices defined by the WHO since 2018, studies on the effectiveness of transitional care programs report inconsistent results, partly as a result of differences in the service of each country and in the characteristics of the world population. Nevertheless, few studies have evaluated the factors that affect the success of the implementation of transitional care, and in existing studies may have inflated the careful selection of people who could benefit from this type of care and reduce their efficiency and effectiveness of care [1].

Continuity and coordination of care have an extraordinary impact when interventions are an integral part of a comprehensive care model, defining primary care as a focus. The evidence suggests that the effective management of the hospital–home transition, in addition to other benefits, speeds up the functional recovery of the person, estimated in functional gains greater than or equal to 35% [1,15,16].

The moment of hospital discharge and return home is also a challenge for the family, as it will be the moment when self-care management will be their responsibility, in need of numerous adaptations to what they were assisting in the hospital context. Hospital discharge planning is therefore one of the strategies for action to optimize this transition, maximize adaptation and reduce the risk of hospital readmissions.

The focus group participants recognize this need and identify gains for the family by participating with the interventions of the rehabilitation nurse in terms of transitional care, reinforcing the idea that, for the transition of care to be successful, it is necessary to plan, prepare, education for the health of the individual and his/her family from the moment of his/her hospitalization [17,18]. However, the changes are not always addressed by health professionals with due relevance, which thus provides a fragmentation of care after discharge. Often, the guidelines for discharge are carried out in an automated and hasty manner, only provided at the time of discharge, without considering the conditions and needs of each client and his family. Even when discharge is properly prepared and the user and family feel confident, they can return home and still experience difficulties and uncertainties regarding their treatment and recovery [17].

Another theme that finds convergent points in scientific production and the focus group is the role of health professionals, over whom the challenge of interaction, coordination, and integration between caregivers at different levels of care, ensuring the planning of discharge and a subsequent safe follow-up, with the involvement of the person and his caregiver, prevails, at all stages of transitional care. The coordination of care should involve the integration of interventions and levels of care (vertical and horizontal integration), using specific mechanisms and instruments for care planning, including the transmission of information, monitoring of needs and therapeutic plans, with the aim of optimising the provision of continuous and comprehensive care, in due place and time [19].

Through the data obtained through the realization of the focus group, rehabilitation nurses condensed their intentions in the development of guidelines for referencing the person to the community, in the standardization of communication between professionals (method and language) and peer formation. They also mention, as a proposal, to improve the standardization of it systems so that it is possible not only to share information, as well as to monitor developments in the care process according to the same health indicators.

Health care needs have evolved and, as such, specialized nursing care, and specifically advanced practice nurses have emerged as an attempt to adapt responses to these needs. A nurse with advanced training is a duly accredited nurse who has acquired specialized knowledge, has a high decision-making capacity and clinical skills for advanced practice [20], as well as for the evaluation and management of care for chronically ill patients, for example after hospital discharge [21].

The qualified performance of nurses is recognized as fundamental for the realization of safe transitions, as well as contributing to the visibility and valorisation of nursing intervention. However, the nurses that participated on the FG state that it is not possible for them to provide exclusively specialized care in rehabilitation, accumulating interventions that could be developed by general care nurses.

Professionals also identifies other barriers to the integration and coordination of care and family involvement, such as the lack of team time for this investment, the complexity of the person's health and their post-discharge care. Some studies also highlight the difficulties of communication and articulation between levels of care as an impediment to an integrated response to the needs of the population with complex health–disease problems [7,9,13,22].

There are some tools and interventions for transitional care, which enhance the participation of the person in his/her discharge planning and rehabilitation, namely: family meetings; preparation of discharge planning; existence of checklist respecting the needs of care identified by the person and caregiver, available community resources, the need for support products, among others; definition of a health education program; and home visits that may include the decision-making process of the person, involving the family and caregivers, facilitating participation in their daily life [23].

Participants advocate the need of strategies and health policies to increase the coordination and vertical integration of community and hospital care. This continues to prove to be a persistent challenge with repercussions already demonstrated in the tendency to reduce hospitalization time, home follow-up and, consequently, in reducing the rate of occupancy of hospital beds. Ensuring this coordination between levels of care, considering the risks at different stages of the cycle, and ensuring transitional care is imperative for the development of a more sustainable health system [24,25].

In other countries, the scientific evidence is clear with regard to successful interventions and implementation strategies for the transition of care, namely the integration of people with change of functionality in policy processes with a view to improving the responsiveness, efficiency and effectiveness, and sustainability of programs, strengthening self-determination and user satisfaction; the collection of statistical data on the development of health information systems, with the aim of supporting a political impulse, decision-making in policy reformulation and equitable allocation of resources; cross-sectorial coordination in the provision of rehabilitation care; and the establishment of a rehabilitation program aligned with pre-existing health programs, supporting its sustainability. It is emphasized as an action strategy, specifically, the development of a community-focused care program (primary health care), promoting home visits after clinical discharge, and the designation of a nurse case manager as the process leader [26,27].

The management and leadership of transitional care programs should undoubtedly be attributed to nurses of advanced nursing practice. The advanced practice nurse is often seen as the clinical specialist, with functions that include understanding and influence on management issues, policy development and clinical leadership. Although the core of the practice is based on advanced technologies, education and knowledge, being flexible according to the reality of each country, the distinction between advanced and generalist nursing practice is clear. Still, the nature of advanced nursing practice concerns a designated function focused on care delivery in the field of prevention and cure, including rehabilitation care and chronic disease management [20].

The leadership of transitional care programmes includes the perception of the rehabilitation nurses who constituted the focus group, who recognise their contribution to improving the quality and access to care [28], and in the gains associated with the person, family and professionals involved in the projects already implemented, namely autonomy at the time of return home, the reduction of the use of the emergency service, the minimization of the caregiver's anxiety, and the articulation between rehabilitation nurses. In short, it is important to emphasize that, although it is imperative to monitor health policies in relation to the care needs of the Portuguese population, there will be no exclusive or unique approach that solves the necessary reform of health systems. In this sense, it is suggested that the general recommendations of the world organizations can be followed, flexibly adopting the practices that can increase the effectiveness of health spending and the efficiency of health systems, adapting to the socio-geopolitical context in which we are integrated.

The limitations of the present study are mainly due to the method itself. For the focus group method, the limitations also stem from the selection of the method, highlighting a small representative sample and limited to a geographical area.

It should be noted that no Portuguese studies on the theme under study have been identified, leading us to believe that the contribution of this study may foster interest in the area of study and development of further studies.

5. Conclusions

The present study allowed the identification of strategies that minimize fragmentation risk of care and promote the participation of the person in transitional care. Ensuring transitional care is imperative to increase the quality of care, the satisfaction of professionals, clients, and the development of a system of sustainable health.

At a macro level, even though the health system has tried to keep up with the evolution of the needs of the Portuguese population, there are still inefficiencies and gaps in the transition of care, often associated with communication, articulation and access to care, harming the general objective of a health system, promoting health care of higher quality, with better health outcomes and associated with a lower cost.

Nevertheless, the lack of formalization of the care transition process is a reality, lacking explicit national policies. The coordination and integration of community care with hospital care is a persistent challenge, demonstrating a tendency to reduce hospitalization time, home follow-up and, consequently, the rate of occupancy of hospital beds. Training, monitoring and coordination between levels of care needs to be ensured.

It is concluded that ensuring transitional care is imperative for the development of a sustainable health system, increasing the quality of care and the satisfaction of professionals and clients.

Author Contributions: Conceptualization, R.P., Ó.F. and C.L.B.; methodology, R.P., Ó.F. and C.L.B.; software, R.P.; validation Ó.F. and C.L.B.; formal analysis, R.P., Ó.F. and C.L.B.; investigation, R.P., Ó.F. and C.L.B.; resources, R.P., Ó.F. and C.L.B.; data curation, R.P., Ó.F. and C.L.B.; writing—original draft preparation, R.P.; writing—review and editing, R.P., Ó.F. and C.L.B.; visualization, R.P., Ó.F. and C.L.B.; supervision, Ó.F. and C.L.B.; project administration, R.P. and C.L.B.; funding acquisition, R.P., Ó.F. and C.L.B. All authors have read and agreed to the published version of the manuscript.

Funding: The present study was funded by the Center for Research, Innovation, and Development in Nursing, in Portugal, by means of grants provided to some of the authors (CIDNUR, Safe2transition_2021).

Institutional Review Board Statement: The present study was carried out according to the guidelines of the Declaration of Helsinki and approved by an Ethics Committee from the Hopital of Vila Franca de Xira.

Informed Consent Statement: Informed consent was obtained from all subjects involved in the study.

Data Availability Statement: Data are available upon request to the authors.

Acknowledgments: The authors express their gratitude to all participants for their contributions to the study.

Conflicts of Interest: The authors declare no conflict of interest.

References

1. Organização Mundial de Saúde. *Continuity and Coordination of Care: A Practice Brief to Support Implementation of the WHO Framework on Integrated People-Centred Health Services*; World Health Organization: Geneva, Switzerland, 2018.
2. Ferreira, E.; Lourenço, O.; Costa, P.; Pinto, S.C.; Gomes, C.; Oliveira, A.P.; Ferreira, Ó.; Baixinho, C.L. Active Life: A project for a safe hospital-community transition after arthroplasty. *Rev. Bras. Enferm.* **2019**, *72*, 147–153. [CrossRef] [PubMed]
3. Menezes, T.M.O.; Oliveira, A.L.B.; Santos, L.B.; Freitas, R.A.; Pedreira, L.C.; Veras, S.M.C.B. Hospital transition care for the elderly: An integrative review. *Rev. Bras. Enferm.* **2019**, *72* (Suppl. 2), 294–301. [CrossRef] [PubMed]
4. Mendes, F.; Gemito, M.; Caldeira, E.; Serra, I.; Casas-Novas, M. A continuidade de cuidados de saúde na perspetiva dos utentes. *Ciênc. Saúde Colet.* **2017**, *22*, 841–853. [CrossRef] [PubMed]
5. Observatório Português dos Sistemas de Saúde. *Relatório Primavera*; OPSS: Lisboa, Portugal, 2019; Available online: https://fronteirasxxi.pt/wp-content/uploads/2020/02/Observat%C3%B3rio-Portugu%C3%AAs-Dos-Sistemas-De-Sa%C3%BAde-2019.pdf (accessed on 8 February 2022).
6. Baixinho, C.L.; Ferreira, Ó. From the hospital to the community: The (un)safe transition. *Rev. Baiana Enferm.* **2019**, *33*, e35797. [CrossRef]
7. Occelli, P.; Touzet, S.; Rabilloud, M.; Ganne, C.; Poupon Bourdy, S.; Galamand, B.; Debray, M.; Dartiguepeyrou, A.; Chuzeville, M.; Comte, B.; et al. Impact of a transition nurse program on the prevention of thirty-day hospital readmissions of elderly patients discharged from short-stay units: Study protocol of the PROUST stepped-wedge cluster randomised trial. *BMC Geriatr.* **2016**, *16*, 57. [CrossRef]
8. Batista, J.; Pinheiro, C.M.; Madeira, C.; Gomes, P.; Ferreira, Ó.R.; Baixinho, C.L. Transitional Care Management from Emergency Services to Communities: An Action Research Study. *Int. J. Environ. Res. Public Health* **2021**, *18*, 12052. [CrossRef]
9. Pedrosa, A.R.; Ferreira, Ó.R.; Baixinho, C.L. Transitional rehabilitation care and patient care continuity as an advanced nursing practice. *Rev. Bras. Enferm.* **2022**, *75*, e20210399. [CrossRef]

10. Moore, T.; McKee, K.; McLoughlin, P. Online focus groups and qualitative research in the social sciences: Their merits and limitations in a study of housing and youth. *People Place Policy* **2015**, *9*, 17–28. [CrossRef]

11. Silva, I.; Veloso, A.; Keating, J. Focus Group: Considerações teóricas e metodológicas. *Rev. Lusófona Educ.* **2014**, *26*, 175–190. Available online: https://revistas.ulusofona.pt/index.php/rleducacao/article/view/4703 (accessed on 8 February 2022).

12. Bardin, L. *Análise de Conteúdo*, 5th ed.; Edições 70: Lisboa, Portugal, 2011.

13. Ferreira, B.; Gomes, T.; Baixinho, C.L.; Ferreira, O. Transitional care to caregivers of dependent older people: An integrative literature review. *Rev. Bras. Enferm.* **2020**, *73* (Suppl. 3), e20200394. [CrossRef]

14. Allen, J.; Hutchinson, A.; Brown, R.; Livingston, P. User experience and care for older people transitioning from hospital to home: Patients' and carers' perspectives. *Health Expect.* **2017**, *21*, 518–527. [CrossRef] [PubMed]

15. Mas, M.; Inzitari, M.; Sabaté, S.; Santaeugènia, S.; Miralles, R. Hospital-at-home Integrated Care Programme for the management of disabling health crises in older patients: Comparison with bed-based Intermediate Care. *Age Ageing* **2017**, *46*, 925–931. [CrossRef] [PubMed]

16. Cations, M.; Lang, C.; Crotty, M.; Wesselingh, S.; Whitehead, C.; Inacio, M.C. Factors associated with success in transition care services among older people in Australia. *BMC Geriatr.* **2020**, *20*, 496. [CrossRef] [PubMed]

17. Sousa, M.; Cabrita, R.; Mamadhussen, S.; Ferrito, C.; Figueiredo, A. Intervenções de enfermagem na transição de cuidados em adultos com acidente vascular cerebral: Uma scoping review. *Cad. Saúde* **2019**, *11*, 5–11. [CrossRef]

18. Hahn-Goldberg, S.; Jeffs, L.; Troup, A.; Kubba, R.; Okrainec, K. "We are doing it together": The integral role of caregivers in a patients' transition home from the medicine unit. *PLoS ONE* **2018**, *13*, e0197831. [CrossRef] [PubMed]

19. De Almeida, P.F.; Medina, M.G.; Fausto, M.C.R.; Giovanella, L.; Bousquat, A.; de Mendonça, M.H.M. Coordenação do cuidado e Atenção Primária à Saúde no Sistema Único de Saúde. *Saúde Debate* **2018**, *42*, 244–260. [CrossRef]

20. International Council of Nurses. *Guidelines on Advanced Practice Nursing*; ICN: Geneva, Switzerland, 2020.

21. Weber, L.; Lima, M.; Acosta, A. Qualidade da transição do cuidado e sua associação com a readmissão hospitalar. *Aquichan* **2019**, *19*, e1945. [CrossRef]

22. Rasmussen, L.F.; Grode, L.B.; Lange, J.; Barat, I.; Gregersen, M. Impact of transitional care interventions on hospital readmissions in older medical patients: A systematic review. *BMJ Open* **2021**, *11*, e040057. [CrossRef]

23. Dyrstad, D.; Testad, I.; Storm, M. A review of the literature on patient participation in transitions of the elderly. *Cogn. Technol. Work* **2014**, *17*, 15–34. [CrossRef]

24. Low, L.L.; Tan, S.Y.; Ng, M.J.; Tay, W.Y.; Ng, L.B.; Balasubramaniam, K.; Towle, R.M.; Lee, K.H. Applying the Integrated Practice Unit Concept to a Modified Virtual Ward Model of Care for Patients at Highest Risk of Readmission: A Randomized Controlled Trial. *PLoS ONE* **2017**, *12*, e0168757. [CrossRef]

25. Swanson, J.; Moger, T. Comparisons of readmissions and mortality based on postdischarge ambulatory follow-up services received by stroke patients discharged home: A register-based study. *BMC Health Serv. Res.* **2019**, *19*, 4. [CrossRef] [PubMed]

26. Naylor, M.D.; Aiken, L.H.; Kurtzman, E.T.; Olds, D.M.; Hirschman, K.B. The care span: The importance of transitional care in achieving health reform. *Health Aff.* **2018**, *30*, 746–754. [CrossRef] [PubMed]

27. McVeigh, J.; MacLachlan, M.; Gilmore, B.; McClean, C.; Eide, A.H.; Mannan, H.; Geiser, P.; Duttine, A.; Mji, G.; McAuliffe, E.; et al. Promoting good policy for leadership and governance of health related rehabilitation: A realist synthesis. *Glob. Health* **2016**, *12*, 49. [CrossRef] [PubMed]

28. Baixinho, C.L.; Presado, M.H.; Ribeiro, J. Qualitative research and the transformation of public health. *Ciênc. Saúde Colet.* **2019**, *24*, 1582. [CrossRef]

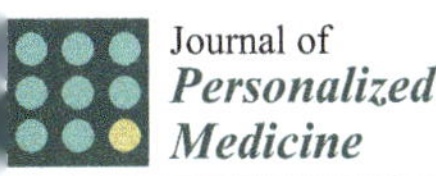
Journal of
Personalized
Medicine

MDPI

Article

Health Promotion and Disease Prevention in the Elderly: The Perspective of Nursing Students

Rogério Ferreira [1,2], Cristina Lavareda Baixinho [3,4,*], Óscar Ramos Ferreira [4], Ana Clara Nunes [2], Teresa Mestre [2] and Luís Sousa [1,5]

[1] Comprehensive Health Research Centre, 1150-082 Lisboa, Portugal; ferrinho.ferreira@ipbeja.pt (R.F.); lmms@uevora.pt (L.S.)
[2] Polytechnic Institute of Beja, 7800-000 Beja, Portugal; ana.nunes@ipbeja.pt (A.C.N.); teresa.mestre@ipbeja.pt (T.M.)
[3] Center for Innovative Care and Health Technology (ciTechCare), Polytechnic of Leiria, 2410-541 Leiria, Portugal
[4] Nursing Research, Innovation and Development Centre of Lisbon (CIDNUR), Nursing School of Lisbon, 1600-190 Lisboa, Portugal; oferreira@esel.pt
[5] S. João de Deus Higher School of Nursing, University of Évora, 7000-811 Évora, Portugal
*   Correspondence: crbaixinho@esel.pt

Citation: Ferreira, R.; Baixinho, C.L.; Ferreira, Ó.R.; Nunes, A.C.; Mestre, T.; Sousa, L. Health Promotion and Disease Prevention in the Elderly: The Perspective of Nursing Students. *J. Pers. Med.* **2022**, *12*, 306. https://doi.org/10.3390/jpm12020306

Academic Editors: Fábio G. Teixeira, Catarina Godinho and Júlio Belo Fernandes

Received: 29 December 2021
Accepted: 16 February 2022
Published: 18 February 2022

Publisher's Note: MDPI stays neutral with regard to jurisdictional claims in published maps and institutional affiliations.

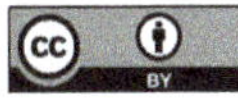

Abstract: Health promotion and disease prevention are closely linked to health literacy. Therefore, intervention to increase individuals' knowledge is essential if action is to be taken to promote a healthy lifestyle with support from health professionals for decision making on choices leading to behavioral change. Taking into account the growing aging population, nurses and nursing students have to develop interventions to promote health and prevent disease in these people, in order to keep them healthy and with quality of life. This study aims to understand how nursing students' experiences in a clinical teaching context contributed to the development of their competencies in the promotion of health and prevention of disease in the elderly. Method: Qualitative, exploratory, and descriptive study carried out with ten students about to finish a graduate nursing course in a higher education institution in the South of Portugal. This study was carried out through narratives, one of the most common data collection procedures in social and health investigations. The content analysis technique, more specifically the thematic categorical analysis, was used for data analysis. The study received authorization from the Ethics Committee of the institution where it took place. Results: Three categories were found: "Strategies to promote health and prevent disease in the elderly", "Health improvements from the implementation of the strategies to promote health and prevent disease in the elderly", and "The impact your participation in these strategies to promote health and prevent disease in the elderly had on your formative process". Conclusion: The students developed competencies during their clinical teaching experiences through the implementation of strategies of health promotion and disease prevention adapted to/focused on the needs of the elderly.

Keywords: aged; disease prevention; health promotion; nursing education; nursing students

1. Introduction

Portugal has one of the oldest populations in the world. Nonetheless, projections show that the Portuguese population may go from 2.1 million elders in 2015 to 2.8 million people in 2080, and the aging index may duplicate, from 147 to 317 elderly people per 100 young people [1]. Demographic aging has been a target of study for authors and students from many fields of knowledge, and it is not uncommon to hear about the "problem of demographic aging" [2]. The aging of the Portuguese population and the increase in mean life expectation suggests that there are improvements in mortality rates in adults and elderlies [1,3]. Therefore, this is not a problem per se but also an advantage, as it mostly reflects improvements in the living conditions and health policies of the so-called developed societies. However, it is undeniable that due to the aging process, i.e., biological aging, gradual changes occur in the human organism's ability to adapt. As a result, people become increasingly likely to acquire acute and chronic diseases and disabilities, with repercussions on their quality of life. This context is coupled with the emergence of new needs that force us to characterize the phenomenon and rethink the roles and rights of the elder. The aging of society is unavoidable, but as it advances, dependence, vulnerability, and weakness also grow [4,5]. These conditions are concerning, and we must carry out interventions in regard to them.

Although the mean life expectancy in Portugal is higher than the mean of the other Organization for Economic Co-operation and Development (OECD) countries [6], the index "number of healthy years of life after 65 years old" is one of the lowest recorded ones. Despite living longer, we live with more comorbidities during our last years of life, which include diabetes, cardiovascular diseases, respiratory diseases, obesity, and cancer [6]. This is why health promotion and disease prevention in the elderly should be promoted to foment and maximize healthy, active, and successful aging [7].

Health promotion and disease prevention are intimately tied with knowledge and, therefore, with health literacy, among other variables. Health promotion treats individuals as active agents, with the power and capacity to control and make decisions about their own health [8]. Therefore, increasing the knowledge of individuals is essential for more assertive and health-promoting measures to be taken. Generally, health education is the chief strategy to train people, groups, or communities. According to studies about this topic, factors that influence an individual's health literacy are static, but knowledge is dynamic. Therefore, knowledge is a modifiable construct that can be changed by interventions appropriate to health literacy [9]. Hence, education in health intends to increase the knowledge of individuals, providing them with tools that allow them to learn better, increasing their knowledge, and developing competencies that favor their own health and that of the community around them [10].

In the scope of their clinical classes, students of the graduate nursing course "learn, within a team which has direct contact with an individual and/or collectivity that may be in a good state of health or ill, to plan, provide, and evaluate the global nursing care required, based on the knowledge and competences acquired" (Norm 2005/36/CE from the European Parliament and from the Council, 7 September 2005, No. 5, article 3°) [11]. Clinical classes are articulated with the other disciplines as it mobilizes knowledge and abilities, consolidating and complementing what was learned—in particular, what was seen in previous clinical teaching classes—to achieve improved health results, ensuring that the learning processes are increasingly complex. The clinical classes in Community Health Nursing of the nursing graduation course at the Instituto Politécnico de Beja (IPBeja), in particular, aim to develop competencies that allow the student to provide nursing care to individuals, including their family and community, leading them to become increasingly thoughtful citizens that can bring improvements in health. The clinical classes take place in Primary Health Care Units, preferably at the family healthcare unit, where students are integrated into the activities of the team/unit, recognizing needs and providing care to persons, their families, and to the community, in the scope of the Primary Health Care. Students also develop, in groups, a community intervention project, using the health-planning methodology to deal with the needs of the unit/community where they carry out their clinical classes [12].

We believe that the results of this study, involving students who had the opportunity to live rich and diversified experiences in clinical settings of community health care delivery and focused on health promotion and disease prevention in the elderly, may be an important contribution to reflection and analysis on health promotion and disease prevention practices in the elderly from the perspective of nursing students in learning environments.

As a result, this study included students who had full and diverse experiences, in a clinical context, of providing health to a community, focusing on the promotion of health and prevention of disease in the elderly. This study aims to understand how nursing students' experiences in a clinical teaching context contributed to the development of their competencies in the promotion of health and prevention of disease in the elderly. We believe that the results of this study may be an important contribution to the reflection on this issue and the relevance of learning experiences in clinical settings, aiming at the development of health promotion and disease prevention skills in older people.

2. Background

The growing number of community-dwelling elderly and the increased risks of adverse health events that accompany aging call for health promotion interventions [13].

The maintenance of the elderly in their social context fits in with the strategies for an active, participatory, healthy aging and is an illustration of true centered care with a holistic and integrative vision, emphasizing self-determination and valorization of individual characteristics, expectations, and potentialities and assigning them an active role as decision-makers as agents of their own lives [8,14–17]. For this to happen, health promotion and disease prevention in this population should involve the adoption of healthy lifestyles and the inclusion of strategies promoting health literacy [9,10], contributing to their learning and development of skills that promote their health. The strengthening of elderly knowledge is primordial for taking more assertive and healthier measures and options. Health Education is the "mother strategy" for the empowerment of people, groups, or communities [8].

This preventive approach is a strategy at the primary health care level and requires significant community participation, with the involvement of multiple partners through mechanisms to improve people's literacy level and the creation of environments conducive to promoting and protecting elderly health [7–9,13–17].

Although health promotion is seen as a major activity of health professionals, it should include the coordination between health institutions and community partners through programs conducive to healthy and successful aging promoting social interaction and mental health, promotion of physical activity, promotion of healthy eating habits, prevention and self-monitoring of chronic diseases, promotion of a medication regimen adjusted to the needs, promotion of safety measures [18], and accident prevention [19].

The provision of proximity health care in the social context where the elderly lives should be a response that promotes healthy, active, and successful aging, with the quality of life that it implies [18]. The principle of aging in place advocates that the elderly should remain in their own place, in their own homes, and in the social context that contributes to their autonomy, according to their preferences [8]. The difficulties and limitations that arise with the advancing age can be minimized with social and health responses, which are compatible with policies for caring elderly at home and are promoters of active and successful aging [8,14,15].

When addressing the subject of training or education aimed preferably at the elderly, we inevitably talk about gerontagogy, an expression advocated by Lemieux in 1997, which in general terms is defined as an interdisciplinary educational discipline that has as its object the study of the elderly in an educational situation [20]. This hybrid scope that combines two specialties, i.e., pedagogy and gerontology, is a category that bets on the renewal of the ways of thinking about education and aging [8]. Gerontagogy constitutes, above all, a paradigm, a concrete way of betting on the education of elderlies with dependencies or not [20].

In their role as "educators" of this population, nurses should always bear in mind that this is a special pedagogy because it is addressed to a population with specific characteristics, but they should also rethink and adjust the teaching methods, which should be as participatory as possible, with the elderly playing an active and leading role [8,13–16]. We agree that in parallel with the increase in the aging population and a change in the disease spectrum, the nurse's role is shifting from the traditionally following physicians' orders to a more expanded role with responsibility for preventive care [8]. Nurses also pay more attention to health promotion advice, lifestyle counseling, educational programs, and the provision of early interventions to prevent exacerbation or complications for persons living with diseases [8–11,13].

These actions should be appropriate to the needs of the elderly and are justified taking into account the existence of risk factors. They should contribute to their ability to manage their lives with functional independence and have an optimistic perception of life associated with their participation in social and leisure activities [8–10,16]. Health gain's studies resulting from the implementation of health promotion programs highlight the increase in functional capacity, quality of life, and social participation, the improvement in knowledge and awareness about lifestyles and their impact on elderly health, the gains in terms of mental health, and the decrease in the number of medical consultations and hospitalizations [14,15,18].

In view of the above, and with this perspective that the promotion of active aging, preserving the elderly's abilities, is one of the aims of the intervention of health professionals, particularly nurses [13–15], it is important that nursing students acquire not only knowledge about health literacy [9,10], health education techniques, and behavioral change but also develop skills to facilitate elderly's access to health information and support decision making, thus achieving better health outcomes [8,16].

3. Materials and Methods

This study was qualitative, exploratory, and descriptive, focused on the relevance of the care provided by the nurse and aiming to promote health and prevent disease in the elderly, from the perspective of nursing students going through the learning process.

The participants are in the last period of the nursing graduation course of a public higher education institution in the South of Portugal. They successfully finished the discipline Nursing Clinical Classes in Community Health. The sample was intentional (non-probabilistic), selected by the investigators. It involved students with rich and diverse experiences in a clinical context of the provision of health care to the community, focusing on the promotion of health and the prevention of disease in the elderly. Inclusion criteria adopted were as follows: being a student in the 4th year of the nursing graduation course of a public higher education institution in the South of Portugal, having been approved in the discipline Nursing Clinical Classes in Community Health, having been involved in practices of health promotion and disease prevention in the elderly, and being willing to participate in the study. There were no exclusion criteria.

Data were collected using narratives since in social and health investigations, this is one of the most used procedures to gather information on the meaning of experiences [21] of students in clinical contexts in regard to the provision of nursing care to the elderly and their families. A script to guide the narratives was created and submitted to the judges to guarantee the content validity of the instrument. The main concern of this project was to guarantee that the guiding questions of the narrative were in accordance with the objectives defined and allowed for a reorganization of the experiences of care to the elderly in a coherent and significant way, giving meaning to the experience and enabling its (re)construction as a process integrated into the context of clinical practice [21]. The script aimed to provoke reflections and analysis about the practices of health promotion and disease prevention in the elderly from the perspective of nursing students in their learning process. When writing/narrating about the care practices, students reconstructed and re-organized their experiences, giving meaning to the events that supported the narrative in a way consistent with their current understanding. This means that its use was based on the assumption of valuing reflection on clinical practice as a strategy that ensures the reconstruction of knowledge based on the reflected knowledge. The script included three guiding questions:

— In what strategies to promote health and prevent disease in the elderly were you involved?
— What health benefits emerged from the implementation of these strategies to promote health and prevent disease in the elderly?
— What was the impact of these strategies in your education process?

All necessary ethical precepts that must guide the elaboration of a study such as this were followed in any contact with the higher education institution and its students. On the institutional level, the study with Process No. 24/2021 received a favorable evaluation on 8 July 2021 from the Ethics Commission of the Instituto Politécnico de Beja. The participating students were assured that their participation in the study would be entirely voluntary and that they could abandon it at any time, with no need to justify their decision or any future consequences. Their anonymity was guaranteed, as well as the confidentiality of their data since professional secrecy is both an obligation and a duty. In addition, they signed the free and informed consent form.

Participants were contacted by the main investigator, who presented the investigation project and explained the goal of the study, its objectives, and the importance of participating. It also involved the expression of availability to clarify doubts and ensure understanding of the guiding questions of the reflection. The study was carried out through e-mail.

The students elaborated their narratives in response to the guiding questions. These were sent via e-mail to the main researcher in a pdf file.

The main researcher was responsible for managing the data collected, ensuring the anonymity and confidentiality of the data. All information that could identify the participants was restricted, and each participant received a name. The names of the participants will be replaced by identification numbers (P1, P2, P3...) in all records and publications. In the topics (content units) presented in the results of the study, measures to protect the identity of the students were taken. Data protection went from the selection of the participants to the collection, analysis, and dissemination of the results of the study.

The information collected and submitted to analysis, in addition to the free and informed consent form documents, was stored in a drive owned by the main researcher responsible for this study and will remain stored for five years. The data were encrypted, including raw data, to prevent access to it by unauthorized third parties. Other people will not have access to this information.

The narratives, more than a document, are a primary source that integrates the reflection of these students [21]. They were analyzed using the content analysis technique, more specifically, the thematic category analysis [22]. Its choice is related to the fact that it is a set of communication analysis techniques, in which systematic and objective procedures to describe the content of messages are used to obtain indicators that allow the inference of knowledge concerning the conditions of production of the messages. In the first stage, the texts were skimmed to verify whether the information collected was in accordance with the objective of the study. The narratives formed the corpus of the analysis, that is, the material produced for the investigation to be analyzed [22]. The second stage was the coding of the data, with the definition of thematic units and context units. Thematic units, according to Bardin [22], are statements about a subject to which a vast range of unique formulations may be associated. Contextual units—the "comprehension units" used to understand the exact meaning of each thematic unit—was the response of each participant to the guiding questions for the narrative. In addition to defining coding units, categories and indicators were defined. In the third stage, the results were treated through inference, attributing meanings to the qualitative analysis of the categories.

For the thematic category analysis, the text was separated into thematic units (themes) and categories, according to analogical regroupings [14]. In this process, semantic categorization criteria were used.

Three categories were found in this study: "Strategies to promote health and prevent disease in the elderly", "Health improvements from the implementation of strategies to promote health and prevent disease in the elderly", and "The impact of the participation in these strategies to promote health and prevent disease in the elderly had on the formative process". In the narratives of the students, several indicators emerged from the analogical and progressive classification of the elements, as expressed in Table 1.

Table 1. Categories and indicators; Beja, 2021.

Category	Indicator
Strategies	— Adequate information and communication — Health education — Home care — Social projects
Health benefits	— Disease prevention — Health promotion — Wellbeing and self-care — Behavioral change — Empowering — Client satisfaction — Management of the therapeutic regime — Expenses — Life expectancy
Impact on the formative process	— Learning and/or development of competencies — Raising awareness of competencies

To guarantee the quality of the investigation, several procedures were developed, among which we point out:

i. Data collection and analysis procedures were explained, as well as the entire theoretical perspective, which was the framework for the study.

ii. Participant review: The results of the analysis carried out by the main investigator were sent back to the participants so they could verify whether the interpretations actually reflected their ideas about the topic.

iii. Peer/judge revision: Judges/experts on the subject were asked for collaboration, so they could validate the content analysis and make suggestions for improvement.

4. Results

This study involved ten students in the last year of the nursing graduation course. Their ages went from 22 to 28 years of age, with a mean of 23.8. Most (7) were female.

The analysis of the narratives of this group of students allowed us to analyze their perspectives about the practice of health promotion and disease prevention in the elderly.

We present the results based on the selected categories and the indicators identified in the content analysis.

4.1. Strategies

In this category, we present the perceptions of the students in regard to the different strategies to promote health and prevent disease in the elderly used in their educational process. The following indicators emerged in the narratives:

4.1.1. Adequate Information and Communication

Adequate information and communication are determinants for the promotion of healthy lifestyles and the prevention of disease in the elderly. In the following registration unit, the information focuses on the promotion of healthy lifestyles.

> *[...] I managed to provide information about the adequate diet people should follow, to encourage the practice of exercise, to encourage vaccination, to encourage them to reduce drinking and smoking (to elders with these habits). (P1)*

> *Proper information and communication focus on creating a therapeutic relationship in this registration unit.*

Some strategies were adopted to promote health and prevent disease in the elders, focusing on the creation of a therapeutic relationship, which is the development of a bond between the elder and the nursing worker; on the daily reality of the elder; on the adoption of active listening, availability, and empathy with the person, that is, on using an adequate and efficient communication. (P3)

4.1.2. Health Education

This strategy was the most mentioned one, both in regard to the number of students who mentioned it (9) and to the number of thematic units (14). It involved the elderly, in general, in encouraging the adoption of healthy lifestyles, people with diabetes and hypertension, and elderly people who attended diabetic foot consultations, as shown in the following registration units.

The strategies selected included a session of education to elders who went to diabetic foot consultations in that health center. To do so, people were invited, a PowerPoint presentation about the topic was created and presented to those who were present in the session before it started. (P2)

[. . .] developing health education groups; elaborating programs targeted at the health of the elder. (P3)

Therefore, these surveillance consultations, specialized and/or general, make it possible for nurses to act in the fields of disease prevention, in people with higher risk for specific pathologies or for health promotion, through the encouragement of the adoption of healthy lifestyles, be it in those who have a specific disease, in those who may develop a certain disease, or in healthy people. (P4)

Health education involved caregivers of the elderly during home visits, as shown in the following registration unit.

I carried out health education sessions on the benefits of exercise; informative pamphlets/discourses during consultations about the importance of the flu vaccine; education in health for the caregivers, during home consultation, about pressure ulcer prevention in bedridden clients; informative discourses about the dangers of polypharmacy and of the non-adherence or incorrect administration of therapy; leaflets and informative discourses about the preventive measures against the dissemination of COVID-19; health education about measures to prevent against MRSA [. . .]. (P4)

Empowering the elderly to be independent in activities of daily living and adopting healthy lifestyles were the focus of health education in the following registration units.

It should be mentioned that I was involved in diverse strategies, and it should be highlighted that most took place in the clinical classes in health centers, where I could carry out health education, provide information to elders on the adoption of healthy lifestyles that they should follow, including the prevention of the use of alcohol and tobacco, encouraging the adherence to vaccination, encouraging the practice of exercise, also being involved with the control of risk factors, such as overweight, arterial hypertension, diabetes mellitus, and dyslipidemia. (P5)

[. . .] intervention directed at promoters of healthy diets, which integrated information about the repercussion of bad dietary habits, the teaching of a balanced diet with no excessive salt, sugar, or fats, and instructions on the correct way to make foods, directed at the caregivers/institutions. (P6)

[. . .] projects of exercise, which implied in fomenting the importance of regularly exercising or walking in an open space and its benefits for health, in addition to physical activities in group, making available informative and illustrative leaflets. (P6)

4.1.3. Home Care

Home care involving the elder and their family was considered to be a health promotion and disease prevention strategy.

The creation and organization of networks of care to be provided at home and at the outpatient clinic, giving support to the specific needs of the elder and their relatives, maintaining the wellbeing and comfort at home, a strategy important to avoid hospitalizations or institutionalization. (P6)

4.1.4. Social Projects

Social projects were mentioned by a student as a strategy used in the promotion of health and prevention of disease in the elder.

[...] the development of social projects [...] (P6)

4.2. Health Benefits

From the perspective of these students, many benefits to their health came from their use of strategies to promote health and prevent disease in the elderly. The several benefits to health, expressed in the narratives of these students, show how they valued the rich strategies used in different contexts of care.

4.2.1. Disease Prevention

The strategies used were determinant to prevent diseases and several complications, as the statements below indicate.

[...] reduction of the number of elders with minor and major complications associated with diabetes, hypertension, obesity, etc. (P4)

[...] the diminution of COVID-19 infections. (P4)

[...] the diminution of complications from the disease, the stabilization of symptoms. (P6)

The health benefit was avoiding ulcers and many complications that could have emerged from this injury. (P9)

4.2.2. Health Promotion

Health promotion, as a health benefit, appears as associated with awareness about the disease.

[...] increased awareness about the disease... P4

4.2.3. Wellbeing and Self-Care

Wellbeing and self-care were the indicator of this category, expressed by a high number of students (6). The frequency of thematic units (10) suggests the importance attributed to these health benefits that resulted from the strategies to promote health and prevent disease in the elderly in a clinical context.

[...] which will consequently improve their quality of life. (P3)

The health benefits resulting from the implementation of these strategies to promote health and prevent disease in the elderly include increased global wellbeing, as well as improved health state and quality of life of the elder [...]. (P5)

[...] weight loss, progressive increase in functional independence. (P6)

[...] the comfort and satisfaction of needs and family harmony. (P6)

Increased autonomy and independence of the elder as they carry out their daily life activities. (P8)

[...] thus allowing an increase in the quality of life. (P9)

[...] in addition to the improvement in their quality of life. (P10)

4.2.4. Behavioral Change

The strategies to promote health and prevent disease caused behavioral changes in the elders, particularly in regard to changes in risk behavior and the adoption of healthy lifestyles.

[...] at the time of the presentation of the education session, the elders were interested and willing to change some risk behaviors they had to improve their health and prevent disease. (P2)

[...] the sessions led to many health benefits; specifically, the adoption of healthy lifestyles, the reduction of polypharmacy, the creation of a calm environment, adapted to each elder [...] (P10)

4.2.5. Empowering

One of the students highlighted the empowering of the elder as a health benefit, which allows elders to be prepared to make decisions for the implementation of strategies connected to their health conditions (Vale et al., 2018).

[...] the empowering of the elder. (P3)

4.2.6. Client Satisfaction

The satisfaction of the elder with the valorization and support provided is evident in the narratives of these students, reflecting on their activities in regard to the workers that intervene in health promotion strategies.

When the elder feels valued and supported, they will be willing to actively listen to the things the professional has to say and teach in regard to the promotion of their health. (P3)

4.2.7. Management of the Therapeutic Regime

One of the benefits from the narratives of the students in regard to the strategies to promote health and prevent disease in the elderly was the management of the therapeutic regime.

[...] correct adherence to the therapy [...] (P4)

Increased adherence to the therapeutic regime. (P8)

4.2.8. Expenses

The reduced economic costs were also highlighted as a health benefit from the strategies to promote health and prevent disease in which these students participated in the clinical context.

[...] the reduction of the costs inherent to the disease process [...] (P3)

[...] will reduce the need to use health services and, therefore, reduce the economic needs related to health. (P5)

4.2.9. Life Expectancy

The increased life expectancy was also mentioned by a student as one of the health benefits resulting from the implementation of strategies to promote health and prevent disease.

In regard to the male population, there have been some life expectancy increases, especially after 60 years old. [...] Portugal has one of the lowest male life expectancies, and the health benefits are not high when compared to other European countries. (P7)

4.3. Impact on the Formative Process

From the perspective of these students, participation in health promotion and disease prevention strategies impacted their learning, the development of competencies, and the awareness about these competencies.

4.3.1. Learning and Developing Competencies

The learning and the development of competencies were indicators that emerged from the narratives of five students. The participation of these students in the strategies to promote health and prevent disease in the elderly helped them to understand the importance of education for health and to develop more efficient and effective health education interventions, as can be seen in the following registration units.

> *[…] it had quite a positive impact on my formation process, as it helped me realize the importance of education in health and the effect it has on the health of people. In this regard, I could understand that if you intervene early, you can change certain risk behaviors and prevent disease, thus avoiding other, more serious issues. (P2)*

> *My participation in the strategies to promote health and prevent disease in the elderly allows me to understand what are the most effective and efficient interventions, as well as to develop technical-scientific competencies in health that directly affect the behavior of the elderly. (P3)*

Building new practices and understanding the importance of empowerment of the elderly person are implicit in the learning and skill development of these students.

> *It also allows for the construction of new practices of health, from the perspective of reflecting and adopting new methods to care for the elder, based on health promotion and disease prevention. (P3)*

> *[…] academic education has an essential role, as it provides us with several qualities, such as creativity, resilience, pragmatism, perseverance, the capacity to deal with the unpredictable, to work and cooperate with other sectors of society, to use research and maximize their importance, etc.… which are paramount tools for us to become competent health professionals and the best facilitators for the promotion of a healthy and active aging, free from prejudice and social stigma. (P6)*

The students' participation in these strategies helped them to acquire new skills and knowledge.

> *My participation in these strategies allowed me to understand that when we encourage and try to strengthen the abilities of the elder, they feel their competency as individuals, valued, and are predisposed for more active participation. The elder feels empowered and capable of taking control of their own lives, thus being more receptive to participation in health care. (P8)*

> *My participation in these strategies to promote health and prevent disease in the elderly allowed me to apprehend new competencies and knowledge, especially in regard to health promotion and disease prevention in the elder, enriching my formation process as it allowed me to carry out correct interventions in the future. (P10)*

4.3.2. Raising Awareness of Competencies

Participating in these strategies with the elders was determinant to raise their awareness about their capabilities, especially in regard to training persons and health promotion, as manifested in the statement below.

> *The fact that we are constantly directly or indirectly connected to the act of caring, instructing, educating, and intervening with the person makes us aware, as our academic formation advances, that, among all tasks a health professional has, in the specific case of the nurse, training and promoting health, which mostly involves behavioral changes, is the most complex one, because it requires continuous, aware, and desirable investment. (P6)*

5. Discussion

The results of this qualitative study reiterated that clinical classes, as a form of teaching, allow for an integration of theory and practice in learning [23], influencing the perception of students about health promotion and disease prevention in the elder. The connection between "school desk" knowledge and practice is vital to support the making of clinical decisions [24], and in this concrete case, for the learning of strategies that allow for the health promotion of the more vulnerable elder population. We corroborated the findings according to which elders with multiple morbidities need more complex health care, and health promotion is still not a priority for this group of people [25]. Aging is still one of the greatest challenges for health and social systems in general and for nursing care in particular. To respond to it with cost-effective solutions, effective strategies are needed that can guarantee a healthy and active life for those who are aging [26]. Evidence-based strategies will only be prescribed and implemented if health professionals have the necessary knowledge and develop competencies to lead this process. However, the results of the research indicate that one of the barriers to the dissemination of health promotion is the shortcoming in the preparation of future nurses [26]. This statement assumes that it is naive to presume that the inclusion of the topic on nursing courses syllabi will be enough to deal with current needs [26].

For future nurses to assume this role, they need to understand and have experience in it as students [26,27]. They must also learn to work in teams that integrate health promotion [24] as a core element of their intervention with the elderly.

As a result, the findings of this investigation allow one to perceive that clinical learning in the community, together with the elders and their families, and with learning results targeted at health promotion and disease prevention contribute to overcoming the afore-mentioned barrier. Therefore, this clinical learning strategy allows for the provision of care that is more focused on people and adjusted to their needs, expectations, and values, with better results in regard to therapeutic regime adherence [28].

In the category "Strategies to promote health and prevent disease in the elderly", the students expressed how much importance they attribute to different strategies to promote health and prevent disease during their formation process. Home care, information, communication, and health education stood out. As other studies have observed, the implementation of health promotion in home care is important to reiterate the self-care abilities of the elder and increase or improve their knowledge about their own health, allowing them better opportunities to decide about their own care [24,29,30].

It should be highlighted that only one student mentioned social projects and their influence on health promotion. Social prescriptions are a recent topic in health and emerge in literature as an approach that promotes the use of non-clinical local activities, such as exercise, social, technological, and touristic activities, as recommended by health professionals. This could help improve one's physical and psychological wellbeing, health behavior, and self-efficacy and reduce expenses [31], treating diseases and complications associated with the reduction of physical activities and social participation. Due to its potential, it should be included in the syllabi of health courses.

Regarding the category "Health benefits from the implementation of the strategies to promote health and prevent disease in the elderly", the students valued, among other elements, wellbeing, self-care, behavioral changes, and empowerment. The transference of knowledge about health and healthy lifestyles to the elder, targeted at their individual needs and using cognitive-behavioral strategies adequate to their level of literacy, reiterates responsibility, promotes self-esteem and feelings of safety, and increases the probability of a person to remain independent at home for longer [24].

On the other hand, the promotion of self-care and the prevention of complications influence the management of the therapeutic regime and the adherence to treatment, also affecting expenses and quality of life, since interventions to promote health and prevent disease may help avoid urgency services, avoiding human suffering, the use of community resources, and probably reducing the risk for errors associated with health care [24], such as increased risks for infection and falls at the urgency services, or hospitalization.

The possibility of observing these "in loco" benefits reaffirms what the student has learned, making them conscious about the importance of these interventions for the quality of life of the elderly, including the management of their therapy, prevention, complications, and their own satisfaction.

The discourse the participants wrote allows one to observe that the articulation between theory and practice and the possibility of working with health promotion elements in the clinical context allows for the learning and/or development of competencies related to them, about which the students become more conscious. Opportunities to plan and implement health education sessions and interventions to promote health and prevent disease, as well as the confront between what was learned and what was implemented in the clinic, lead to the development of competencies related to communication and transmission of information, which is in accordance with aspects related to behavioral changes, which are paramount to improve adherence to the therapeutic regime.

Research with nursing students, aiming to analyze the knowledge of students from the last year of the nursing course about the concepts of health promotion and disease prevention, found that the students knew the concepts and that the relation between theory and practice is important [27] since most of them understand the concepts, but show difficulties to apply them in the daily practice of health services.

It is important to highlight the importance of nursing educators in this process. They can create a syllabus based on the principles of health promotion, which, later, are reflected in clinical experience [26]. The other aspect that should be taken into consideration is the use of information and communication technologies in the care of isolated elderly people in a pandemic context. Its use may be a solution to be considered, but it is important to prepare students for its application [32].

In this line of thought, we believe that the findings of this study have important implications for the teaching of nursing and for health and education policies, as they allow for the understanding of the strategies used in the promotion of health and prevention of disease in the elderly, in addition to the benefits obtained from the implementation of these strategies.

Limitations

This research has limitations related to the method, the narratives, and the eligibility criteria of the participants, that is, with regard to sample size, the e-mail methodology applied in data collection, and the "intentional" selection of respondents. Further studies, with more participants, should delve deeper into strategies that allow for the development of competencies in the provision of care to elders, especially focusing on health promotion and disease prevention strategies in the context of the community.

6. Conclusions

Our findings allowed us to understand how students developed competencies in the promotion of health and prevention of diseases in the context of clinical classes. The analysis of the discourses led to the emergence of topics such as "Strategies to promote health and prevent disease in the elderly", "Health improvements from the implementation of the strategies to promote health and prevent disease in the elderly", and "The impact your participation in these strategies to promote health and prevent disease in the elderly had on your formative process". These findings can contribute to the construction of syllabi in nursing graduation courses, focusing on strategies of health promotion and disease prevention that revolve around the needs and expectations of the elderly, aiming to improve their adherence to therapy.

Author Contributions: Conceptualization, R.F., C.L.B. and A.C.N.; methodology, R.F., C.L.B. and A.C.N.; formal analysis, R.F., L.S. and C.L.B.; investigation, R.F., L.S. and C.L.B.; resources, R.F., C.L.B. and A.C.N.; data curation, R.F. and A.C.N.; writing—original draft preparation, R.F., C.L.B. and A.C.N.; writing—review and editing, R.F., C.L.B., Ó.R.F., A.C.N., T.M. and L.S.; visualization, R.F., C.L.B., Ó.R.F., A.C.N., T.M. and L.S.; supervision, R.F., C.L.B. and A.C.N.; project administration, R.F., C.L.B., A.C.N. and L.S.; funding acquisition, R.F., C.L.B. and L.S. All authors have read and agreed to the published version of the manuscript.

Funding: The present study was funded by Instituto Politécnico de Beja—Project 4IE+.

Institutional Review Board Statement: The present study was carried out according to the guidelines of the Declaration of Helsinki and approved by an Ethics Committee.

Informed Consent Statement: Informed consent was obtained from all individuals who participated in the study.

Data Availability Statement: Data are available only upon request to the authors.

Acknowledgments: The authors express their gratitude to all participants for their contributions to the study.

Conflicts of Interest: The authors declare no conflict of interest.

References

1. Instituto Nacional de Estatística. Projeções de População Residente em Portugal. 2017. Available online: https://www.ine.pt/xportal/xmain?xpid=INE&xpgid=ine_destaques&DESTAQUESdest_boui=277695619&DESTAQUESmodo=2 (accessed on 27 November 2021).
2. Nunes, A.C.; Costa, P.M. Envelhecimento ativo: Desafios, oportunidades e políticas. In *Desafios e Oportunidades do Envelhecimento*; Faria, M.C., Ramalho, J.P., Nunes, A.C., Eds.; International Press: Lisboa, Portugal, 2020; pp. 463–480.
3. Ferreira, E.M.; Lourenço, O.M.; da Costa, P.V.; Pinto, S.C.; Gomes, C.; Oliveira, A.P.; Ferreira, Ó.; Baixinho, C.L. Active Life: A project for a safe hospital-community transition after arthroplasty. *Rev. Bras. Enferm.* **2019**, *72*, 147–153. [CrossRef] [PubMed]
4. Fonseca, C.; de Pinho, L.G.; Lopes, M.J.; do Céu Marques, M.; Garcia-Alonso, J. The Elderly Nursing Core Set and the cognition of Portuguese older adults: A cross-sectional study. *BMC Nurs.* **2021**, *20*, 1–8. [CrossRef] [PubMed]
5. Reis, G.M.; Sousa, L.M.; Silva, P.; Pereira, P.; Sim-Sim, M. Frailty in the Elderly and Interventions Supported by Information and Communication Technologies: A Systematic Review. In *Exploring the Role of ICTs in Healthy Aging*; Mendes, D., Fonseca, C., Lopes, M.J., García-Alonso, J., Murillo, J.M., Eds.; IGI Global: Hershey, PA, USA, 2020; pp. 120–137. [CrossRef]
6. Ministério da Saúde. Retrato da Saúde, Lisboa, Portugal, 2018. Available online: https://www.sns.gov.pt/wpcontent/uploads/2018/04/RETRATODASAUDE_2018_compressed.pdf (accessed on 27 November 2021).
7. Reis, M.; Casas-Novas, M.V.; Serra, I.; Magalhães, M.D.; Sousa, L. The importance of a training program on active aging from the perspective of elderly individuals. *Rev. Bras. Enferm.* **2021**, *74* (Suppl. 2), e20190843. [CrossRef]
8. Ferreira, R.; Nunes, A.C.; Baixinho, C.L.; Sousa, L. Promoção da Saúde e Prevenção da Doença em Pessoa Idosa. In *Competências em Enfermagem, Gerontogeriátrica: Uma Exigência para a Qualidade do Cuidado. Série Monográfica Educação e Investigação em Saúde*; Em Almeida, M.L., Tavares, J., Ferreira, J.S.S., Eds.; Unidade de Investigação em Ciências da Saúde, Enfermagem (UICISA:E)/Escola Superior de Enfermagem de Coimbra (ESEnfC): Coimbra, Portugal, 2021; p. 141154.
9. Nouri, S.S.; Barnes, D.E.; Volow, A.M.; McMahan, R.D.; Kushel, M.; Jin, C.; Boscardin, J.; Sudore, R.L. Health literacy matters more than experience for advance care planning knowledge among older adults. *JAGS* **2019**, *67*, 2151–2156. [CrossRef] [PubMed]
10. Nutbeam, D.; McGill, B.; Premkumar, P. Improving health literacy in community populations: A review of progress. *Health Promot. Int.* **2018**, *33*, 901–911. [CrossRef] [PubMed]
11. Directive 2005/36/ec of the European Parliament and of the Council of 7 September 2005 on the Recognition of Professional Qualifications. *Off. J. Eur. Union. L* **2005**, *L 255*, 22–52. Available online: https://wwwcdn.dges.gov.pt/sites/default/files/directiva36_2005.pdf (accessed on 28 November 2021).
12. Instituto Politécnico de Beja. *Descritor da Unidade Curricular Ensino Clínico em Enfermagem em Saúde Comunitária*; IPB: Beja, Portugal, 2018; Available online: https://www.ipbeja.pt/cursos/ess-enf/Paginas/UnidadesCurriculares.aspx (accessed on 27 November 2021).
13. Marcus-Varwijk, A.E.; Madjdian, D.S.; de Vet, E.; Mensen, M.W.M.; Visscher, T.L.S.; Ranchor, A.V.; Slaets, J.P.J.; Smits, C.H.M. Experiences and views of older people on their participation in a nurse-led health promotion intervention: "Community Health Consultation Offices for Seniors". *PLoS ONE* **2019**, *14*, e0216494. [CrossRef] [PubMed]
14. Karlsson, S. Looking for elderly people´s needs: Teaching critical reflection in Swedish social work education. *Soc. Work Educ.* **2020**, *39*, 227–240. [CrossRef]
15. Wu, F.; Drevenhorn, E.; Carlsson, G. Nurses' Experiences of Promoting Healthy Aging in the Municipality: A Qualitative Study. *Healthcare* **2020**, *8*, 131. [CrossRef]
16. Delamaire, M.; Lafortune, G. Nurses in advanced roles: A description and evaluation of experiences in 12 developed countries. In *OECD Health Working Paper*; OECD: Paris, France, 2010.
17. Maier, C.B.; Aiken, L.H. Task shifting from physicians to nurses in primary care in 39 countries: A cross-country comparative study. *Eur. J. Public Health* **2016**, *26*, 927–934. [CrossRef]
18. Cardoso, T.; Martins, M.; Monteiro, M. Community care unit and elderly health promotion: An intervention programe. *Rev. De Enferm. Ref.* **2017**, *IV*, 103–114. [CrossRef]
19. Baixinho, C.L.; Dixe, M.; Madeira, C.; Alves, S.; Henriques, M.A. Falls in institutionalized elderly with and without cognitive decline: A study of some factors. *Dement. Neuropsychol.* **2019**, *13*, 116–121. [CrossRef] [PubMed]

20. Martínez, M.S. Haciendo Avanzar la Gerontagogía: Aprendiendo de la Experiencia Canadiense. *Pedagog. Social. Rev. Inteniniversitaria* **2001**, *6–7*, 243–262. Available online: https://www.researchgate.net/publication/28221576_Haciendo_avanzar_la_gerontagogia_aprendiendo_de_la_experiencia_canadiense (accessed on 27 November 2021).
21. Silva, I.B.; Amendoeira, J. O uso da narrativa no paradigma da investigação qualitativa. *Ciênc. Vida Saúde* **2018**, *6*, 29–40. Available online: http://ojs.ipsantarem.pt/index.php/REVUIIPS (accessed on 24 October 2021).
22. Bardin, L. *Análise de Conteúdo: Edição Revista e Ampliada*, 70th ed.; São Paulo: São Paulo, Brazil, 2016.
23. Shoghi, M.; Sajadi, M.; Oskuie, F.; Dehnad, A.; Borimnejad, L. Strategies for bridging the theory-practice gap from the perspective of nursing experts. *Heliyon* **2019**, *5*, e02503. [CrossRef]
24. Karlsson, S.; Ridbäck, A.; Brobeck, E.; Pejner, M.N. Health Promotion Practices in Nursing for Elderly Persons in Municipal Home Care: An Integrative Literature Review. *Home Health Care Manag. Pract.* **2020**, *32*, 53–61. [CrossRef]
25. Duplaga, M.; Grysztar, M.; Rodzinka, M.; Kopec, A. Scoping review of health promotion and disease prevention interventions addressed to elderly people. *BMC Health Serv. Res.* **2016**, *16* (Suppl. 5), 278. [CrossRef]
26. Mooney, B.; Timmins, F.; Byrne, G.; Corroon, A.M. Nursing students' attitudes to health promotion to: Implications for teaching practice. *Nurse Educ. Today* **2011**, *31*, 841–848. [CrossRef]
27. Gurgel, K.F.; Santos, A.D.B.; Monteiro, A.I.; Lima, K.Y.N. Health promotion and disease prevention: The knowledge of nursing students. *Rev. De Enferm. UFPE-Line* **2015**, *9*, 368–375. [CrossRef]
28. Lyu, C.M.; Zhang, L. Concept analysis of adherence. *Front. Nurs.* **2018**, *6*, 81–86. [CrossRef]
29. Ferreira, R.F.; Nunes, A.C.; Canhestro, A.M. Models and Politics of Cares of the Elderly in the Home. In *Gerontechnology*; García-Alonso, J., Fonseca, C., Eds.; First International Workshop: Cáceres, Spain; Évora, Portugal, 2018. [CrossRef]
30. Baixinho, C.L.; Presado, M.H.; Ribeiro, J. Qualitative research and the transformation of public health. *Cien Saude Colet* **2019**, *24*, 1583. [CrossRef]
31. Costa, A.; Sousa, C.J.; Seabra, P.R.C.; Virgolino, A.; Santos, O.; Lopes, J.; Henriques, A.; Nogueira, P.; Alarcão, V. Effectiveness of Social Prescribing Programs in the Primary Health-Care Context: A Systematic Literature Review. *Sustainability* **2021**, *13*, 2731. [CrossRef]
32. Woo, B.F.; Poon, S.N.; Tam, W.W.; Zhou, W. The impact of COVID19 on advanced practice nursing education and practice: A qualitative study. *Int. Nurs. Rev.* **2021**, *in press*. [CrossRef] [PubMed]

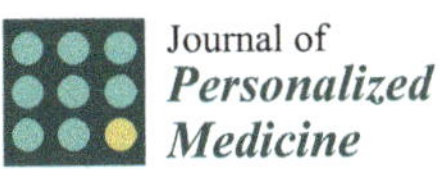

Journal of *Personalized Medicine*

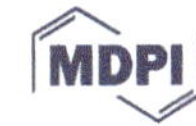

Article

Patients' Characterization of Medication, Emotions, and Incongruent Perceptions around Adherence

Pikuei Tu [1], Danielle Smith [1], Rachel Clark [1], Laura Bayzle [2], Rungting Tu [3,*] and Cheryl Lin [1,*]

[1] Policy and Organizational Management Program, Duke University, Durham, NC 27705, USA; pikuei.tu@duke.edu (P.T.); danielle.c.smith@duke.edu (D.S.); tanjaclark@gmail.com (R.C.)

[2] The Link Group, Durham, NC 27713, USA; lbayzle@tlg.com

[3] College of Management, Shenzhen University, Shenzhen 518060, China

* Correspondence: rungting2@gmail.com (R.T.); c.lin@duke.edu (C.L.)

Abstract: Medication nonadherence is prevalent among patients with chronic diseases. Previous research focused on patients' beliefs in medication or illness and applied risk-benefit analyses when reasoning their behavior. This qualitative study examined rheumatoid arthritis (RA) patients' perceptions and feelings toward medication in parallel with attitudes about their own adherence. We conducted four 90-min focus groups and seven 60-min interviews with a diverse sample of RA patients ($n = 27$). Discussions covered dilemmas encountered, emotions, and thought process concerning medication, and included application of projective techniques. Transcripts were analyzed in NVivo-12 using a thematic coding framework through multiple rounds of deduction and categorization. Three themes emerged, each with mixed sentiments. (1) *Ambivalent feelings toward medication*: participants experienced internal conflicts as their appreciation of drugs for relief contradicted worries about side effects or "toxicity" and desire to not identify as sick, portraying medications as "best friend" and "evil". (2) *Struggles in taking medication*: participants "hated" the burden of managing regimen and resented the reliance and embarrassment. (3) *Attitudes and behavior around adherence*: most participants self-reported high adherence yet also described frequently self-adjusting medications, displaying perception-action incongruency. Some expressed nervousness and resistance while others felt empowered when modifying dosage, which might have motivated or helped them self-justify nonadherence. Only a few who deviated from prescription discussed it with their clinicians though most participants expressed the desire to do so; open communication with providers reinforced a sense of confidence and control of their own health. Promoting personalized care with shared decision-making that empowers and supports patients in managing their long-term treatment could encourage adherence and improve overall health outcome.

Keywords: compliance; qualitative; empowerment; medication acceptability; intentional nonadherence; decision; self esteem; pharmacology; rheumatology; autoimmune

Citation: Tu, P.; Smith, D.; Clark, R.; Bayzle, L.; Tu, R.; Lin, C. Patients' Characterization of Medication, Emotions, and Incongruent Perceptions around Adherence. *J. Pers. Med.* **2021**, *11*, 975. https://doi.org/10.3390/jpm11100975

Academic Editors: Fábio G. Teixeira, Catarina Godinho and Júlio Belo Fernandes

Received: 2 September 2021
Accepted: 27 September 2021
Published: 29 September 2021

Publisher's Note: MDPI stays neutral with regard to jurisdictional claims in published maps and institutional affiliations.

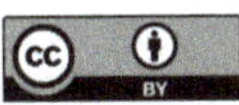

1. Introduction

Rheumatoid arthritis (RA) is a chronic autoimmune disease characterized by inflammation and synovitis that result in joint pain, stiffness, and difficult mobility that can last for prolonged periods of time [1,2]. RA patients often experience decreased quality of life as their symptoms interfere with daily activities and impact job productivity [3,4]. Treatment of RA typically starts with one or more disease-modifying antirheumatic drugs (DMARDs) [5,6]. Biologics are added if standard-of-care DMARDs alone are ineffective [7]. As with most chronic illnesses, nonadherence is common amongst RA patients, with rates ranging from 20% to 70% [8–10]. In addition to an increased risk to patient safety and poorer health outcomes, nonadherence results in growing healthcare costs and the overuse of healthcare resources [11,12]. However, the effects of many interventions have been nonsignificant or short-term [13,14], and reviews found that most of the studies evaluating these programs to be low-quality or difficult to replicate [14,15].

Medication adherence is a complex behavior with hundreds of variables documented as indicators including patient-, medication-, and illness-specific and contextual factors [16,17]. It is defined as the extent to which a patient's behavior "corresponds with agreed recommendations from a healthcare provider" [12], highlighting shared-decision making and patients' active participation in determining their health. Compliance, commonly used interchangeably yet with a passive connotation, more specifically denotes patients following regimens including prescribed dosage, frequency, and duration [18,19]. Self-efficacy, patient-provider relationship, beliefs in medication, social support, and age were among the most frequently cited adherence factors in rheumatology [20]. Nonadherence is prevalent when patients are worried about or deterred by side-effects [21,22], false online information [23], or costs [24]. Studies often use a necessity-concerns or benefit-risk differential framework to compare facilitators and barriers to adherence quantitatively [25–27]. Qualitative research, which is fewer in number of publications [28,29], has described more in depth the reasoning for not complying with treatment instruction, the impact taking chronic medication has on RA patients, and the feelings of shame, uncertainty, stress, or anxiety accompanying medication-taking [30,31]. Pharmaceutics has advanced to improve the ease of consuming medication and tailored to a more personalized approach [32–34]. At the same time, patients' willingness to accept regimens also relies on their perceptions toward medication and persistent behavior to complete the therapy process [16,19,35]. Few studies have concurrently considered patients' characterization of medications beyond the risk-benefit deliberation and their interpretation of adherence to examine how these views manifest in or influence medication behavior.

Innovation and development in medicine cannot materialize their full value if patients do not take the medication. The objectives of this study, which focused on patient-related attributes, were to (a) analyze patient attitudes—including cognitive disposition and emotions—on medications in parallel with feelings regarding their own nonadherence, (b) understand triggers or motivators for self-adjusting their prescribed regimen, and (c) present a holistic view of the psychological profile of RA patients' medication decision process via their own narratives to inform personalized care that could instill confidence in managing their chronic therapy, encouraging adherence and improving health outcomes.

2. Methods

2.1. Recruitment

We conducted four 90-min focus groups (FG 1–4) and seven 60-min individual in-depth interviews (IDI) with RA patients ($n = 27$) in the greater Raleigh-Durham area of North Carolina. Participants in the groups and interviews did not overlap. All participants were recruited through a regional research database and flyers in local rheumatology clinics. Eligibility criteria included: age 18 to 75, have been diagnosed and prescribed medication for RA for at least 6 months, and not currently or planning to become pregnant or breastfeed in the next 12 months (as these individuals may have distinctive reasons for nonadherence not applicable during regular time or to other patient population). To gather data from diverse experiences and perspectives, potential participants were contacted, screened, and selected for a purposive sample of different age, ethnicity, household income, number of years from first diagnosis, and self-reported adherence.

2.2. Measure

There is a number of validated scales aimed to assess patients' adherence, such as Morisky Medication Adherence Scale (MMAS), Medication Adherence Rating Scale (MARS), Hill-Bone Scale, and Compliance Questionnaire for Rheumatology (CQR) [36–39]. These measures have been used primarily in quantitative research and clinical trials. Because this study's objective was to appraise patients' self-perceived adherence in relation to their actual behavior of taking medication, we posed a direct question "how would you describe how often you follow the prescription in taking all your RA medications, including the dosage, timing, and frequency as instructed?" with the intention to capture possible bias or misconception in a self-reported measure. Answers ranging from never, not often, sometimes, most of the time, and always were recorded as 1 to 5; these numbers were noted below when presenting the participants' quotes to reflect each individual's own view for context.

2.3. Procedure

We developed a semi-structured discussion guide centered around the study objectives, considering questions employed in past qualitative research and gaps identified in the literature. The guide was used for both FG and IDI to probe patients' perceptions, experiences, and behavior related to RA medication. Discussions covered their emotions, dilemmas encountered, personal and professional relationships as a chronic patient, and thought process concerning RA disease and treatment. In one segment of each discussion, we used projective interviewing technique to gain a deeper understanding of participants' perspectives that may not be revealed or expressed fully in direct questioning (e.g., "if your RA medication was a person, what would they be like?" instead of "what do you think of your medication?" which may render a simple answer such as "my medication is alright") [40,41]. This technique has been widely utilized in psychology and consumer research to encourage interviewees to share their true feelings or opinions more freely rather than respond in a presumably socially acceptable or expected way [42,43]. A trained moderator facilitated the focus groups and two researchers conducted each interview. Written informed consent was obtained prior to all discussions. Recordings were transcribed by one researcher and quality checked by a second researcher.

2.4. Data Analysis

We performed deductive, thematic analysis [44,45] to develop a codebook. Research team members first went through all the recordings and/or transcripts individually and brainstormed the categorization of potential themes observed from the FG and IDI, initially with two general domains of patient attitudes or emotions pertaining to medication and perceptions toward non/adherence. Via multiple discourses and iterations, the team then together identified feelings toward medication itself and the action of taking medication as separate aspects, and subsequently decided on three themes most relevant to the study objectives. Two researchers independently coded all FG and IDI transcriptions using NVivo-12; disagreements in coding were discussed with and mediated by a third researcher. Representative quotes were chosen from each theme and subtheme to illustrate participants' narratives in managing their medication. Less prominent categories considered during the coding process, such as satisfaction with provider, denial or helplessness during initial diagnosis, and social support were not presented in the Results. The study protocol was approved by Duke University Institutional Review Board.

3. Results

A total of 27 RA patients were interviewed in groups or individually. Participants ranged from ages 18 to 71, and time of RA diagnosis ranged from 2 to 43 years ago. The majority of participants identified as Non-Hispanic Caucasian and 25.9% were minorities. When describing how often they follow their prescriptions, three participants said sometimes, eight said most of the time, and sixteen (59.3%) said always (Table 1).

Table 1. Participant Demographics, Time of Diagnosis, and Self-Reported Adherence.

n = 27	*n* (%)	Mean (SD)
Gender		
Woman	21 (77.8%)	
Man	6 (22.2%)	
Age (years)		46.4 (14.56)
18–29	4 (14.8%)	
30–49	13 (48.1%)	
50–64	7 (25.9%)	
65+	3 (11.1%)	
Ethnicity		
Caucasian	20 (74.0%)	
African American	3 (11.1%)	
Hispanic	4 (14.8%)	
First diagnosed (years ago)		11.0 (8.1)
1–4	4 (14.8%)	
5–9	8 (29.6%)	
10–14	8 (29.6%)	
15–19	5 (18.5%)	
20–24	1 (3.7%)	
25+	1 (3.7%)	
Self-reported adherence		4.5 (0.7)
1 = never	0	
2 = not often	0	
3 = sometimes	3 (11.1%)	
4 = most of the time	8 (29.6%)	
5 = always	16 (59.3%)	

Through thematic analysis of the group and individual interviews, three themes were identified: (1) conflicting feelings toward medication, (2) concerns and complexity in medication-taking, and (3) manifestations of and attitudes toward self-adjusting medications. The first theme considered participants' perceptions of their medications while the second depicted how they felt during or about the physical act of taking chronic medications. The third highlighted how participants viewed and conveyed their own adherence or non-compliance.

3.1. Ambivalent Feelings toward Medication

Many participants had negative feelings toward their medication. Some viewed it with worry and apprehension due to the many side effects of the drug; these side effects could be either personally experienced or anticipated. While appreciating the benefit medication brought in reducing or even eliminating their pain or disability, participants expressed bitterness concerning their reliance.

> *"I drink gallons of water a day because I've got to flush that out of my system, that stuff is toxic. . . . my organs are probably just screaming on the inside."* (FG 1, SRA 5)

> *"I'm a little concerned because the medication which seems to be working well, you know, can kind of damage your liver or kidneys."* (FG 1, SRA 5)

> *"I hate prednisone. It's like the most evil but it helps."* (FG 4, SRA 4)

For some participants, medication was associated with increased freedom, as the relief received from taking it enabled them to carry out more daily activities. However, sometimes the drug's power to determine their capability seemed intimidating. This conflicting perception was vividly represented in the way participants personified their medication when prompted with the projective technique to portray their relationship with or attachment to RA medication.

"[My medication] feels like the annoying person in junior high that's always there . . . [I'm] like 'can you leave me alone?' . . . I know my medication is helping me; it's good to have that friend." (FG 4, SRA 5)

"I guess you'd say [the medicine is my] best friend . . . I can't say it makes you feel perfect, but I think without it I would feel much worse." (FG 1, SRA 5)

"It's a Viking. So, it's strong and fights for me and defends me. But if I'm on the bad side of my Viking, it might hurt me." (FG 2, SRA 5)

"I have a 'date' with (drug name) once a week. Nobody likes needles but I do love the (drug name) needle because . . . I promise you by, like the second day, you can feel it; I can breathe and move. It's $3500 [for a three-month supply]—it's like the most expensive thing in my home. But I will sell things so I can get it . . . [However], every time I take this needle out I'm like, oh my God, don't let five years from now I grow an extra ear or anything." (FG 1, SRA 5)

3.2. Struggles in Taking Medication

More than just the medication itself, participants also had repellant feelings toward the physical act of taking medication and responsibility of managing the often-complex regimens. The need to keep track of and self-administer medication was stressful and burdensome, particularly for the few who were prescribed self-injection biologics. This forced participants to identify as an ailing patient, which they struggled to accept and felt embarrassed by.

"I really hated it because it meant that I was sick, and I was the only one that had to take medicine in my family. Even my grandmother is healthier than me." (IDI 2, SRA 4)

"I'm embarrassed when I go places, or even when our kids would have friends over . . . I feel like a druggie taking all this medicine when I'm 40 years old." (FG 4, SRA 5)

Participants writhed to decide whether or not to take their medication and frequently considered if their desire for relief was stronger than their resentment or fears toward the medication. Some participants focused on the positives; the medicine could be a "miracle" in reducing symptoms and improving mobility, bringing back a sense of independence. Moreover, the reality of having to get injections or take pills for the rest of one's lifetime was difficult to reconcile for participants. In the end, even participants with overwhelmingly negative feelings toward medication still described having no choice but to take it for those benefits.

"I was able to write and function and forget about my arthritis." (IDI 7, SRA 5)

"It's like an internal battle with myself, and I go back and forth for a couple of days before I just break down and say it's easier just to take it." (IDI 3, SRA 5)

"I know it's like that evil thing . . . You know you would be better if you could get off of it, but I cannot get off of it." (FG 4, SRA 5)

3.3. Actions and Attitudes around Non/Adherence

3.3.1. In/Congruence between Perceptions and Behavior

Unless there were serious side effects, almost all participants resigned to taking the medication. However, while some participants took the medication exactly as instructed, often noting the seriousness of the drugs, others described adjusting the dosage up or down to tailor the prescription to their own symptoms and the side effects they were experiencing at the time.

"I take them exactly as prescribed. It's strong medication, and if you start self-regulating, I just can't imagine the side effects . . . that really scares me." (FG 2, SRA 4)

"It upset my stomach, so I started taking less and less, and trying to find that edge where it was healthy, but I wasn't getting sick." (FG 3, SRA 5)

When asked whether, when, and how they adjusted their medication, participants' responses revealed discrepancies between their self-perception of adherence and actions. While a few participants who frequently adjusted their medication were aware of their nonadherence, most participants had reported taking their medication as prescribed most of the time or always (SRA 4 or 5).

> *"Sometimes on a bad day, I will get frustrated because I feel like my medication is not working anyways, so then I don't want the side effects as well if I take it. So, perhaps on bad days, I'm less compliant."* (IDI 6, SRA 3)

> *"[My doctors] would prescribe that, but I would take half of that when I feel like I need it or more if I felt like I needed it."* (FG 1, SRA 5)

> *"I just took one extra one, and it worked, so I guess I need to talk to the doctor about me having to take a little bit more than just that one pill when I am having an episode."* (FG 2, SRA 4)

3.3.2. Emotions and Empowerment from Self-Adjusting Medication

Participants described a wide spectrum of feelings towards adjusting their own treatment regimens. Some felt anxious and risky and revealed being nervous about doctors' reactions and potentially experiencing more symptoms or side effects, though this was not always enough to stop them from "tweaking" or experimenting. Participants also expressed worry and unsettlement when intentionally not adhering to their prescription.

> *"I would say uneasy … because if I skip a dosage, or if I'm kind of playing around with it, I'm not sure what the outcome is going to be. So, it's like a risk I'm taking."* (FG 3, SRA 4)

> *"[I feel] like I'm a disappointment sometimes to [my care team]."* (FG 4, SRA 4)

> *"I'll get paranoid that my joints are secretly, you know quietly getting damaged and that I'm not helping them."* (FG 4, SRA 5)

On the other hand, over a third of participants discussed the upside of self-adjusting medication. They felt strength in regaining control as they were able to make their own treatment decisions when they felt necessary or helpful.

> *"I would say [I feel] empowered to be able to decide if I was able to take it or not whereas before I felt reliant."* (IDI 2, SRA 4)

> *"Empowered. I mean, it's in my hands … I feel like I'm taking charge of my own health."* (FG 1, SRA 5)

> *"In control. It makes you feel like you're doing a little bit of something on your own and not being told exactly, 'You got to do this'."* (FG 4, SRA 5)

Compounding this was the confidence that they knew their bodies, and in particular, knew their bodies more than their clinicians did. For some participants, the longer they were on the medication and the more experience they had, the more they trusted themselves to self-adjust their dosages.

> *"I make decisions based on my side-effects. If they are intolerable, I figure [my doctor] is not in my body, he doesn't know."* (FG 4, SRA 4)

> *"The doctor put us on a dosage, but because we know our own bodies, we know that we may feel better. So maybe we don't need as much medication as they actually prescribed."* (FG 1, SRA 5)

> *"I know my body, and I know by experience … At the beginning I wouldn't do it [self-adjust my medication) and I followed the instructions of the doctor and [it] got me really in a bad spot … But then [I felt] in control because now I learned how to manage my own body, right."* (FG 2, SRA 5)

Only a few participants who adjusted their medications discussed it with their clinicians, though most others expressed the desire to. Open and supportive communication with their care team also made these participants feel more secure in their dosage decisions and reinforced a sense of control over their own health.

"I think empowered and in control definitely applied later when [my doctor] started communicating with me and asking me what I wanted to do." (IDI 1, SRA 4)

"I feel in control because if [there is] something that's not right [when I take my medication differently] I know I can always pick up the phone and call the nurse and they'll send a message to my PA nurse, and they'll call me back. So, I can kind of govern my own self." (FG 2, SRA 5)

These narrated feelings and attitudes are synthesized in Figure 1.

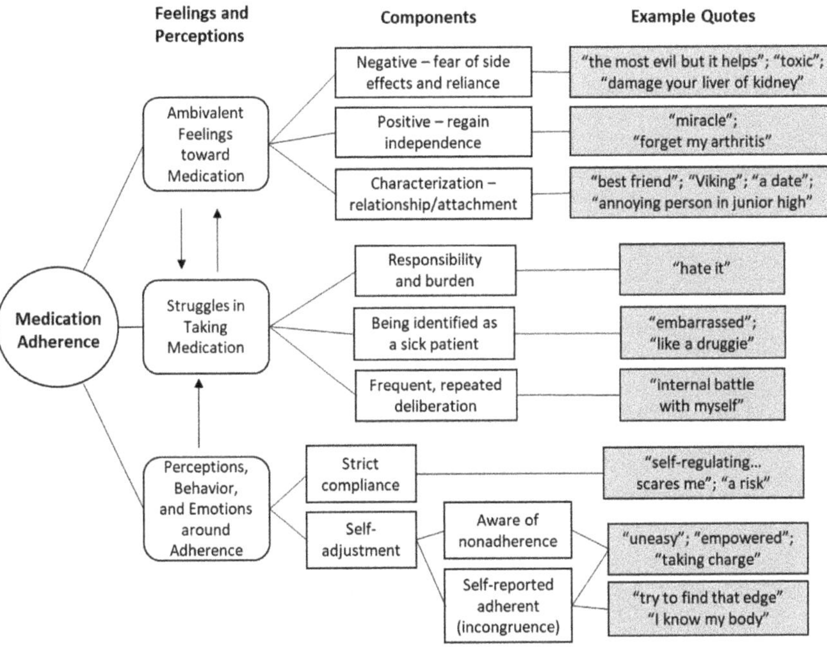

Figure 1. Emerged Themes of Medication Adherence from RA Patiens' Perspective.

4. Discussion

This study portrayed RA patients' perceptions and psychological processes concerning three key components of their medication-taking behavior to help inform personalized care. The qualitative methods illustrated the paradox in their feelings toward the medication as well as the views and decisions regarding the self-adjusting of their medication. While almost all participants expressed negative feelings about the RA medication itself and about taking the medication, they still relied on it for relief and were grateful for its effects, despite the annoyance, restraint, and lack of freedom medication can cause. These findings are in line with previous studies of patients with chronic diseases and reflect the balancing act patients often wrestle with when accepting and staying compliant with a treatment regimen [46–48]. The projective interview technique brought out additional sentiments and struggles that were intimate to RA patients but sparsely presented in the existing literature [41,42,49]. Participants' elaboration on their perspectives offered rich insights for evaluating medication acceptability and treatment fit beyond logistical and biological indicators.

Though discontinuation of a drug was uncommon (other than when switching medications), many participants adjusted their doses up or down if and when medications were not meeting their expectations, did not feel necessary, or had intolerable side effects. Research similarly has identified common concerns or complaints RA patients have when taking their medication [50–52]. Our study further pointed out the restlessness patients also have when not taking their medication, as well as the worry of other side effects from modifying the regimen, distinctive from the literature which predominantly discusses the negative view of side effects patients have when following prescriptions.

Such noncompliance was described even by participants who claimed to always be adherent. This highlights that all patients, even those with seemingly high medication acceptability or adherence rates, are at risk of intentionally deviating from prescriptions, calling for continual attention in personalized care. The evidence also helps explain the trend of overestimation in self-reporting compared to objective measures by biochemical level, pharmacy data, or monitoring devices [13,53–55]. The discrepancy in adherence rates or incongruency between perceptions and action in some cases may be due to different interpretations of adherence, in which the patients believed they were following the prescription, rather than due to recall bias or an attempt to appear compliant to please the provider or researchers.

Moreover, our observations exemplify how indefinite and constant the risk-benefit conflict is for patients as they had to decide if and how to adjust their dosages on a day-by-day basis depending on symptoms. Adherence programs should be tailored to address this thin balance and move towards more patient-centric interventions that not only elicit patients' input but also understand and allow the need for modifying dosage at varied times under clinician's guidance. Earlier studies have shown that an integrated, individualized approach is especially favorable for patients with changing needs due to unpredictable disease status such as Parkinson's and autoimmune diseases, including RA [56–59].

Having to take chronic medication in order to function encroached on independence and self-esteem, especially if a patient wanted to reduce or avoid a medication from his or her regimen but was too dependent on it for relief to act on that desire. On the other hand, having the ability to make adjustments based on feelings and experience with the treatment or disease restored a level of self-control that they felt they had lost as their lives became overwhelmed and defined by RA and medication [60]. The feelings of empowerment and confidence may have helped participants legitimize or even incentivized their deviating behavior. Our reporting of the possible self-rationalization or self-justification and dual-view about adjusting medication suggests valuable implications to address the issue. Future research could examine the relationships between patients' medication acceptability/tolerability, feeling of losing control, beliefs in the legitimacy or risk of modifying dosage, and changes in their adherence.

While many studies on adherence have discussed measurements and identified factors influencing patient behavior [23,46,51,52,60], we elucidated how adherence looks and feels when patients self-adjust their medication. It is important to note the complexity around the term "adherence" or "compliance" in RA research here. In contrast to other chronic diseases and though few of our participants reported it, some RA patients may be directed by their clinicians to self-adjust certain medications depending on their symptoms and side effects, blurring the line between what is considered adherent or nonadherent. Because of this complexity and variation in practice, asking RA patients whether they are adherent or taking their medications as prescribed may not sufficiently determine whether patients are accepting or appropriately using their medication. More research should be done to resolve and set a standard on how adherence is defined among RA patients. By all definitions, open discussion with patients about how they are taking their medication is crucial. Previous studies have demonstrated the benefits of patient-centered care and the association it has with empowerment and adherence [13,60–63]. Healthcare and research teams could explore ways to provide individual patients with appropriate parameters for adjusting or strategically managing treatment regimens as needed. Such practices could offer patients that sense of control and authority over their own bodies, while motivating long-term adherence.

The study is subject to limitations. The findings may not be generalizable to other patient populations given the relatively small sample size as well as the unique and fluctuating nature of RA disease activity. Additionally, there is a potential for bias in the focus groups as participants may change or withhold information in an effort to conform with the group. This limitation was mitigated by the seven in-depth interviews completed with single participants as the consistency of findings between the focus groups and interviews adds validity to our results. Future research could include interviews with physicians to discuss the appropriate adjustment of RA medications. Exploring physicians' perspectives and understanding of how patients' RA experiences impact adherence may also help customize care and interventions.

5. Conclusions

Shared decision making in healthcare suggests that physicians must understand the expectations and concerns patients have regarding their treatment [58,64,65]. Personalized care, at a higher level, requires continued attention to patients' experiences with the disease and medication as well as their needs and preferences in therapy. This is especially important to maintain with chronic patients and over time because, concurrent with other studies [23,66], we found that as participants became more experienced with taking their medications they were more confident in adjusting their treatment regimens. Understanding how patients view and act on their own nonadherence can better inform the complexity of this behavior and ways to prevent or address it. These findings offer a more holistic view of patients' attitudes towards adherence, considering the feelings that result from it in parallel with those that induce it. Considering the high portion of interventions with unsatisfactory results, future studies could design and assess the long-term effectiveness of programs aiming to empower patients early in the treatment process through honest discussions with clinicians in order to reduce nonadherence and achieve better disease management and outcomes.

Author Contributions: Conceptualization, P.T., R.T. and C.L.; methodology, P.T., L.B. and C.L.; data analysis, P.T., D.S., R.C., R.T. and C.L.; visualization, C.L.; writing—draft preparation, P.T., D.S. and C.L.; writing—revision, P.T., D.S., R.C., L.B., R.T. and C.L.; supervision, C.L. All authors have read and agreed to the published version of the manuscript.

Funding: This research was partially supported by Bass Connections, Duke University.

Institutional Review Board Statement: This research was approved by the Duke University Institutional Review Board. The study was conducted according to the guidelines of the Declaration of Helsinki.

Informed Consent Statement: Informed consent was obtained from all participants involved in the study.

Data Availability Statement: The portion of the transcript data pertaining to this paper are available from the corresponding author for one year from publication upon reasonable request with a methodologically sound proposal.

Acknowledgments: The authors want to thank their research teams' assistance during the data collection process, the participants' time and willingness to share their experiences, and The Link Group experts' support and advice on focus group and interview design and administration.

Conflicts of Interest: The authors declare no conflict of interest.

References

1. Scott, D.L.; Wolfe, F.; Huizinga, T.W. Rheumatoid Arthritis. *Lancet* **2010**, *376*, 1094–1108. [CrossRef]
2. Birch, J.T.; Bhattacharya, S. Emerging Trends in Diagnosis and Treatment of Rheumatoid Arthritis. *Prim. Care Clin. Off. Pract.* **2010**, *37*, 779–792. [CrossRef]
3. Ahlstrand, I.; Björk, M.; Thyberg, I.; Börsbo, B.; Falkmer, T. Pain and Daily Activities in Rheumatoid Arthritis. *Disabil. Rehabil.* **2012**, *34*, 1245–1253. [CrossRef]
4. Miagoux, Q.; Singh, V.; de Mézquita, D.; Chaudru, V.; Elati, M.; Petit-Teixeira, E.; Niarakis, A. Inference of an Integrative, Executable Network for Rheumatoid Arthritis Combining Data-Driven Machine Learning Approaches and a State-of-the-Art Mechanistic Disease Map. *J. Pers. Med.* **2021**, *11*, 785. [CrossRef]
5. Donahue, K.E.; Gartlehner, G.; Jonas, D.E.; Lux, L.J.; Thieda, P.; Jonas, B.L.; Hansen, R.A.; Morgan, L.C.; Lohr, K.N. Systematic Review: Comparative Effectiveness and Harms of Disease-Modifying Medications for Rheumatoid Arthritis. *Ann. Intern. Med.* **2008**, *148*, 124. [CrossRef]
6. Choy, E.H.S.; Smith, C.; Doré, C.J.; Scott, D.L. A Meta-Analysis of the Efficacy and Toxicity of Combining Disease-Modifying Anti-Rheumatic Drugs in Rheumatoid Arthritis Based on Patient Withdrawal. *Rheumatology* **2005**, *44*, 1414–1421. [CrossRef]
7. Aletaha, D.; Smolen, J.S. Diagnosis and Management of Rheumatoid Arthritis: A Review. *JAMA* **2018**, *320*, 1360–1372. [CrossRef] [PubMed]
8. Van den Bemt, B.J.; van Lankveld, W.G. How Can We Improve Adherence to Therapy by Patients with Rheumatoid Arthritis? *Nat. Clin. Pract. Rheumatol.* **2007**, *3*, 681. [CrossRef] [PubMed]
9. Van den Bemt, B.J.F.; van den Hoogen, F.H.J.; Benraad, B.; Hekster, Y.A.; van Riel, P.L.C.M.; van Lankveld, W. Adherence Rates and Associations with Nonadherence in Patients with Rheumatoid Arthritis Using Disease Modifying Antirheumatic Drugs. *J. Rheumatol.* **2009**, *36*, 2164–2170. [CrossRef]
10. Scheiman-Elazary, A.; Duan, L.; Shourt, C.; Agrawal, H.; Ellashof, D.; Cameron-Hay, M.; Furst, D.E. The Rate of Adherence to Antiarthritis Medications and Associated Factors among Patients with Rheumatoid Arthritis: A Systematic Literature Review and Metaanalysis. *J. Rheumatol.* **2016**, *43*, 512–523. [CrossRef]
11. Hovstadius, B.; Petersson, G. Non-Adherence to Drug Therapy and Drug Acquisition Costs in a National Population—A Patient-Based Register Study. *BMC Health Serv. Res.* **2011**, *11*, 326. [CrossRef]
12. Sabaté, E.; World Health Organization (Eds.) *Adherence to Long-Term Therapies: Evidence for Action*; World Health Organization: Geneva, Switzerland, 2003; ISBN 978-92-4-154599-0.
13. Costa, E.; Giardini, A.; Savin, M.; Menditto, E.; Lehane, E.; Laosa, O.; Pecorelli, S.; Monaco, A.; Marengoni, A. Interventional Tools to Improve Medication Adherence: Review of Literature. *Patient Prefer. Adherence* **2015**, *9*, 1303–1314. [CrossRef]
14. Anderson, L.J.; Nuckols, T.K.; Coles, C.; Le, M.M.; Schnipper, J.L.; Shane, R.; Jackevicius, C.; Lee, J.; Pevnick, J.M.; Members of the PHARM-DC Group. A Systematic Overview of Systematic Reviews Evaluating Medication Adherence Interventions. *Am. J. Health Syst. Pharm.* **2020**, *77*, 138–147. [CrossRef]
15. Pinho, S.; Cruz, M.; Ferreira, F.; Ramalho, A.; Sampaio, R. Improving Medication Adherence in Hypertensive Patients: A Scoping Review. *Prev. Med.* **2021**, *146*, 106467. [CrossRef]
16. Kvarnström, K.; Westerholm, A.; Airaksinen, M.; Liira, H. Factors Contributing to Medication Adherence in Patients with a Chronic Condition: A Scoping Review of Qualitative Research. *Pharmaceutics* **2021**, *13*, 1100. [CrossRef]
17. Kardas, P.; Lewek, P.; Matyjaszczyk, M. Determinants of Patient Adherence: A Review of Systematic Reviews. *Front. Pharmacol.* **2013**, *4*, 91. [CrossRef] [PubMed]
18. Hugtenburg, J.G.; Timmers, L.; Elders, P.J.; Vervloet, M.; van Dijk, L. Definitions, Variants, and Causes of Nonadherence with Medication: A Challenge for Tailored Interventions. *Patient Prefer. Adherence* **2013**, *7*, 675–682. [CrossRef] [PubMed]
19. Vrijens, B.; De Geest, S.; Hughes, D.A.; Przemyslaw, K.; Demonceau, J.; Ruppar, T.; Dobbels, F.; Fargher, E.; Morrison, V.; Lewek, P.; et al. A New Taxonomy for Describing and Defining Adherence to Medications. *Br. J. Clin. Pharmacol.* **2012**, *73*, 691–705. [CrossRef]
20. Salt, E.; Frazier, S.K. Adherence to Disease-Modifying Antirheumatic Drugs in Patients with Rheumatoid Arthritis: A Narrative Review of the Literature. *Orthop. Nurs.* **2010**, *29*, 260–275. [CrossRef]
21. Burmester, G.R.; Pope, J.E. Novel Treatment Strategies in Rheumatoid Arthritis. *Lancet* **2017**, *389*, 2338–2348. [CrossRef]
22. Villa-Hermosilla, M.-C.; Fernández-Carballido, A.; Hurtado, C.; Barcia, E.; Montejo, C.; Alonso, M.; Negro, S. Sulfasalazine Microparticles Targeting Macrophages for the Treatment of Inflammatory Diseases Affecting the Synovial Cavity. *Pharmaceutics* **2021**, *13*, 951. [CrossRef]
23. Pasma, A.; van 't Spijker, A.; Luime, J.J.; Walter, M.J.M.; Busschbach, J.J.V.; Hazes, J.M.W. Facilitators and Barriers to Adherence in the Initiation Phase of Disease-Modifying Antirheumatic Drug (DMARD) Use in Patients with Arthritis Who Recently Started Their First DMARD Treatment. *J. Rheumatol.* **2015**, *42*, 379–385. [CrossRef]
24. Harrold, L.R.; Briesacher, B.A.; Peterson, D.; Beard, A.; Madden, J.; Zhang, F.; Gurwitz, J.H.; Soumerai, S.B. Cost-Related Medication Nonadherence in Older Rheumatoid Arthritis Patients. *J. Rheumatol.* **2013**, *40*, 137–143. [CrossRef]
25. Clifford, S.; Barber, N.; Horne, R. Understanding Different Beliefs Held by Adherers, Unintentional Nonadherers, and Intentional Nonadherers: Application of the Necessity–Concerns Framework. *J. Psychosom. Res.* **2008**, *64*, 41–46. [CrossRef]

26. Zwikker, H.E.; van Dulmen, S.; den Broeder, A.A.; van den Bemt, B.J.; van den Ende, C.H. Perceived Need to Take Medication Is Associated with Medication Non-Adherence in Patients with Rheumatoid Arthritis. *Patient Prefer. Adherence* **2014**, *8*, 1635–1645. [CrossRef] [PubMed]

27. Kumar, K.; Raza, K.; Nightingale, P.; Horne, R.; Chapman, S.; Greenfield, S.; Gill, P. Determinants of Adherence to Disease Modifying Anti-Rheumatic Drugs in White British and South Asian Patients with Rheumatoid Arthritis: A Cross Sectional Study. *BMC Musculoskelet. Disord.* **2015**, *16*, 396. [CrossRef] [PubMed]

28. Quandt, S.A.; Arcury, T.A. Qualitative Methods in Arthritis Research: Overview and Data Collection. *Arthritis Rheum.* **1997**, *10*, 273–281. [CrossRef] [PubMed]

29. Kelly, A.; Tymms, K.; Fallon, K.; Sumpton, D.; Tugwell, P.; Tunnicliffe, D.; Tong, A. Qualitative Research in Rheumatology: An Overview of Methods and Contributions to Practice and Policy. *J. Rheumatol.* **2021**, *48*, 6–15. [CrossRef] [PubMed]

30. Bala, S.-V.; Samuelson, K.; Hagell, P.; Fridlund, B.; Forslind, K.; Svensson, B.; Thomé, B. Living with Persistent Rheumatoid Arthritis: A BARFOT Study. *J. Clin. Nurs.* **2017**, *26*, 2646–2656. [CrossRef] [PubMed]

31. Shaw, Y.; Metes, I.D.; Michaud, K.; Donohue, J.M.; Roberts, M.S.; Levesque, M.C.; Chang, J.C. Rheumatoid Arthritis Patients' Motivations for Accepting or Resisting Disease-Modifying Antirheumatic Drug Treatment Regimens. *Arthritis Care Res.* **2018**, *70*, 533–541. [CrossRef]

32. Shariff, Z.; Kirby, D.; Missaghi, S.; Rajabi-Siahboomi, A.; Maidment, I. Patient-Centric Medicine Design: Key Characteristics of Oral Solid Dosage Forms That Improve Adherence and Acceptance in Older People. *Pharmaceutics* **2020**, *12*, 905. [CrossRef] [PubMed]

33. Baumgartner, A.; Drame, K.; Geutjens, S.; Airaksinen, M. Does the Polypill Improve Patient Adherence Compared to Its Individual Formulations? A Systematic Review. *Pharmaceutics* **2020**, *12*, 190. [CrossRef] [PubMed]

34. Direito, R.; Rocha, J.; Sepodes, B.; Eduardo-Figueira, M. Phenolic Compounds Impact on Rheumatoid Arthritis, Inflammatory Bowel Disease and Microbiota Modulation. *Pharmaceutics* **2021**, *13*, 145. [CrossRef]

35. Ruiz, F.; Vallet, T.; Pensé-Lhéritier, A.; Aoussat, A. Standardized Method to Assess Medicines' Acceptability: Focus on Paediatric Population. *J. Pharm. Pharmacol.* **2017**, *69*, 406–416. [CrossRef]

36. Morisky, D.E.; Ang, A.; Krousel-Wood, M.; Ward, H.J. Predictive Validity of A Medication Adherence Measure in an Outpatient Setting. *J. Clin. Hypertens.* **2008**, *10*, 348–354. [CrossRef]

37. Carl, T. The Hill-Bone Scales. Available online: https://nursing.jhu.edu/faculty_research/research/projects/hill-bone/hill-bone-scales.html (accessed on 25 September 2021).

38. Hughes, L.D.; Done, J.; Young, A. A 5 Item Version of the Compliance Questionnaire for Rheumatology (CQR5) Successfully Identifies Low Adherence to DMARDs. *BMC Musculoskelet. Disord.* **2013**, *14*, 286. [CrossRef]

39. Lam, W.Y.; Fresco, P. Medication Adherence Measures: An Overview. *BioMed Res. Int.* **2015**, *2015*, e217047. [CrossRef]

40. Blatt, S.J. The Validity of Projective Techniques and Their Research and Clinical Contribution. *J. Pers. Assess.* **1975**, *39*, 327–343. [CrossRef]

41. Bell, J.E. *Projective Techniques: A Dynamic Approach to the Study of the Personality*; Longmans, Green & Co.: Oxford, UK, 1948.

42. Haire, M. Projective Techniques in Marketing Research. *J. Mark.* **1950**, *14*, 649–656. [CrossRef]

43. Mesías, F.J.; Escribano, M. Projective Techniques–Chapter 4. In *Methods in Consumer Research*; Ares, G., Varela, P., Eds.; Woodhead Publishing Series in Food Science, Technology and Nutrition; Woodhead Publishing: Sawston, UK, 2018; Volume 1, pp. 79–102. ISBN 978-0-08-102089-0.

44. Fereday, J.; Muir-Cochrane, E. Demonstrating Rigor Using Thematic Analysis: A Hybrid Approach of Inductive and Deductive Coding and Theme Development. *Int. J. Qual. Methods* **2006**, *5*, 80–92. [CrossRef]

45. Arcury, T.A.; Quandt, S.A. Qualitative Methods in Arthritis Research: Sampling and Data Analysis. *Arthritis Rheum.* **1998**, *11*, 66–74. [CrossRef] [PubMed]

46. Müller, R.; Kallikorm, R.; Põlluste, K.; Lember, M. Compliance with Treatment of Rheumatoid Arthritis. *Rheumatol. Int.* **2012**, *32*, 3131–3135. [CrossRef] [PubMed]

47. Carder, P.C.; Vuckovic, N.; Green, C.A. Negotiating Medications: Patient Perceptions of Long-Term Medication Use. *J. Clin. Pharm. Ther.* **2003**, *28*, 409–417. [CrossRef] [PubMed]

48. Popa-Lisseanu, M.G.G.; Greisinger, A.; Richardson, M.; O'Malley, K.J.; Janssen, N.M.; Marcus, D.M.; Tagore, J.; Suarez-Almazor, M.E. Determinants of Treatment Adherence in Ethnically Diverse, Economically Disadvantaged Patients with Rheumatic Disease. *J. Rheumatol.* **2005**, *32*, 913–919.

49. Jones, B.; Hunt, A.; Hewlett, S.; Harcourt, D.; Dures, E. Rheumatology Patients' Perceptions of Patient Activation and the Patient Activation Measure: A Qualitative Interview Study. *Musculoskeletal Care* **2021**. [CrossRef]

50. National Collaborating Centre for Primary Care. Patients' experience of medicine-taking. In *Medicines Adherence: Involving Patients in Decisions About Prescribed Medicines and Supporting Adherence*; Royal College of General Practitioners: London, UK, 2009.

51. Li, L.; Cui, Y.; Yin, R.; Chen, S.; Zhao, Q.; Chen, H.; Shen, B. Medication Adherence Has an Impact on Disease Activity in Rheumatoid Arthritis: A Systematic Review and Meta-Analysis. *Patient Prefer. Adherence* **2017**, *11*, 1343–1356. [CrossRef]

52. Salt, E.; Frazier, S.K. Predictors of Medication Adherence in Patients with Rheumatoid Arthritis. *Drug Dev. Res.* **2011**, *72*, 756–763. [CrossRef]

53. Shi, L.; Liu, J.; Koleva, Y.; Fonseca, V.; Kalsekar, A.; Pawaskar, M. Concordance of Adherence Measurement Using Self-Reported Adherence Questionnaires and Medication Monitoring Devices. *Pharmacoeconomics* **2010**, *28*, 1097–1107. [CrossRef]

54. Foley, L.; Larkin, J.; Lombard-Vance, R.; Murphy, A.W.; Hynes, L.; Galvin, E.; Molloy, G.J. Prevalence and Predictors of Medication Non-Adherence among People Living with Multimorbidity: A Systematic Review and Meta-Analysis. *BMJ Open* **2021**, *11*, e044987. [CrossRef]

55. Varallo, G.; Scarpina, F.; Giusti, E.M.; Suso-Ribera, C.; Cattivelli, R.; Guerrini Usubini, A.; Capodaglio, P.; Castelnuovo, G. The Role of Pain Catastrophizing and Pain Acceptance in Performance-Based and Self-Reported Physical Functioning in Individuals with Fibromyalgia and Obesity. *J. Pers. Med.* **2021**, *11*, 810. [CrossRef]

56. Van Munster, M.; Stümpel, J.; Thieken, F.; Pedrosa, D.J.; Antonini, A.; Côté, D.; Fabbri, M.; Ferreira, J.J.; Růžička, E.; Grimes, D.; et al. Moving towards Integrated and Personalized Care in Parkinson's Disease: A Framework Proposal for Training Parkinson Nurses. *J. Pers. Med.* **2021**, *11*, 623. [CrossRef]

57. Metta, V.; Batzu, L.; Leta, V.; Trivedi, D.; Powdleska, A.; Mridula, K.R.; Kukle, P.; Goyal, V.; Borgohain, R.; Chung-Faye, G.; et al. Parkinson's Disease: Personalized Pathway of Care for Device-Aided Therapies (DAT) and the Role of Continuous Objective Monitoring (COM) Using Wearable Sensors. *J. Pers. Med.* **2021**, *11*, 680. [CrossRef] [PubMed]

58. Taylor, P.C.; Betteridge, N.; Brown, T.M.; Woolcott, J.; Kivitz, A.J.; Zerbini, C.; Whalley, D.; Olayinka-Amao, O.; Chen, C.; Dahl, P.; et al. Treatment Mode Preferences in Rheumatoid Arthritis: Moving Toward Shared Decision-Making. *Patient Prefer. Adherence* **2020**, *14*, 119–131. [CrossRef]

59. De Belvis, A.G.; Pellegrino, R.; Castagna, C.; Morsella, A.; Pastorino, R.; Boccia, S. Success Factors and Barriers in Combining Personalized Medicine and Patient Centered Care in Breast Cancer. Results from a Systematic Review and Proposal of Conceptual Framework. *J. Pers. Med.* **2021**, *11*, 654. [CrossRef]

60. Lin, C.; Tu, R.; Bier, B.; Tu, P. Uncovering the Imprints of Chronic Disease on Patients' Lives and Self-Perceptions. *J. Pers. Med.* **2021**, *11*, 807. [CrossRef]

61. Castro, E.M.; Van Regenmortel, T.; Vanhaecht, K.; Sermeus, W.; Van Hecke, A. Patient Empowerment, Patient Participation and Patient-Centeredness in Hospital Care: A Concept Analysis Based on a Literature Review. *Patient Educ. Couns.* **2016**, *99*, 1923–1939. [CrossRef]

62. Bartkeviciute, B.; Lesauskaite, V.; Riklikiene, O. Individualized Health Care for Older Diabetes Patients from the Perspective of Health Professionals and Service Consumers. *J. Pers. Med.* **2021**, *11*, 608. [CrossRef] [PubMed]

63. Menditto, E.; Orlando, V.; De Rosa, G.; Minghetti, P.; Musazzi, U.M.; Cahir, C.; Kurczewska-Michalak, M.; Kardas, P.; Costa, E.; Sousa Lobo, J.M.; et al. Patient Centric Pharmaceutical Drug Product Design—The Impact on Medication Adherence. *Pharmaceutics* **2020**, *12*, 44. [CrossRef]

64. Taylor, P.; Manger, B.; Alvaro-Gracia, J.; Johnstone, R.; Gomez-Reino, J.; Eberhardt, E.; Wolfe, F.; Schwartzman, S.; Furfaro, N.; Kavanaugh, A. Patient Perceptions Concerning Pain Management in the Treatment of Rheumatoid Arthritis. *J. Int. Med. Res.* **2010**, *38*, 1213–1224. [CrossRef]

65. Elwyn, G.; Frosch, D.; Thomson, R.; Joseph-Williams, N.; Lloyd, A.; Kinnersley, P.; Cording, E.; Tomson, D.; Dodd, C.; Rollnick, S.; et al. Shared Decision Making: A Model for Clinical Practice. *J. Gen. Intern. Med.* **2012**, *27*, 1361–1367. [CrossRef] [PubMed]

66. Mathews, A.L.; Coleska, A.; Burns, P.B.; Chung, K.C. The Evolution of Patient Decision-Making Regarding Medical Treatment of Rheumatoid Arthritis. *Arthritis Care Res.* **2016**, *68*, 318–324. [CrossRef] [PubMed]

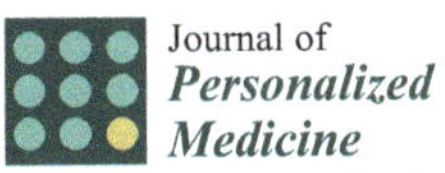

Journal of
Personalized
Medicine

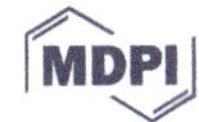

Review

Virtual Reality-Based Therapy Reduces the Disabling Impact of Fibromyalgia Syndrome in Women: Systematic Review with Meta-Analysis of Randomized Controlled Trials

Irene Cortés-Pérez [1,2], Noelia Zagalaz-Anula [2], María del Rocío Ibancos-Losada [2], Francisco Antonio Nieto-Escámez [3,4], Esteban Obrero-Gaitán [2,*] and María Catalina Osuna-Pérez [2]

[1] Granada Northeast Health District, Andalusian Health Service, Street San Miguel 2, 18500 Guadix, Spain; icp00011@red.ujaen.es
[2] Department of Health Sciences, University of Jaén, Campus Las Lagunillas s/n, 23071 Jaén, Spain; nzagalaz@ujaen.es (N.Z.-A.); mril0001@red.ujaen.es (M.d.R.I.-L.); mcosuna@ujaen.es (M.C.O.-P.)
[3] Department of Psychology, University of Almería, Ctra. Sacramento s/n, 04120 Almería, Spain; pnieto@ual.es
[4] Center for Neuropsychological Assessment and Rehabilitation (CERNEP), Ctra. Sacramento s/n, 04120 Almeria, Spain
* Correspondence: eobrero@ujaen.es; Tel.: +34-953212918

Citation: Cortés-Pérez, I.; Zagalaz-Anula, N.; Ibancos-Losada, M.d.R.; Nieto-Escámez, F.A.; Obrero-Gaitán, E.; Osuna-Pérez, M.C. Virtual Reality-Based Therapy Reduces the Disabling Impact of Fibromyalgia Syndrome in Women: Systematic Review with Meta-Analysis of Randomized Controlled Trials. *J. Pers. Med.* **2021**, *11*, 1167. https://doi.org/10.3390/jpm11111167

Academic Editors: Fábio G. Teixeira, Catarina Godinho and Júlio Belo Fernandes

Received: 18 October 2021
Accepted: 6 November 2021
Published: 9 November 2021

Publisher's Note: MDPI stays neutral with regard to jurisdictional claims in published maps and institutional affiliations.

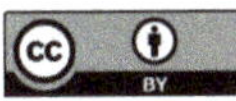

Abstract: Background: Virtual reality-based therapy (VRBT) is a novel therapeutic approach to be used in women with fibromyalgia syndrome (FMS). The aim of our study is to assess the effect of VRBT to reduce the impact of FMS in outcomes such as pain, dynamic balance, aerobic capacity, fatigue, quality of life (QoL), anxiety and depression. Methods: Systematic review with meta-analysis was conducted from a bibliographic search in PubMed, Scopus, PEDro, Web of Science and CINAHL until April 2021 in accordance with PRISMA guidelines. We included randomized controlled trials (RCTs) that compare VRBT versus others to assess the mentioned outcomes in women with FMS. Effect size was calculated with standardized mean difference (SMD) and its 95% confidence interval (95% CI). Results: Eleven RCTs involving 535 women with FMS were included. Using the PEDro scale, the mean methodological quality of the included studies was moderate (6.63 ± 0.51). Our findings showed an effect of VRBT on the impact of FMS (SMD −0.62, 95% CI −0.93 to −0.31); pain (SMD −0.45, 95% CI −0.69 to −0.21); dynamic balance (SMD −0.76, 95% CI −1.12 to −0.39); aerobic capacity (SMD 0.32, 95% CI 0.004 to 0.63); fatigue (SMD −0.58, 95% CI −1.02 to −0.14); QoL (SMD 0.55, 95% CI 0.3 to 0.81); anxiety (SMD −0.47, 95% CI −0.91 to −0.03) and depression (SMD −0.46, 95% CI −0.76 to −0.16). Conclusions: VRBT is an effective therapy that reduces the impact of FMS, pain, fatigue, anxiety and depression and increases dynamic balance, aerobic capacity and quality of life in women with FMS. In addition, VRBT in combination with CTBTE showed a large effect in reducing the impact of FMS and fatigue and increasing QoL in these women.

Keywords: fibromyalgia; virtual reality; physiotherapy; pain; fatigue; quality of life; meta-analysis

1. Introduction

Fibromyalgia syndrome (FMS) is a chronic disease of unknown etiology that courses with generalized and diffuse non-inflammatory pain and hyperalgesia in different human body points [1]. Other FMS symptoms are joint stiffness [2], generalized fatigue [3], impaired balance [4], anxiety and depression [5], and emotional overload [6] that reduces functional capacity [7] personal autonomy, social relationships [8] and quality of life (QoL) [9,10]. The global prevalence of FMS ranges between 2% and 8% of the population [11], mainly affects women (61–90%) [12] aged 50 years and over [13] and involve a large consumption of social and health resources [14]. The negative impact of FMS has turned FMS into a public health problem that requires the search for a therapeutic approach to reduce the negative impact of FMS symptoms [15].

Although the pathogenesis of FMS is unknown, the mechanisms responsible for dysfunctional pain in FMS, without having identifiable tissue lesions, are mainly related to disorders of the central nervous system (CNS) that may explain diffuse musculoskeletal pain [16]. Several studies have reported numerous changes in the brain cortex and spinal cord descending tracts (i.e., descending pain modulatory system) in patients with FMS producing central sensitization (CS) [17] and deficits in pain inhibitory mechanisms [18]. Several studies have shown that patients with FMS present hyperactivity and hyperexcitability of their CNS, suggesting that it is supported by continuous nociceptive peripheral inputs [19]. Recent neuroimaging and biochemical studies have shown a reduction in serotonin (5HT) and noradrenalin (NA) in cerebrospinal fluid [20] that may support continuous and widespread pain in FMS due to dysfunction in the descending inhibitory systems [21]. In addition, the activity of the insula lobe was shown to increase, producing higher levels of the neurotransmitter glutamate in the posterior insula, which has been associated with chronic pain [22]. Studies have reported evidence regarding peripheral neurogenic inflammation in patients with FMS, compared to healthy subjects, due to the presence of different proinflammatory peptides from the nerve terminals of peptidergic C-fibers, including substance P, calcitonin gene-related protein and neurokinin A [22], all of which are related to vasodilatation and an increase in vascular permeability responsible for maintaining pain in FMS [23].

In recent years, numerous therapeutic proposals have been implemented in an attempt to reduce the symptoms and the impact of FMS [14]. In addition to pharmacotherapy, conservative non-pharmacological interventions based on physiotherapy, conventional therapy (CT), or physical exercise are another modality in the treatment of FMS [24]. Recent studies have highlighted active physical training as an effective therapy to improve balance [25], pain [26], muscle fatigue [27], anxiety [28] and QoL [29], among others, in patients with FMS. However, with the aim to get an increasing in the effect of CT, new technologies have been used. For example, virtual reality-based therapy (VRBT) has experienced growth as a method for physical and cognitive training, showing benefits in different contexts [30]. Virtual reality (VR) technology enables patients to be included in a virtual environment similar to the real world through a computer and interact with it [31]. Immersive VR (iVR) uses headsets to display 3D digital images at 360° that simulate any scenario with high realism, allowing patients to interact with this virtual environment using a hand controller or their own hands [32]. Non-immersive VR (niVR) is considered more accessible and inexpensive than iVR and enables patients to visualize virtual environments in 2D projected onto a screen and interact with them through the use of a mouse, keyboard or joysticks [33,34]. VRBT is considered a useful intervention along with CT for neurological [35] or musculoskeletal disorders [36] that can be used at home, thereby favoring patient accessibility to physiotherapy protocols (telephysiotherapy), which has been especially important during the COVID-19 pandemic [37].

The usability and feasibility of VRBT in CT protocols with promising results in the management of pain, anxiety or mood states have been shown [38]. For example, in patients with FMS, VRBT has allowed specific, intensive, multisensory and active therapies with quick feedback in different environments and situations to be performed that increased the motivation of the patient [39] and adherence to the therapy [40]. However, the absence of a systematic review (SR) that unifies the available knowledge on the use and effects of VRBT in patients with FMS may limit the impact of VRBT use. Therefore, the aim of our research is to assess the effect of virtual reality-based therapy (VRBT) reduce the disabling impact of fibromyalgia syndrome (FMS). In addition, to know if the effect shown by VRBT is greater when VRBT is used alone or in combination with other therapies on FMS.

2. Materials and Methods

2.1. Protocol Design

This systematic review is reported in accordance with the preferred reporting items for systematic reviews and meta-analyses (PRISMA) statement [41] and it was, previously registered in PROSPERO: CRD42021225635.

2.2. Search Strategy and Data Sources

Two authors (I.C.-P. and M.C.O.-P.), independently, performed a bibliographical search in PubMed Medline, Web of Science (WOS), Scopus, CINAHL Complete and PEDro (Physiotherapy Evidence Database) to select articles published up to April 2021. The authors reviewed the reference lists from retrieved full-text studies and previously published grey literature, expert documents and congress abstracts. Based on Medical Subjects Headings (MeSH) the keywords used in the search strategy were "fibromyalgia", "virtual reality" and "virtual reality exposure therapy" with its synonyms. Based on the particular database, the Boolean operators "AND"/"OR" were used to combine the keywords and entry terms, according to PICOS tool of Cochrane Collaboration [42], for the retrieval of reports of randomized controlled trials (RCTs). Language and publication date filters were not used. A third expertise author (E.O.-G.) revised the bibliographic search and resolved doubts. Table 1 shows the search strategy used in each database.

Table 1. Search strategy used in each database.

Databases	Search Strategy
PubMed Medline	(fibromyalgia[mh] OR fibromyalgia[tiab] OR fibromyalgia syndrome[tiab] OR fibromyalgia*[tiab] OR chronic, fatigue syndrome[tiab]) AND (virtual reality[mh] OR virtual reality[tiab] OR virtual reality exposure therapy[mh] OR virtual reality exposure therapy[tiab] OR exergam*)
Web of Science	TOPIC: (*fibromyalgia* OR *chronic, fatigue syndrome*) AND TOPIC: (*virtual reality* OR *exergame*)
SCOPUS	(TITLE-ABS-KEY ("fibromyalgia" OR "fibromyalgia syndrome" OR "chronic fatigue syndrome") AND TITLE-ABS-KEY ("virtual reality" OR "exercises" OR "videogames"))
PEDro	Fibromyalgia AND virtual reality Fibromyalgia AND exergames
CINAHL Complete	AB (fibromyalgia OR fibromyalgia syndrome OR chronic fatigue syndrome) AND AB (virtual reality OR exergames OR videogames)

2.3. Study Selection and Inclusion Criteria

Two blinded reviewers (N.Z.-A. and F.A.N.-E.), independently, screened the titles and abstracts of all references retrieved in each database. When one of these authors selected an article during the inclusion phase based on the title and abstract, it was examined in detail. All disagreements were resolved by a third author (M.C.O.-P.). A study was included in the present SR when it met all the following inclusion criteria: (1) RCTS or RCT pilot study; (2) comprised by women with FMS; (3) with at least two groups; (4) of which one group received VRBT; (5) compared with controls; (6) and reported quantitative data of different outcomes related with FMS impact (see Section 2.5). The exclusion criteria that were established included (1) experimental studies without a comparison group and (2) studies comprising patients with a variety of musculoskeletal disorders (i.e., not only FMS).

2.4. Data Extraction

Two authors (I.C.-P. and E.O.-G.) independently collected data from the included studies in a standardized Microsoft Excel data-collection form. To resolve disagreements, a third author was consulted (M.C.O.-P.). We extracted the following data: (1) overall characteristics of the study (authorship and publication date, study design, number of groups, total sample size and time since FMS diagnosis); (2) characteristics of the intervention and control groups (number of participants, mean age, sex, body mass index, intervention and duration of the intervention in weeks, number of sessions per week and duration of each session in minutes); (3) data related to the post-intervention outcomes (outcomes assessed, mean and SD of each outcome in each study and group); and (4) evaluation time sequence (right at the end of the therapy or follow-period). When a study did not provide statistics appropriate for performing the meta-analysis, we extracted the median, standard error, range or interquartile range to be transformed into a SD [42].

2.5. Outcomes

The main outcome assessed in this SR was the impact of FMS, which was assessed in patients with FMS after receiving VRBT in comparison to other interventions (such as conventional therapy-based therapeutic exercise (CTBTE) or stretching [ST]) or no intervention (NI). The Fibromyalgia Impact Questionnaire (FIQ) was selected to assess the impact of FMS in the selected studies. In addition, other variables assessed in this SR were pain, dynamic balance, aerobic capacity, fatigue, QoL, anxiety and depression. Different assessments examining the same outcome were grouped together for analysis (see results of meta-analyses section).

2.6. Risk of Bias and Methodological Quality Assessment

The PEDro Scale was used to assess the risk of bias of the included studies [43]. The PEDro Scale comprised 11 items with two answer options ("yes" if the criterion was clearly satisfied and "no" if the criterion was not satisfied) [44]. The total score could vary across a range from 0 (high risk of bias) to 10 (low risk of bias), and item 1 was not used for its relationship with external validity [45].

The Grading of Recommendations Assessment, Development, and Evaluation (GRADE) assessment [46] was used to analyze the quality evidence of the findings. This scale assesses the risk of bias in each study, inconsistency, indirectness, precision and the risk of publication bias. All these items, except the risk of bias, were assessed using the GRADE checklist of Meader et al. (2014) [47] Inconsistency was assessed based on heterogeneity level [48]; precision was assessed through the number of participants per study (large > 300 participants, moderate 300–100 participants and low < 100 participants) and with the number of studies included (large >10 studies, moderate 10–5 studies and low < 5 studies) [46]; and indirect evidence was considered to exist in those articles in which the results were indirectly measured and was scored as "yes" or "no". Risk of publication bias is explained in statistical analysis Section 2.7.

Two authors (N.Z.-A. and M.d.R.I.-L.) independently assessed the risk of bias, and quality evidence and doubts related to this assessment were resolved in consultation with a third researcher (M.C.O.-P.). The quality evidence of each meta-analysis was downgraded from high quality by one level for each factor that was found. In the case of the presence of several limitations, the overall quality level was downgraded by two levels. Finally, the level of evidence in each meta-analysis was categorized as (1) high: the findings are robust; (2) moderate: it is possible that new research may change our results; (3) low; the level of confidence in our pooled effect is very slight; or (4) very low: any estimate of effect is very uncertain.

2.7. Statistical Analysis

Two authors (E.O.-G. and I.C.-P.) carried out the meta-analysis using Comprehensive Meta-Analysis version 3.0 (Biostat, Englewood, NJ, USA) [49]. Meta-analysis was conducted only if an outcome measure was provided by at least two studies. To perform the meta-analysis, we followed the recommendations of Cooper et al. (2009) [50] and to estimate the effect of VRBT, Cohen's standardized mean difference (SMD) [51] and its 95% confidence interval (95% CI) in a random effects model proposed by DerSimonian and Laird [52] were used. Cohen's SMD can be interpreted as one of four effect strength levels:

no effect (SMD 0), small (SMD 0.2–0.4), medium (SMD 0.4–0.7) and large (SMD > 0.8) [53]. In addition, when an outcome was assessed with the same test, we calculated the mean difference (MD) with the aim of comparing our results to the minimal clinically important difference (MCID) value for each assessed outcome. The pooled effect of each meta-analysis is displayed using forest plots [54]. The risk of publication bias was assessed through the visualization of symmetric (low risk) or asymmetric (high risk) funnel plots [55] using Egger's test (where if the p-value < 0.1, there exists a risk of publication bias) [56]. In addition, the trim-and-fill method was used to estimate the adjusted SMD, taking into account any possible risk of publication bias [57]. Based on Rothman's recommendations for the effect size variation limit in the assessment of confusion bias, when the adjusted SMD varied more than 10% with respect to the original and raw pooled effects, the quality level of evidence was downgraded one level, although the funnel plot was slightly asymmetrical [58]. Finally, the level of heterogeneity was assessed with the Q-test and the degree of inconsistency (I^2) from Higgins et al. [48]. Heterogeneity may be present when the p-value < 0.1, and it can be categorized as low ($I^2 < 25\%$), moderate (I^2 between 25–50%) or large ($I^2 > 50\%$) [59,60].

2.8. Additional Analyses

To assess the effect of the use of VRBT alone or combined with CTBTE on the impact of FMS, we performed a subgroup analysis (VRBT + CTBTE vs. CTBTE or VRBT vs. NI) using data from RCTs. In addition, a sensitivity analysis was performed using the leave-one-out method [42,50] that shows how each individual study affected the overall estimate based on the remaining studies. Finally, a qualitative synthesis was carried out for those variables that did not report data that could be meta-analyzed but were analyzed in the studies included in the review.

3. Results
3.1. Study Selection

The PRISMA flow chart (Figure 1) displays the study selection process. One hundred forty-nine records were retrieved from the initial bibliographical search (145 from databases and 4 in others additional sources). Seventy-five studies were excluded for duplication, and 74 references were initially screened by title and abstract. Ten studies were removed based on title/abstract, and 53 studies did not meet the inclusion criteria. Finally, 11 RCTs [61–71] were included. Specifically, 10 RCTs [61,62,64–71] were included in the quantitative synthesis, and 2 RCTs [63,67] were included in the qualitative synthesis. One RCT [67] provided information for quantitative and qualitative synthesis.

3.2. Characteristics of the Studies Included in the Review

All included RCTs were carried out between 2015 and 2021 (2015 [65], 2017 [62,64], 2019 [63,68,70,71], 2020 [61,66,67] and 2021 [69]) in Spain [62–65,67,68,70,71], Turkey [66,69] and Brazil [61]. The included studies reported data from 535 participants with FMS (100% women) with a mean age of 51.11 ± 4.2 years old, a mean BMI of 27.27 ± 1.6 kg/m^2 and a mean duration of FMS symptoms of 10.49 ± 5.4 years. Two hundred seventy-nine women (51.68 ± 3.9 years old) were in the experimental intervention groups receiving VRBT, and 256 participants (50.54 ± 4.6 years old) were in the control intervention groups. In the experimental group, 10 RCTs used non-immersive VRBT [61–65,67–71] and 1 RCT [66] used immersive VRBT. In addition, VRBT was used alone in 9 RCTs [61–65,67,68,70,71] and in combination with CTBTE in another 2 RCTs [66,69]. Regarding the control groups, in 2 RCTs, women received CTBTE (aerobic exercise [69] and Pilates therapy [66]); in one RCT [61], women received ST; and in 8 RCTs [62–65,67,68,70,71] participants did not receive any therapy. The duration of VRBT in weeks was heterogeneous at 3 [65], 7 [61], 8 [62,64,66,69] and 24 weeks [63,67,68,70,71]; the number of sessions per week was 2 [62–68,70,71] and 3 [61,69] and finally, the duration of each session in minutes was 60 min [61,62,64,65,67,68,70,71], 35 min [69] or 80 min [66]. All assessments were carried out to the end of the intervention. Table 2 shows the characteristics of the studies included in this SR.

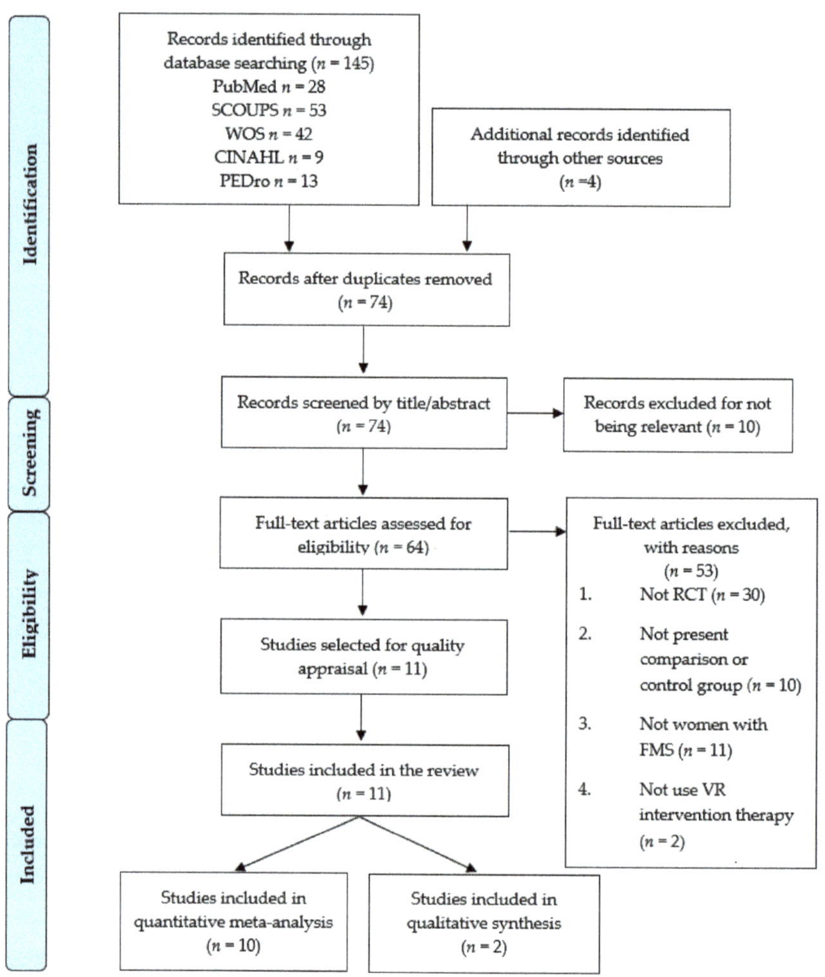

Figure 1. Preferred reporting items for systematic reviews and meta-analyses (PRISMA) flow chart for the systematic literature search and study selection process. Note: One study (León-Llamas, JL et al. 2020) [67] provided information for quantitative and qualitative synthesis.

3.3. Risk of Bias Assessment of the Studies Included in the Review

The risk of bias scores for 7 RCTs [61–64,68,70,71] were obtained on the PEDro website, and for four RCTs [65–67,69] it was assessed manually. All included RCTs obtained a score of at least 5 points. The mean PEDro score was 6.63 ± 0.51 points. The impossibility of blinding the participants and the therapist and participants' concealed allocation were the items involved in the high risk of bias. Table 3 shows the PEDro assessment.

Table 2. Characteristics of the studies included in the review.

Authorship and Date	Country	K	N	N_e	Age	BMI	Evol. Years	Type	Weeks	Ses/WeekMin	N_c	Age	BMI	Evol. Years	Type Control	Variable	Test	Follow-Up
					Experimental Group							**Control Group**					**Outcomes**	
				Sample Characteristics				**Intervention Characteristics**				**Sample Characteristics**						
Collado-Mateo, D. et al., 2017a [62]	Spain	6	76	41	52.52	25.79	9.6	ni VRBT	8	2	60	35	52.47	27.75	11.02	NI	FMS Impact	FIQ	Inm. Effect
																	Quality of Life	EuroQol-5D	
																	Fatigue	FIQ-Fatigue	
																	Pain	FIQ-Pain	
																	Anx/Dep	VAS	
Collado-Mateo, D. et al., 2017b [64]	Spain	1	76	41	52.43	25.79	10.36	ni VRBT	8	2	60	35	52.58	27.75	12.48	NI	Dynamic Balance	TGUGT	Inm. Effect
García-Palacios, A. et al., 2015 [65]	Spain	4	59	30	50.48	NR	9.32	ni VRBT	3	2	60	29	50.48	NR	9.32	NI	FMS Impact	FIQ	Inm. Effect
																	Quality of Life	QLI-SP	
																	Pain	BPI	
																	Depression	BDI-II	
Gulsen, C. et al., 2020 [66]	Turkey	5	16	8	46.5	26.81	4	iVRBT + CTBTE	8	2	80	8	38.5	22.85	4	CTBTE	FMS Impact	FIQ	Inm. Effect
																	Pain	VAS	
																	Fatigue	FSS	
																	Aerobic capacity	6-MWT	
																	Quality of Life	SF-36	

Table 2. *Cont.*

| | | | | Experimental Group | | | | | | | | | Control Group | | | | | Outcomes | | |
| | | | | Sample Characteristics | | | | Intervention Characteristics | | | | | Sample Characteristics | | | | | | | |
Authorship and Date	Country	K	N	N_e	Age	BMI	Evol. Years	Type	Weeks	Ses/WeekMin		N_c	Age	BMI	Evol. Years	Type Control	Variable	Test	Follow-Up
León-Llamas, J.L. et al., 2020 [67]	Spain	1/ QS	50	25	54	27	8.5	ni VRBT	24	2	60	25	53	28.5	11	NI	Aerobic capacity	PVO$_2$	Inm. Effect
Martín-Martínez, J.P. et al., 2019 [68]	Spain	1	55	28	54.04	27.36	19.2	ni VRBT	24	2	60	27	53.41	28.84	16.76	NI	Dynamic Balance	TGUGT	Inm. Effect
Polat, M. et al., 2021 [69]	Turkey	7	40	20	42.6	26.6	1.5	ni VRBT + CTBTE	8	3	35	20	47	27.9	1.4	CTBTE	FMS Impact	FIQ	Inm. Effect
																	Aerobic capacity	6-MWT	
																	Pain	VAS	
																	Fatigue	FSS	
																	Quality of Life	EQ-5D-5L	
																	Anx/Dep	HADS-A/-D	
Silva de Carvalho, M. et al., 2020 [61]	Brasil	4	21	11	55.64	30.28	9.91	ni VRBT	7	3	60	10	47.7	26.09	14.65	ST	FMS Impact	FIQ	Inm. Effect
																	Aerobic capacity	6-MWT	
																	Fatigue	FIQ-Fatigue	
																	Pain	FIQ-Pain	

Table 2. *Cont.*

Authorship and Date	Country	K	N	Ne	Age	BMI	Evol. Years	Type	Weeks	Ses/WeekMin	Nc	Age	BMI	Evol. Years	Type Control	Variable	Test	Follow-Up
				Experimental Group								**Control Group**				**Outcomes**		
				Sample Characteristics				Intervention Characteristics				Sample Characteristics						
Villafaina, S. et al., 2019a [63]	Spain	2	55	28	54.04	27.36	19.2	ni VRBT	24	2	60	27	53.41	28.84	16.74	NI	Pain	VAS	Inm. Effect
																	Quality of Life	EQ-5D-5L	
Villafaina, S. et al., 2019b [70]	Spain	3	37	22	54.27	27.1	NR	ni VRBT	24	2	60	15	53.44	28.19	NR	NI	FMS Impact	FIQ	Inm. Effect
																	Dynamic Balance	TGUGT	
																	Aerobic capacity	6-MWT	
Villafaina, S. et al., 2019c [71]	Spain	QS	50	25	52	NR	16	ni VRBT	24	2	60	25	54	NR	16	NI	Brain Dynamics	EEG Signals	Inm. Effect

Abbreviations: K, Number of comparisons provided; N, total sample size; Ne, experimental group sample size; BMI, body mass index; Evol, evolution; Ses, sSessions; Min, minutes; Nc, control group sample size; niVRBT, non-immersive virtual reality; iVR, immersive virtual reality; CTBTEM, conventional therapy based virtual training; ST, stretching exercise; FMS, fibromyalgia syndrome; FIQ, Fibromyalgia Impact Questionnaire; Anx, anxiety; Dep, depression; VAS, Visual Analogue Scale; TGUGT, Timed Get Up and Go Test; QLI-SP, Quality of Life Index; BPI, Brief Pain Inventory; BDI-II, Beck Depression Inventory II; FSS, Fatigue Severity Scale; EQ-5D-5L, The Euro Quality of Life Five Dimensions; HADS, Hospital Anxiety and Depression Scale-Anxiety Dimension; HADS-D, Hospital Anxiety and Depression Scale-Depression Dimension; EEG Signals, electroencephalographic signals.

Table 3. Methodological quality and risk of bias (PEDro Scores) of the studies included in the review.

Items Authorship	1	2	3	4	5	6	7	8	9	10	11	TOTAL
Collado-Mateo, D. et al., 2017a [62]	N	Y	N	Y	N	N	Y	Y	Y	Y	Y	7
Collado-Mateo, D. et al., 2017b [64]	Y	Y	Y	Y	N	N	Y	Y	N	Y	Y	7
García-Palacios, A. et al., 2015 [65]	Y	Y	N	Y	N	N	Y	Y	Y	Y	Y	7
Gulsen, C. et al. 2020 [66]	Y	Y	N	Y	N	N	N	Y	Y	Y	Y	6
León-Llamas, J.L. et al., 2020 [67]	Y	Y	N	Y	N	N	Y	Y	Y	Y	Y	7
Martín-Martínez, J.P. et al., 2019 [68]	Y	Y	N	Y	N	N	Y	Y	Y	Y	Y	7
Polat, M. et al., 2021 [69]	Y	Y	N	Y	N	N	Y	Y	Y	Y	Y	7
Silva de Carvalho, M. et al., 2020 [61]	Y	Y	N	Y	N	N	Y	N	Y	Y	Y	6
Villafaina, S. et al., 2019a [63]	Y	Y	N	Y	N	N	Y	Y	Y	Y	Y	7
Villafaina, S. et al., 2019b [70]	Y	Y	N	Y	N	N	Y	N	Y	Y	Y	6
Villafaina, S. et al., 2019c [71]	Y	Y	N	N	N	N	Y	Y	Y	Y	Y	6

Abbreviations: 1 = eligibility criteria, 2 = random allocation, 3 = concealed allocation, 4 = baseline comparability, 5 = blind subjects, 6 = blind therapists, 7 = blind assessors = 8, adequate follow-up, 9 = intention-to-treat analysis, 10 = between-group comparisons, 11 = point estimates and variability, Note = eligibility criteria item does not contribute to total score, Y = Yes, N = No.

3.4. Quantitative Synthesis

Ten RCTs [61,62,64–71] with 34 independent comparisons providing data for 485 women with FMS (50.92 ± 4.4 years old, mean BMI of 27.27 ± 1.59 kg/m^2 and a mean duration of symptoms of 10.49 years) were included in the quantitative synthesis. Table 4 shows the main findings of each meta-analysis.

3.4.1. Impact of FMS Symptoms

Six RCTs [61,62,65,66,69,71] provided data from 249 women with FMS (49.3 ± 5.06 years old), in which the impact of FMS was assessed using the FIQ-total score. Moderate-quality evidence suggested a medium effect of VRBT on FIQ scores (SMD −0.62, 95% CI −0.93 to −0.31; $p < 0.001$) (Figure 2) showing a reduction of FIQ of −9.96 (95% CI −13.64 to −6.28) compared to control, favored VRBT. No risk of publication bias (Egger $p = 0.9$) or heterogeneity (I^2 5.18%) were found. Sensitivity analysis did not reported variation.

Subgroup analysis showed a reduction in FIQ scores favors VRBT (MD −9.01, 95% CI −14.13 to −3.88) compared to NI and in the combined use of VRBT + CTBTE (MD −9.86, 95% CI −17.65 to −2.06) in comparison to CTBTE, with low- and very low-quality evidence, respectively.

Table 4. Main findings in meta-analyses.

Outcomes				Summary of Findings								Quality of Evidence (Grade)					
			Pooled Effect Het				Publication Bias										
									Trim and Fill								
	K	N	N_s	SMD	95% CI	I^2 (p for Q-test)	Funnel Plot (p for Egger)	Adj SMD	% of Var	Risk of Bias	Incons	Indirect	Imprec	Pub. Bias	Quality
Impact of FMS Symptoms	6	249	41.5	−0.62	−0.93 to −0.31	5.2% ($p = 0.4$)	Sym ($p = 0.9$)	−0.62	0%	Medium	No	No	Yes	No	Moderate
Pain	6	267	44.5	−0.45	−0.69 to −0.21	0% ($p = 0.52$)	Asym ($p = 0.2$)	−0.72	28%	Medium	No	No	Yes	Yes	Low
Dynamic Balance	3	168	56	−0.76	−1.12 to −0.39	4.4% ($p = 0.35$)	Sym ($p = 0.52$)	−0.75	0%	Medium	No	No	Yes	No	Low
Aerobic Capacity	5	164	32.8	0.32	0.004 to 0.63	0% ($p = 0.57$)	Asym ($p = 0.31$)	0.36	12%	Medium	No	No	Yes	Yes	Low
Fatigue	4	153	38.5	−0.58	−1.02 to −0.14	5.4% ($p = 0.37$)	Asym ($p = 0.09$)	−0.48	20%	Medium	No	No	Yes	Yes	Low
Quality of Life	5	246	49.2	0.55	0.3 to 0.81	0% ($p = 0.73$)	Sym ($p = 0.9$)	0.52	0%	Medium	No	No	Yes	No	Moderate
Anxiety	3	137	45.7	−0.47	−0.91 to −0.03	0% ($p = 0.32$)	Asym ($p =0.2$)	−0.57	22%	Medium	No	No	Yes	Yes	Very-Low
Depression	4	196	49	−0.46	−0.76 to −0.16	4.6% ($p = 0.4$)	Asym ($p =0.14$)	−0.52	13%	Medium	No	No	Yes	Yes	Low

Abbreviations: GRADE = grading of recommendations assessment, development, and evaluation, Het = heterogeneity, K = number of comparisons, N = total sample size, Ns = Participants per study, SMD = Cohen's standardized mean difference, 95% CI = 95% confidence interval, I^2 = degree of inconsistency p = p-value; Adj = adjusted, % of var = percentage of variation, Indirect = indirectness, Imprec = imprecision, Pub bias = publication bias, Sym = symmetric, Asym = asymmetric.

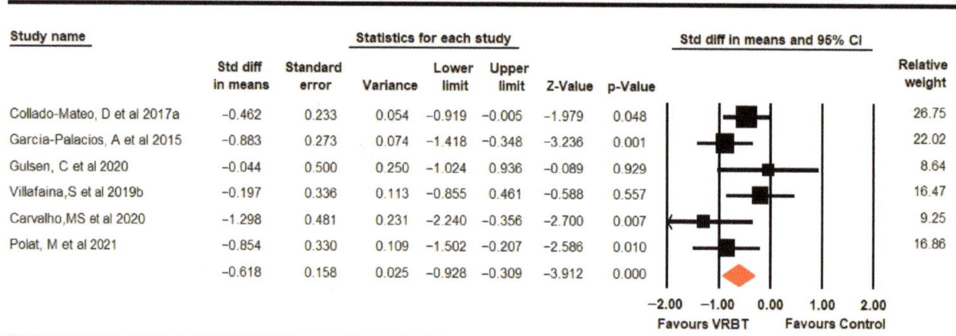

Study name	Std diff in means	Standard error	Variance	Lower limit	Upper limit	Z-Value	p-Value	Relative weight
Collado-Mateo, D et al 2017a	−0.462	0.233	0.054	−0.919	−0.005	−1.979	0.048	26.75
Garcia-Palacios, A et al 2015	−0.883	0.273	0.074	−1.418	−0.348	−3.236	0.001	22.02
Gulsen, C et al 2020	−0.044	0.500	0.250	−1.024	0.936	−0.089	0.929	8.64
Villafaina,S et al 2019b	−0.197	0.336	0.113	−0.855	0.461	−0.588	0.557	16.47
Carvalho,MS et al 2020	−1.298	0.481	0.231	−2.240	−0.356	−2.700	0.007	9.25
Polat, M et al 2021	−0.854	0.330	0.109	−1.502	−0.207	−2.586	0.010	16.86
	−0.618	0.158	0.025	−0.928	−0.309	−3.912	0.000	

Figure 2. Forest plot of the effect of virtual reality-based therapy from the Fibromyalgia Impact Questionnaire.

3.4.2. Pain

Six RCTs [61,62,65,66,69,70] provided data on 267 women with FMS (49.28 ± 5.04 years old) using the VAS, the pain dimension on the FIQ and the Brief Pain Inventory (BPI). Low-quality evidence showed a moderate effect of VRBT (SMD −0.45, 95% CI −0.69 to −0.21; p < 0.001) compared to controls (Figure 3). The risk of publication bias may be considered (Egger p = 0.2 and trim-and-fill variation of 28%) without heterogeneity (I^2 0%). Sensitivity analysis showed a variation of 17% when Collado-Mateo [62] was removed.

Study name	Std diff in means	Standard error	Variance	Lower limit	Upper limit	Z-Value	p-Value	Relative weight
Collado-Mateo, D et al 2017a	−0.653	0.236	0.056	−1.115	−0.190	−2.763	0.006	27.71
Garcia-Palacios, A et al 2015	−0.173	0.261	0.068	−0.685	0.338	−0.664	0.507	22.70
Gulsen, C et al 2020 (2)	−0.227	0.502	0.252	−1.210	0.756	−0.453	0.650	6.14
Villafaina, S et al 2019a	−0.556	0.275	0.076	−1.095	−0.017	−2.022	0.043	20.45
Carvalho, MS et al 2020	−0.437	0.442	0.195	−1.304	0.429	−0.989	0.322	7.91
Polat, M et al 2021	−0.438	0.320	0.102	−1.065	0.189	−1.368	0.171	15.09
	−0.448	0.124	0.015	−0.692	−0.205	−3.607	0.000	

Figure 3. Forest plot of the effect of virtual reality-based therapy on pain.

Subgroup analysis showed low-quality evidence of a medium effect of VRBT in comparison with NI (SMD −0.64, 95% CI −1.18 to −0.11), favored VRBT.

3.4.3. Dynamic Balance

Three RCTs [64,68,71] reported data from 168 women with FMS (53.36 ± 0.74 years old), which assessed dynamic balance using the Timed Get Up and Go Test (TGUGT) and the 10-Step Chair Test (SCT). Low-quality evidence of a medium-high effect of VRBT (SMD −0.76, 95% CI −1.12 to −0.39; p < 0.001) on dynamic balance in comparison with NI was found (Figure 4). No risk of publication bias (Egger p = 0.52) and low heterogeneity were present (I^2 4.35%). There was an estimated variation of 20% with respect to the original SMD when Villafaina was excluded [71]. In this outcome, subgroup analysis was not performed due to lack of studies for other comparisons.

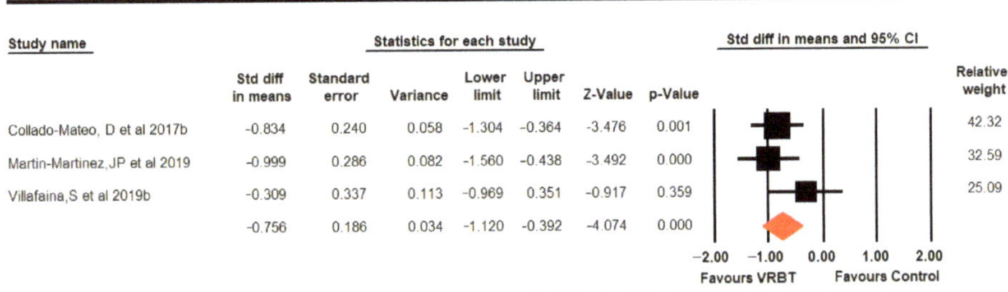

Figure 4. Forest plot of the effect of virtual reality-based therapy on dynamic balance.

3.4.4. Aerobic Capacity

Five RCTs [61,66,67,69,71] provided data from 164 women with FMS (49.26 ± 5.72 years old) to assess aerobic capacity with the 6-minute walk test (6-MWT) and oxygen volume partial pressure (PVO$_2$). Low-quality evidence of a small effect of VRBT (SMD 0.32, 95% CI 0.004 to 0.63; p = 0.047) on aerobic capacity was shown compared to other therapies or NI (Figure 5) without heterogeneity (I^2 0%). The risk of publication bias was low (Egger p = 0.31 and trim-and-fill variation of 12%). Sensitivity analysis showed a variation of 41% with respect to the original pooled effect when excluding Polat [69].

Study name	Std diff in means	Standard error	Variance	Lower limit	Upper limit	Z-Value	p-Value		Relative weight
Gulsen, C et al 2020	−0.130	0.501	0.251	−1.111	0.851	−0.261	0.794		10.03
Leon-Llamas,JL et al 2020	0.233	0.284	0.081	−0.323	0.790	0.822	0.411		31.19
Villafaina,S et al 2019b	0.133	0.335	0.112	−0.524	0.790	0.397	0.691		22.36
Carvalho,MS et al 2020	0.400	0.441	0.195	−0.465	1.265	0.906	0.365		12.90
Polat, M et al 2021	0.739	0.327	0.107	0.099	1.380	2.262	0.024		23.52
	0.315	0.159	0.025	0.004	0.626	1.986	0.047		

−2.00 −1.00 0.00 1.00 2.00
Favours Others   Favours VRBT

Figure 5. Forest plot of the effect of virtual reality-based therapy on aerobic capacity.

Subgroup analysis was performed for the comparison VRBT vs. NI, without find statistical significant between therapies (SMD 0.18; 95% CI −0.17 to 0.54; p = 0.31).

3.4.5. Fatigue

Four RCTs [61,62,66,69] reported data from 153 women with FMS (47.86 ± 5.62 years old) that assessed fatigue through the FIQ fatigue domain and Fatigue Severity Scale (FSS). Low-quality evidence showed a medium effect of VRBT (SMD −0.58, 95% CI −1.02 to −0.14; p = 0.01) on fatigue compared with other interventions or NI (Figure 6) with low heterogeneity (I^2 5.4%). Risk of publication bias was present (Egger p = 0.09 and variation of 20% with the trim-and-fill method). Sensitivity analysis showed a variation of 31% when excluding Polat [69].

Subgroup analysis showed low-quality evidence of a reduction in fatigue (MD −2.21 95% CI −4.33 to −0.1) when VRBT was used in combination with CTBTE compared to CTBTE alone, favored VRBT intervention.

3.4.6. Quality of Life

Five RCTs [62,65,66,69,70] provided data from 246 women with FMS (48.8 ± 5.1 years old) that assessed QoL with the EuroQol-5D, QoL Index and SF-36. Moderate-quality evidence of a medium effect of VRBT (SMD 0.55, 95% CI 0.3 to 0.81; p < 0.001) on QoL was shown in comparison to CTBTE or NI (Figure 7). No risk of publication bias or heterogeneity was found (I^2 0%). Sensitivity analysis did not show variation.

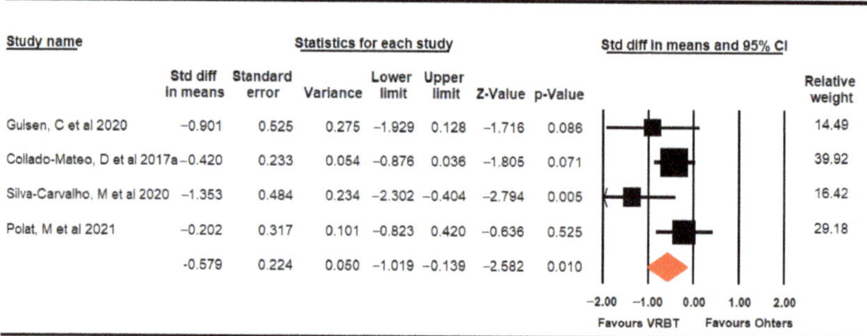

Study name	Std diff in means	Standard error	Variance	Lower limit	Upper limit	Z-Value	p-Value		Relative weight
Gulsen, C et al 2020	−0.901	0.525	0.275	−1.929	0.128	−1.716	0.086		14.49
Collado-Mateo, D et al 2017a	−0.420	0.233	0.054	−0.876	0.036	−1.805	0.071		39.92
Silva-Carvalho, M et al 2020	−1.353	0.484	0.234	−2.302	−0.404	−2.794	0.005		16.42
Polat, M et al 2021	−0.202	0.317	0.101	−0.823	0.420	−0.636	0.525		29.18
	−0.579	0.224	0.050	−1.019	−0.139	−2.582	0.010		

Favours VRBT — Favours Ohters

Figure 6. Forest plot of the effect of virtual reality-based therapy on fatigue.

Study name	Std diff in means	Standard error	Variance	Lower limit	Upper limit	Z-Value	p-Value		Relative weight
Collado-Mateo, D et al 2017a	0.572	0.235	0.055	0.112	1.032	2.437	0.015		30.90
Polat, M et al 2021	0.785	0.328	0.108	0.141	1.428	2.391	0.017		15.81
Garcia-Palacios, A et al 2015	0.610	0.266	0.071	0.088	1.132	2.291	0.022		24.00
Gulsen, C et at 2020	0.359	0.504	0.254	−0.629	1.347	0.713	0.476		6.70
Villafaina, S et al 2019a	0.367	0.275	0.075	−0.171	0.905	1.337	0.181		22.58
	0.554	0.131	0.017	0.299	0.810	4.248	0.000		

Favours Others — Favours VRBT

Figure 7. Forest plot of the effect of virtual reality-based therapy on quality of life.

Subgroup analysis showed a medium effect (SMD 0.48, 95% CI 0.19 to 0.78) of VRBT and VRBT + CTBTE (SMD 0.66, 95% CI 0.12 to 1.2) compared to NI and CTBTE, respectively, with low-quality evidence.

3.4.7. Anxiety and Depression

Anxiety was assessed in 3 RCTs [61,62,69] that provided data from 137 women with FMS (49.65 ± 4.74 years old) using the FIQ anxiety domain and Hospital Anxiety and Depression Scale, anxiety dimension (HADS-A). Very low-quality evidence of a medium effect of VRBT (SMD −0.47, 95% CI −0.91 to −0.03; p = 0.037) in comparison to other interventions or NI (Figure 8) without heterogeneity (I^2 0%) and with a possible risk of publication bias (trim-and-fill variation of 22%). Sensitivity analysis showed a variation of 36% when excluding Polat [69]. In this outcome, subgroup analysis was not performed due to lack of studies for other comparisons (only one study was included per specific comparison).

Four RCTs [61,62,65,69] provided data from 196 women with FMS (49.86 ± 4.02 years old) in which depression was assessed using the FIQ depression domain, HADS depression dimension and Beck Depression Inventory (BDI-II). Low-quality evidence of a medium effect of VRBT (SMD −0.46, 95% CI −0.76 to −0.16; p = 0.003) was shown compared to other interventions or NI (Figure 9). A possible risk of publication bias would be considered due to a variation of 13% with the trim-and-fill method (Egger p = 0.14) and low heterogeneity (I^2 4.59%). Sensitivity analysis displayed a variation of 19% with respect to the original pooled effect when Silva-Carvalho was excluded [61]. A subgroup analysis could only be performed in the comparison VRBT vs. NI, showing a medium effect (SMD −0.56; 95% CI −0.97 to 0.15; *p* = 0.008).

Study name	Std diff in means	Standard error	Variance	Lower limit	Upper limit	Z-Value	p-Value		Relative weight
Collado-Mateo, D et al 2017a	−0.558	0.235	0.055	−1.017	−0.098	−2.377	0.017		47.56
Silva-Carvalho, MS et al 2020	−0.964	0.462	0.213	−1.869	−0.059	−2.088	0.037		19.08
Polat, M et al 2021	−0.059	0.316	0.100	−0.679	0.561	−0.187	0.852		33.36
	−0.469	0.224	0.050	−0.908	−0.029	−2.089	0.037		

Figure 8. Forest plot of the effect of virtual reality-based therapy on anxiety.

Study name	Std diff in means	Standard error	Variance	Lower limit	Upper limit	Z-Value	p-Value		Relative weight
Collado-Mateo, D et al 2017a	−0.386	0.232	0.054	−0.841	0.069	−1.661	0.097		37.88
Silva-Carvalho, MS et al 2020	−1.281	0.480	0.230	−2.220	−0.341	−2.671	0.008		9.97
Polat, M et al 2021	−0.390	0.319	0.102	−1.015	0.236	−1.221	0.222		21.49
Garcia-Palacios, A et al 2015	−0.337	0.262	0.069	−0.851	0.177	−1.286	0.198		30.65
	−0.461	0.154	0.024	−0.764	−0.158	−2.986	0.003		

Figure 9. Forest plot of the effect of virtual reality-based therapy on depression.

3.5. Qualitative Synthesis

Two RCTs [63,67] assessed changes in brain structures but did not report data appropriate for performing a meta-analysis, so a qualitative synthesis was made. León-Llamas, J.L. et al., 2020 [67] evaluated the effects of VRBT on grey matter volume in different brain structures in 50 women with FMS through magnetic resonance imaging (MRI). Significant relationships (*p* < 0.05) between PVO2 and the left and right regions of the hippocampus and the left and right regions of the amygdala were found with VRBT compared to NI. Villafaina, S. et al., 2019a [63] evaluated the effects of VRBT on resting brain dynamics in 55 women with FMS. Significant differences in measured electroencephalographic (EEG) signals were found in some frontal, parietal, temporal and occipital areas (*p* < 0.05) in the VRBT group. VRBT was more effective in the group with a shorter duration of symptoms, showing between-group differences in some frontal and temporal areas.

4. Discussion

FMS is a chronic disease characterized by widespread muscle pain that reduces functional capability and QoL. In addition to other therapies, such as pharmacotherapy [72], balneotherapy [73] or physical exercise [74,75], VRBT has emerged as a new therapy that can reduce the impact of FMS symptoms. The present study proposed to compile the scientific evidence published to date to analyze the effectiveness of VRBT on the impact of FMS and in other related outcomes.

One of the most important impairments of FMS is its impact on ADLs, which is mainly assessed with the FIQ [76]. Our results suggested that VRBT is effective to reduce the impact of FMS symptoms on ADLs. The significant decrease in FIQ scores (approximately 10% of the total score both with VRBT alone or combined with CTBTE) would be related to the fact that VRBT is an active therapy that requires continuous body movements, which can combine the effect of multisensory stimulation and physical exercise. VRBT is considered a positive, different and motivating experience that directly impacts well-being and reduces the perception of the severity of symptoms. These results support the fact that VRBT may be considered a real therapeutic option to reduce the impact of FMS. In addition, subgroup analysis according to specific comparisons, showed that to VRBT is better than or NI (also called, UC) and the combined use of VRBRT with CTBTE is better that to perform only CTBTE. Between these two comparisons, VRBT with CTBTE is the best therapeutic option to improve the FIQ in women with FMS. It can allow personalize therapies combining different VR videogames and CTBTE protocols adapted for each women with FMS.

Some studies have suggested that VRBT is a novel approach in the field of orthopedic rehabilitation [77], in the management of acute or chronic pain [78] and in neuropathic pain control [79], among others. Our findings showed that VRBT could be effective as a non-pharmacological alternative intervention to reduce pain in women with FMS. Subgroup analysis revealed that in comparison with UC, VRBT is effective to reduces the pain level. The high levels of body pain that patients with FMS suffer from are supported by CS, which can be enhanced or maintained by supraspinal processes involving cognitions and focused attention on the sensation of pain [80]. It has been described that emotions that are directly connected to the limbic system can modulate pain through descending pathways [81]. To interact with VRBT as a method of distraction in which many neurophysiological connections occur between the visual and somatosensory systems might divert attention, leading to a slower response to incoming pain signals [78,81]. Likewise, a pleasant playful experience would lead to positive emotions capable of improving endogenous nociceptive inhibition. The continuous pain experience in patients with FMS produces muscle debility that together with negative emotions when moving can favor the appearance of kinesiophobia that reduces active movement and muscle tone, thereby increasing fatigue and pain [82]. VRBT requires autonomous movement of different body parts that can increase muscle tone and the perception of pain-free movement favoring the elimination of restrictions to movement included in the cerebral body scheme due to continued pain. Performing CTBTE through VR devices could provide greater adherence by using exercises adapted to different levels of progression. VR-based exercises could be more enjoyable and stimulating, facilitating implementation in subjects with FMS who have difficulty adhering to CTBTE.

Balance disorders appear in women with FMS, increasing the risk of falls [4]. A recent meta-analysis showed that women with FMS develop balance disorders [83] resulting in a high risk of falls. Some studies have found a reduction in brain grey matter in which vestibular, visual and somatosensory information is processed and integrated to produce a balanced response [84]. For this, it is necessary to implement therapies that provide the patient with multisensory stimulation at the same time that the patients are forced to actively work. Our results suggested that VRBT improves dynamic balance in subjects with FMS. VRBT is an active therapy that requires engaging in physical activities during the sessions, and the findings obtained were similar to those in different reviews that assessed the effects of physical exercise or Tai Chi to increase the balance in FMS women [25,85]. According to Villafaina, S. et al., 2019 [63], VRBT produces changes in different brain areas and increases the grey matter and EEG signals in the frontal, parietal, temporal and occipital lobes, some of which are responsible for integrating the balance information needed to respond to a destabilizing stimulus or Earth's gravitational force. The continued and active work in the standing position with a high level of multisensory stimulation by VR devices improve the neuromuscular efferent responses to maintain balance. Finally, some patients with FMS take anxiety and depression drugs, such as antipsychotics, that can increase the risk of falls [86]. VRBT includes virtual physical exercise to improve muscle tone, postural afferences and neuromotor responses to an antigravitational stimulus, reducing the risk of falls.

Women with FMS reported a decreased aerobic capacity, which could have a negative impact on functional capacity and consequently on QoL. Our findings showed an improvement in aerobic capacity in women who were exposed to VRBT. VRBT could provide the training of representative tasks included in ADLs that require less muscle strength and allow individuals to perform the activity for longer periods of time, which increases the cardiorespiratory fitness of these patients [7].

Generalized fatigue induces a sedentary lifestyle in women with FMS, which reduces aerobic capacity [87]. For this reason, women with FMS can perceive higher levels of fatigue during the performance of ADLs. Our results suggested that VRBT is useful for reducing fatigue in women with FMS, and there was a greater effect when combined with exercise. Our results are in line with a recent review in which VRBT has been postulated to be an effective method to reduce fatigue in different groups of patients [88]. In recent years, numerous therapies have emerged for the treatment of fatigue in FMS; however, the provided evidence has not been sufficient to unify criteria regarding the most appropriate treatment [89]. In this sense, VRBT may be an effective therapy to reduce fatigue because it is a customized method that increases distraction and prevents patients from being aware of fatigue.

In our study, we report that QoL improves after to use of VRBT. Restoring and balancing physical activity is a challenge in patients with FMS and chronic pain. Low mood, pain, and fatigue decrease the willingness to perform ADLs, causing low motivation and a poor sense of self-efficacy and QoL. Recent studies have shown that VRBT improves mood states, positive emotions, motivation, and self-efficacy in FMS patients [39], which should have a positive impact on QoL. A recent review postulated that the regulation of emotions through VRBT could be an effective method to increase QoL and personal well-being [90]. In addition, several studies have analyzed the efficacy of VRBT in combination with other therapies on QoL in different pathologies, such as rheumatic and orthopedic diseases, finding beneficial effects [77].

Our results showed that the levels of anxiety and depression improved after the use of VRBT in women with FMS, although a major effect was found on depression outcomes. Physical exercise in FMS patients has previously been shown to improve anxiety [91] and depression [92]. In recent years, VRBT has been considered a new and cost-effective tool to complement psychological treatments [93]. Our findings are consistent with a recent meta-analysis that assessed the effect of VRBT on anxiety and depression, finding a reduction in anxiety and depression after the application of VRBT in comparison to control conditions (e.g., waitlist, placebo, relaxation or NI) [94].

One study included in our review found significant relationships between pVO_2 and the left and right regions of the hippocampus and the left and right regions of the amygdala after training with VRBT [67]. These findings may be in line with the results of a study that analyzed neural activity and respiratory frequency in anticipation of anxiety. The activation of this area participates in the enhancement of respiratory frequency. Electric current sources were found in the left amygdala in the most anxious subjects [95]. The authors pointed out the need to study the relationship between the aerobic system and the amygdala, since women with FMS constitute a population associated with anxiety symptoms [96,97]. Findings from Villafaina, S et al. 2019 [63] indicated that VRBT can produce changes in the dynamics of the brain that could be related to an increase in cerebral blood flow. These results are particularly relevant to FMS patients because they frequently have altered cerebral blood flow variability and velocity [98,99], as well as impaired cognitive function [100]. Thus, VRBT in FMS patients could increase cerebral blood flow and, consequently, cognitive function. Additionally, the intervention in this study was more effective in the group with a shorter duration of symptoms, showing between-group differences in some frontal and temporal areas. Previous studies have shown that a longer duration of FMS symptoms predicts lower FIQ scores, which shows that patients who have suffered from FMS symptoms for short periods of time may be more severely affected by the disease [101]. These results suggested that VRBT could counteract severe FMS symptoms.

Our results may be considered to have some limitations. First, the low number of studies included may make generalization of our findings difficult. Related with the generalization of our findings a limitation is that our findings are applied to women with an age that varied between 38 and 55 years old (mean of 51.4 years old) and BMI between 25 to 28 (mean of 27.7). It would be important to perform new studies in all groups of age. Second, the impossibility of blinding the therapy to participants increased the risk of selection bias. Third, it is important to consider the possible risk of publication bias that may have reduced the reported effects of therapy. Another limitation was the low number of participants per study, which reduced the precision level of our findings. Besides, it is important to highlight that the large variations in sensitivity analysis may have affected the quality of our findings. Finally, it is important to remark that all studies were performed in Spain, Turkey or Brazil and it can affect to the generalization of our findings. It would be necessary to perform studies in more countries to increase the application of our findings.

5. Conclusions

This is the first SR with meta-analysis that demonstrates the effect of VRBT in women with FMS in reducing the health impact of symptoms of FMS, in short-term follow up. Our results showed an effect of VRBT in comparison to other interventions or NI and favored VRBT intervention based on the impact of FMS, pain, dynamic balance, aerobic capacity, fatigue, QoL, anxiety and depression. In addition, when VRBT was combined with CTBTE and compared to CTBTE alone, our findings showed a large effect of VRBT + CTBTE intervention on the measures of the impact of FMS fatigue and QoL. However, it is necessary to conduct further research on this topic, while increasing the sample size and extending the assessments to the long term.

Author Contributions: Conceptualization, I.C.-P., E.O.-G. and M.C.O.-P.; Methodology, E.O.-G., M.C.O.-P., N.Z.-A. and F.A.N.-E.; Data Curation, I.C.-P., E.O.-G., N.Z.-A. and F.A.N.-E.; Methodological Quality Assessment, N.Z.-A. and M.d.R.I.-L.; Software, I.C.-P. and E.O.-G.; Writing—Original Draft Preparation, I.C.-P., E.O.-G. and M.C.O.-P.; Supervision: M.d.R.I.-L., N.Z.-A. and F.A.N.-E.; Visualization: I.C.-P., E.O.-G., M.C.O.-P., M.d.R.I.-L., N.Z.-A. and F.A.N.-E.; Writing—Review and Editing: I.C.-P., E.O.-G., M.C.O.-P. and N.Z.-A.; Project Administration: M.C.O.-P. All authors have read and agreed to the published version of the manuscript.

Funding: This research received no external funding.

Institutional Review Board Statement: Not applicable.

Informed Consent Statement: Not applicable.

Conflicts of Interest: The authors declare no conflict of interest.

References

1. Wolfe, F.; Clauw, D.J.; Fitzcharles, M.-A.; Goldenberg, D.L.; Katz, R.S.; Mease, P.; Russell, A.S.; Russell, I.J.; Winfield, J.B.; Yunus, M.B. The American College of Rheumatology Preliminary Diagnostic Criteria for Fibromyalgia and Measurement of Symptom Severity. *Arthritis Rheum.* **2010**, *62*, 600–610. [CrossRef] [PubMed]
2. Lomas-Vega, R.; Rodríguez-Almagro, D.; Peinado-Rubia, A.B.; Zagalaz-Anula, N.; Molina, F.; Obrero-Gaitán, E.; Ibáñez-Vera, A.J.; Osuna-Pérez, M.C. Joint Assessment of Equilibrium and Neuromotor Function: A Validation Study in Patients with Fibromyalgia. *Diagnostics* **2020**, *10*, 1057. [CrossRef]
3. Montoro, C.I.; del Paso, G.A.R.; Duschek, S. Alexithymia in fibromyalgia syndrome. *Pers. Individ. Differ.* **2016**, *102*, 170–179. [CrossRef]
4. Peinado-Rubia, A.; Osuna-Pérez, M.C.; Rodríguez-Almagro, D.; Zagalaz-Anula, N.; López-Ruiz, M.C.; Lomas-Vega, R. Impaired Balance in Patients with Fibromyalgia Syndrome: Predictors of the Impact of This Disorder and Balance Confidence. *Int. J. Environ. Res. Public Health* **2020**, *17*, 3160. [CrossRef]
5. Sechi, C.; Lucarelli, L.; Vismara, L. Depressive Symptoms and Quality of Life in a Sample of Italian Women with a Diagnosis of Fibromyalgia: The Role of Attachment Styles. *Depress. Res. Treat.* **2021**, *2021*, 5529032. [CrossRef]
6. Kaleycheva, N.; Cullen, A.E.; Evans, R.; Harris, T.; Nicholson, T.; Chalder, T. The role of lifetime stressors in adult fibromyalgia: Systematic review and meta-analysis of case-control studies. *Psychol. Med.* **2021**, *51*, 177–193. [CrossRef]

7. Gaudreault, N.; Boulay, P. Cardiorespiratory fitness among adults with fibromyalgia. *Breathe* **2018**, *14*, e25–e33. [CrossRef]
8. Sechi, C.; Vismara, L.; Brennstuhl, M.J.; Tarquinio, C.; Lucarelli, L. Adult attachment styles, self-esteem, and quality of life in women with fibromyalgia. *Health Psychol. Open* **2020**, *7*, 2055102920947921. [CrossRef]
9. Offenbaecher, M.; Kohls, N.; Ewert, T.; Sigl, C.; Hieblinger, R.; Toussaint, L.L.; Sirois, F.; Hirsch, J.; Vallejo, M.A.; Kramer, S.; et al. Pain is not the major determinant of quality of life in fibromyalgia: Results from a retrospective "real world" data analysis of fibromyalgia patients. *Rheumatol. Int.* **2021**, *41*, 1995–2006. [CrossRef] [PubMed]
10. MacDougall, P. In fibromyalgia, some therapies may provide small improvements in pain and quality of life. *Ann. Intern. Med.* **2021**, *174*, JC32. [CrossRef] [PubMed]
11. Clauw, D.J. Fibromyalgia: A clinical review. *JAMA* **2014**, *311*, 1547–1555. [CrossRef] [PubMed]
12. Wolfe, F.; Walitt, B.; Perrot, S.; Rasker, J.J.; Häuser, W. Fibromyalgia diagnosis and biased assessment: Sex, prevalence and bias. *PLoS ONE* **2018**, *13*, e0203755. [CrossRef]
13. Queiroz, L.P. Worldwide Epidemiology of Fibromyalgia. *Curr. Pain Headache Rep.* **2013**, *17*, 356. [CrossRef] [PubMed]
14. Okifuji, A.; Hare, B.D. Management of Fibromyalgia Syndrome: Review of Evidence. *Pain Ther.* **2013**, *2*, 87–104. [CrossRef] [PubMed]
15. Cabral, C.M.N.; Miyamoto, G.C.; Franco, K.F.M.; Bosmans, J.E. Economic evaluations of educational, physical, and psychological treatments for fibromyalgia. *Pain* **2021**, *162*, 2331–2345. [CrossRef] [PubMed]
16. Casas-Barragán, A.; Molina, F.; Tapia-Haro, R.M.; García-Ríos, M.C.; Correa-Rodríguez, M.; Aguilar-Ferrándiz, M.E. Association of core body temperature and peripheral blood flow of the hands with pain intensity, pressure pain hypersensitivity, central sensitization, and fibromyalgia symptoms. *Ther. Adv. Chronic Dis.* **2021**, *12*, 2040622321997253. [CrossRef]
17. Rehm, S.; Sachau, J.; Hellriegel, J.; Forstenpointner, J.; Jacobsen, H.B.; Harten, P.; Gierthmühlen, J.; Baron, R. Pain matters for central sensitization: Sensory and psychological parameters in patients with fibromyalgia syndrome. *PAIN Rep.* **2021**, *6*, e901. [CrossRef]
18. Pidal-Miranda, M.; González-Villar, A.J.; Carrillo-De-La-Peña, M.T. Pain Expressions and Inhibitory Control in Patients with Fibromyalgia: Behavioral and Neural Correlates. *Front. Behav. Neurosci.* **2019**, *12*, 323. [CrossRef]
19. Russell, I.J.; Larson, A.A. Neurophysiopathogenesis of Fibromyalgia Syndrome: A Unified Hypothesis. *Rheum. Dis. Clin. North Am.* **2009**, *35*, 421–435. [CrossRef]
20. Harte, S.E.; Harris, R.E.; Clauw, D.J. The neurobiology of central sensitization. *J. Appl. Biobehav. Res.* **2018**, *23*, e12137. [CrossRef]
21. Uygur-Kucukseymen, E.; Castelo-Branco, L.; Pacheco-Barrios, K.; Luna-Cuadros, M.A.; Cardenas, A.; Giannoni-Luza, S.; Zeng, H.; Gianlorenco, A.C.; Gnoatto-Medeiros, M.; Shaikh, E.S.; et al. Decreased neural inhibitory state in fibromyalgia pain: A cross-sectional study. *Neurophysiol. Clin. Neurophysiol.* **2020**, *50*, 279–288. [CrossRef] [PubMed]
22. Littlejohn, G.; Guymer, E. Neurogenic inflammation in fibromyalgia. *Semin. Immunopathol.* **2018**, *40*, 291–300. [CrossRef] [PubMed]
23. Chiu, I.; Von Hehn, C.A.; Woolf, C.J. Neurogenic inflammation and the peripheral nervous system in host defense and immunopathology. *Nat. Neurosci.* **2012**, *15*, 1063–1067. [CrossRef]
24. Macfarlane, G.J.; Kronisch, C.; Dean, L.; Atzeni, F.; Häuser, W.; Flüß, E.; Choy, E.; Kosek, E.; Amris, K.; Branco, J.; et al. EULAR revised recommendations for the management of fibromyalgia. *Ann. Rheum. Dis.* **2016**, *76*, 318–328. [CrossRef] [PubMed]
25. Del-Moral-García, M.; Obrero-Gaitán, E.; Rodríguez-Almagro, D.; Rodríguez-Huguet, M.; Osuna-Pérez, M.C.; Lomas-Vega, R. Effectiveness of Active Therapy-Based Training to Improve the Balance in Patients with Fibromyalgia: A Systematic Review with Meta-Analysis. *J. Clin. Med.* **2020**, *9*, 3771. [CrossRef]
26. Sosa-Reina, M.D.; Nunez-Nagy, S.; Gallego-Izquierdo, T.; Pecos-Martín, D.; Monserrat, J.; Álvarez-Mon, M. Effectiveness of Therapeutic Exercise in Fibromyalgia Syndrome: A Systematic Review and Meta-Analysis of Randomized Clinical Trials. *BioMed. Res. Int.* **2017**, *2017*, 2356346. [CrossRef]
27. Berardi, G.; Senefeld, J.W.; Hunter, S.K.; Bement, M.K.H. Impact of isometric and concentric resistance exercise on pain and fatigue in fibromyalgia. *Graefe's Arch. Clin. Exp. Ophthalmol.* **2021**, *121*, 1389–1404. [CrossRef]
28. Izquierdo-Alventosa, R.; Inglés, M.; Cortés-Amador, S.; Gimeno-Mallench, L.; Chirivella-Garrido, J.; Kropotov, J.; Serra-Añó, P. Low-Intensity Physical Exercise Improves Pain Catastrophizing and Other Psychological and Physical Aspects in Women with Fibromyalgia: A Randomized Controlled Trial. *Int. J. Environ. Res. Public Health* **2020**, *17*, 3634. [CrossRef]
29. Caglayan, B.C.; Keskin, A.; Kabul, E.G.; Calik, B.B.; Aslan, U.B.; Karasu, U. Effects of clinical Pilates exercises in individuals with fibromyalgia: A randomized controlled trial. *Eur. J. Rheumatol.* **2021**, *8*, 150–155. [CrossRef]
30. Costa, M.T.S.; Vieira, L.P.; Barbosa, E.D.O.; Oliveira, L.M.; Maillot, P.; Vaghetti, C.A.O.; Carta, M.G.; Machado, S.; Gatica-Rojas, V.; Monteiro-Junior, R.S. Virtual Reality-Based Exercise with Exergames as Medicine in Different Contexts: A Short Review. *Clin. Pract. Epidemiol. Ment. Health* **2019**, *15*, 15–20. [CrossRef]
31. Corbetta, D.; Imeri, F.; Gatti, R. Rehabilitation that incorporates virtual reality is more effective than standard rehabilitation for improving walking speed, balance and mobility after stroke: A systematic review. *J. Physiother.* **2015**, *61*, 117–124. [CrossRef]
32. Palacios-Navarro, G.; Hogan, N. Head-Mounted Display-Based Therapies for Adults Post-Stroke: A Systematic Review and Meta-Analysis. *Sensors* **2021**, *21*, 1111. [CrossRef]
33. Montoro-Cárdenas, D.; Cortés-Pérez, I.; Zagalaz-Anula, N.; Osuna-Pérez, M.C.; Obrero-Gaitán, E.; Lomas-Vega, R. Nintendo Wii Balance Board therapy for postural control in children with cerebral palsy: A systematic review and meta-analysis. *Dev. Med. Child Neurol.* **2021**, *63*, 1262–1275. [CrossRef] [PubMed]

34. Cortés-Pérez, I.; Zagalaz-Anula, N.; Montoro-Cárdenas, D.; Lomas-Vega, R.; Obrero-Gaitán, E.; Osuna-Pérez, M. Leap Motion Controller Video Game-Based Therapy for Upper Extremity Motor Recovery in Patients with Central Nervous System Diseases. A Systematic Review with Meta-Analysis. *Sensors* **2021**, *21*, 2065. [CrossRef] [PubMed]

35. Zhang, B.; Li, D.; Liu, Y.; Wang, J.; Xiao, Q. Virtual reality for limb motor function, balance, gait, cognition and daily function of stroke patients: A systematic review and meta-analysis. *J. Adv. Nurs.* **2021**, *77*, 3255–3273. [CrossRef] [PubMed]

36. Ahern, M.M.; Dean, L.V.; Stoddard, C.C.; Agrawal, A.; Kim, K.; Cook, C.E.; Garcia, A.N. The Effectiveness of Virtual Reality in Patients with Spinal Pain: A Systematic Review and Meta-Analysis. *Pain Pract.* **2020**, *20*, 656–675. [CrossRef] [PubMed]

37. Hwang, R.; Elkins, M.R. Telephysiotherapy. *J. Physiother.* **2020**, *66*, 143–144. [CrossRef]

38. Darnall, B.D.; Krishnamurthy, P.; Tsuei, J.; Minor, J.D. Self-Administered Skills-Based Virtual Reality Intervention for Chronic Pain: Randomized Controlled Pilot Study. *JMIR Form. Res.* **2020**, *4*, e17293. [CrossRef]

39. Herrero, R.; García-Palacios, A.; Castilla, D.; Molinari, G.; Botella, C. Virtual Reality for the Induction of Positive Emotions in the Treatment of Fibromyalgia: A Pilot Study over Acceptability, Satisfaction, and the Effect of Virtual Reality on Mood. *Cyberpsychology Behav. Soc. Netw.* **2014**, *17*, 379–384. [CrossRef]

40. Mortensen, J.; Kristensen, L.Q.; Brooks, E.P.; Brooks, A.L. Women with fibromyalgia's experience with three motion-controlled video game consoles and indicators of symptom severity and performance of activities of daily living. *Disabil. Rehabil. Assist. Technol.* **2013**, *10*, 61–66. [CrossRef]

41. Moher, D.; Liberati, A.; Tetzlaff, J.; Altman, D.G. Preferred Reporting Items for Systematic Reviews and Meta-Analyses: The PRISMA Statement. *J. Clin. Epidemiol.* **2009**, *62*, 1006–1012. [CrossRef] [PubMed]

42. Higgins, J.P.T.; Green, S. *Cochrane Handbook for Systematic Reviews of Intervention Version 5.1.0*; The Cochrane Collaboration: London, UK, 2011.

43. Maher, C.G.; Sherrington, C.; Herbert, R.D.; Moseley, A.M.; Elkins, M. Reliability of the PEDro Scale for Rating Quality of Randomized Controlled Trials. *Phys. Ther.* **2003**, *83*, 713–721. [CrossRef] [PubMed]

44. Macedo, L.G.; Elkins, M.; Maher, C.; Moseley, A.M.; Herbert, R.; Sherrington, C. There was evidence of convergent and construct validity of Physiotherapy Evidence Database quality scale for physiotherapy trials. *J. Clin. Epidemiol.* **2010**, *63*, 920–925. [CrossRef] [PubMed]

45. Elkins, M.R.; Moseley, A.M.; Sherrington, C.; Herbert, R.D.; Maher, C.G. Growth in the Physiotherapy Evidence Database (PEDro) and use of the PEDro scale. *Br. J. Sports Med.* **2012**, *47*, 188–189. [CrossRef]

46. Atkins, D.; Best, D.; Briss, P.; Eccles, M.; Falck-Ytter, Y.; Flottorp, S.; Guyatt, G.; Harbour, R.; Haugh, M.; Henry, D.; et al. Grading quality of evidence and strength of recommendations. *BMJ* **2004**, *328*, 1490. [CrossRef]

47. Meader, N.; King, K.; Llewellyn, A.; Norman, G.; Brown, J.; Rodgers, M.; Moe-Byrne, T.; Higgins, J.P.; Sowden, A.; Stewart, G. A checklist designed to aid consistency and reproducibility of GRADE assessments: Development and pilot validation. *Syst. Rev.* **2014**, *3*, 82. [CrossRef]

48. Higgins, J.P.T.; Thompson, S.G.; Deeks, J.; Altman, D.G. Measuring inconsistency in meta-analyses. *BMJ* **2003**, *327*, 557–560. [CrossRef]

49. Borenstein, M.; Hedges, L.; Higgins, J.; Rothstein, H. *Comprehensive Meta-Analysis Software Version 3*; Biostat: Washington, DC, USA, 2020.

50. Cooper, H.; Hedges, L.V.; Valentine, J.C. *The Handbook of Research Synthesis and Meta-Analysis*; Russell Sage Foundation: Manhattan, NY, USA, 2009.

51. Cohen, J. *Statistical Power Analysis for the Behavioral Sciences*; Academic Press: New York, NY, USA, 1977.

52. Der Simonian, R.; Laird, N. Meta-analysis in clinical trials. *Control. Clin. Trials* **1986**, *7*, 177–188. [CrossRef]

53. Faraone, S.V. Interpreting estimates of treatment effects: Implications for managed care. *Pharm. Ther.* **2008**, *33*, 700–711.

54. Rücker, G.; Schwarzer, G. Beyond the forest plot: The drapery plot. *Res. Synth. Methods* **2020**, *12*, 13–19. [CrossRef]

55. Sterne, J.A.; Egger, M. Funnel plots for detecting bias in meta-analysis: Guidelines on choice of axis. *J. Clin. Epidemiol.* **2001**, *54*, 1046–1055. [CrossRef]

56. Egger, M.; Smith, G.D.; Schneider, M.; Minder, C. Bias in meta-analysis detected by a simple, graphical test. *BMJ* **1997**, *315*, 629–634. [CrossRef] [PubMed]

57. Duval, S.; Tweedie, R. Trim and Fill: A Simple Funnel-Plot-Based Method of Testing and Adjusting for Publication Bias in Meta-Analysis. *Biometrics* **2000**, *56*, 455–463. [CrossRef] [PubMed]

58. Rothman, K.J.; Greenland, S.; Lash, T.L. *Modern Epidemiology*; Lippincott Williams & Wilkins: Philadelphia, PA, USA, 2008.

59. Higgins, J.; Thompson, S.; Deeks, J.; Altman, D. Statistical heterogeneity in systematic reviews of clinical trials: A critical appraisal of guidelines and practice. *J. Health Serv. Res. Policy* **2002**, *7*, 51–61. [CrossRef]

60. Siddaway, A.P.; Wood, A.M.; Hedges, L.V. How to Do a Systematic Review: A Best Practice Guide for Conducting and Reporting Narrative Reviews, Meta-Analyses, and Meta-Syntheses. *Annu. Rev. Psychol.* **2019**, *70*, 747–770. [CrossRef] [PubMed]

61. de Carvalho, M.S.; Carvalho, L.C.; Menezes, F.D.S.; Frazin, A.; Gomes, E.D.C.; Iunes, D.H. Effects of Exergames in Women with Fibromyalgia: A Randomized Controlled Study. *Games Health J.* **2020**, *9*, 358–367. [CrossRef] [PubMed]

62. Collado-Mateo, D.; Dominguez-Muñoz, F.J.; Adsuar, J.C.; Garcia-Gordillo, M.A.; Gusi, N. Effects of Exergames on Quality of Life, Pain, and Disease Effect in Women with Fibromyalgia: A Randomized Controlled Trial. *Arch. Phys. Med. Rehabil.* **2017**, *98*, 1725–1731. [CrossRef]

63. Villafaina, S.; Collado-Mateo, D.; Fuentes, J.P.; Rohlfs-Domínguez, P.; Gusi, N. Effects of Exergames on Brain Dynamics in Women with Fibromyalgia: A Randomized Controlled Trial. *J. Clin. Med.* **2019**, *8*, 1015. [CrossRef]

64. Collado-Mateo, D.; Dominguez-Muñoz, F.J.; Adsuar, J.C.; Merellano-Navarro, E.; Gusi, N. Exergames for women with fibromyalgia: A randomised controlled trial to evaluate the effects on mobility skills, balance and fear of falling. *PeerJ* **2017**, *5*, e3211. [CrossRef]
65. Garcia-Palacios, A.; Herrero, R.; Vizcaíno, Y.; Belmonte, M.A.; Castilla, D.; Molinari, G.; Baños, R.M.; Botella, C. Integrating Virtual Reality with Activity Management for the Treatment of Fibromyalgia. *Clin. J. Pain* **2015**, *31*, 564–572. [CrossRef]
66. Gulsen, C.; Soke, F.; Eldemir, K.; Apaydin, Y.; Ozkul, C.; Guclu-Gunduz, A.; Akcali, D.T. Effect of fully immersive virtual reality treatment combined with exercise in fibromyalgia patients: A randomized controlled trial. *Assist. Technol.* **2020**. [CrossRef] [PubMed]
67. Leon-Llamas, J.; Villafaina, S.; Murillo-Garcia, A.; Dominguez-Muñoz, F.; Gusi, N. Effects of 24-Week Exergame Intervention on the Gray Matter Volume of Different Brain Structures in Women with Fibromyalgia: A Single-Blind, Randomized Controlled Trial. *J. Clin. Med.* **2020**, *9*, 2436. [CrossRef] [PubMed]
68. Martín-Martínez, J.P.; Villafaina, S.; Collado-Mateo, D.; Pérez-Gómez, J.; Gusi, N. Effects of 24-week exergame intervention on physical function under single- and dual-task conditions in fibromyalgia: A randomized controlled trial. *Scand. J. Med. Sci. Sports* **2019**, *29*, 1610–1617. [CrossRef] [PubMed]
69. Polat, M.; Kahveci, A.; Muci, B.; Günendi, Z.; Karataş, G.K. The Effect of Virtual Reality Exercises on Pain, Functionality, Cardiopulmonary Capacity, and Quality of Life in Fibromyalgia Syndrome: A Randomized Controlled Study. *Games Health J.* **2021**, *10*, 165–173. [CrossRef] [PubMed]
70. Villafaina, S.; Collado-Mateo, D.; Domínguez-Muñoz, F.J.; Fuentes-García, J.P.; Gusi, N. Benefits of 24-Week Exergame Intervention on Health-Related Quality of Life and Pain in Women with Fibromyalgia: A Single-Blind, Randomized Controlled Trial. *Games Health J.* **2019**, *8*, 380–386. [CrossRef]
71. Villafaina, S.; Borrega-Mouquinho, Y.; Fuentes-García, J.P.; Collado-Mateo, D.; Gusi, N. Effect of Exergame Training and Detraining on Lower-Body Strength, Agility, and Cardiorespiratory Fitness in Women with Fibromyalgia: Single-Blinded Randomized Controlled Trial. *Int. J. Environ. Res. Public Health* **2019**, *17*, 161. [CrossRef]
72. Cipolletta, S.; Tomaino, S.C.M.; Magno, E.L.; Faccio, E. Illness Experiences and Attitudes towards Medication in Online Communities for People with Fibromyalgia. *Int. J. Environ. Res. Public Health* **2020**, *17*, 8683. [CrossRef]
73. Cao, C.-F.; Ma, K.-L.; Li, Q.-L.; Luan, F.-J.; Wang, Q.-B.; Zhang, M.-H.; Viswanath, O.; Myrcik, D.; Varrassi, G.; Wang, H.-Q. Balneotherapy for Fibromyalgia Syndrome: A Systematic Review and Meta-Analysis. *J. Clin. Med.* **2021**, *10*, 1493. [CrossRef]
74. Masquelier, E.; D'Haeyere, J. Physical activity in the treatment of fibromyalgia. *Jt. Bone Spine* **2021**, *88*, 105202. [CrossRef]
75. Busch, A.J.; Webber, S.; Richards, R.S.; Bidonde, J.; Schachter, C.L.; Schafer, L.; Danyliw, A.; Sawant, A.; Bello-Haas, V.D.; Rader, T.; et al. Resistance exercise training for fibromyalgia. *Cochrane Database Syst. Rev.* **2013**, *2013*, CD010884. [CrossRef]
76. Bennett, R.M.; Friend, R.; Jones, K.D.; Ward, R.; Han, B.K.; Ross, R.L. The Revised Fibromyalgia Impact Questionnaire (FIQR): Validation and psychometric properties. *Arthritis Res. Ther.* **2009**, *11*, R120. [CrossRef] [PubMed]
77. Gumaa, M.; Youssef, A.R. Is Virtual Reality Effective in Orthopedic Rehabilitation? A Systematic Review and Meta-Analysis. *Phys. Ther.* **2019**, *99*, 1304–1325. [CrossRef] [PubMed]
78. Ahmadpour, N.; Randall, H.; Choksi, H.; Gao, A.; Vaughan, C.; Poronnik, P. Virtual Reality interventions for acute and chronic pain management. *Int. J. Biochem. Cell Biol.* **2019**, *114*, 105568. [CrossRef] [PubMed]
79. Dunn, J.; Yeo, E.; Moghaddampour, P.; Chau, B.; Humbert, S. Virtual and augmented reality in the treatment of phantom limb pain: A literature review. *NeuroRehabilitation* **2017**, *40*, 595–601. [CrossRef] [PubMed]
80. Zusman, M. Forebrain-mediated sensitization of central pain pathways: 'non-specific' pain and a new image for MT. *Man. Ther.* **2002**, *7*, 80–88. [CrossRef]
81. Goldman-Rakic, P.S. The prefrontal landscape: Implications of functional architecture for understanding human mentation and the central executive. *Philos. Trans. R. Soc. B Biol. Sci.* **1996**, *351*, 1445–1453. [CrossRef]
82. Koçyiğit, B.F.; Akaltun, M.S. Kinesiophobia Levels in Fibromyalgia Syndrome and the Relationship Between Pain, Disease Activity, Depression. *Arch. Rheumatol.* **2020**, *35*, 214–219. [CrossRef]
83. Núñez-Fuentes, D.; Obrero-Gaitán, E.; Zagalaz-Anula, N.; Ibáñez-Vera, A.; Achalandabaso-Ochoa, A.; López-Ruiz, M.; Rodríguez-Almagro, D.; Lomas-Vega, R. Alteration of Postural Balance in Patients with Fibromyalgia Syndrome—A Systematic Review and Meta-Analysis. *Diagnostics* **2021**, *11*, 127. [CrossRef]
84. Cagnie, B.; Coppieters, I.; Denecker, S.; Six, J.; Danneels, L.; Meeus, M. Central sensitization in fibromyalgia? A systematic review on structural and functional brain MRI. *Semin. Arthritis Rheum.* **2014**, *44*, 68–75. [CrossRef]
85. Cheng, C.-A.; Chiu, Y.-W.; Wu, D.; Kuan, Y.-C.; Chen, S.-N.; Tam, K.-W. Effectiveness of Tai Chi on fibromyalgia patients: A meta-analysis of randomized controlled trials. *Complement. Ther. Med.* **2019**, *46*, 1–8. [CrossRef]
86. Walitt, B.; Klose, P.; Üçeyler, N.; Phillips, T.; Häuser, W. Antipsychotics for fibromyalgia in adults. *Cochrane Database Syst. Rev.* **2016**, CD011804. [CrossRef] [PubMed]
87. Dailey, D.L.; Law, L.A.F.; Vance, C.G.T.; Rakel, B.A.; Merriwether, E.N.; Darghosian, L.; Golchha, M.; Geasland, K.M.; Spitz, R.; Crofford, L.J.; et al. Perceived function and physical performance are associated with pain and fatigue in women with fibromyalgia. *Arthritis Res.* **2016**, *18*, 68. [CrossRef]
88. Ioannou, A.; Papastavrou, E.; Avraamides, M.N.; Charalambous, A. Virtual Reality and Symptoms Management of Anxiety, Depression, Fatigue, and Pain: A Systematic Review. *SAGE Open Nurs.* **2020**, *6*, 2377960820936163. [CrossRef] [PubMed]

89. Vance, C.G.; Zimmerman, M.B.; Dailey, D.L.; Rakel, B.A.; Geasland, K.M.; Chimenti, R.L.; Williams, J.M.; Golchha, M.; Crofford, L.J.; Sluka, K.A. Reduction in movement-evoked pain and fatigue during initial 30-minute transcutaneous electrical nerve stimulation treatment predicts transcutaneous electrical nerve stimulation responders in women with fibromyalgia. *Pain* **2020**, *162*, 1545–1555. [CrossRef] [PubMed]

90. Montana, J.I.; Matamala-Gomez, M.; Maisto, M.; Mavrodiev, P.A.; Cavalera, C.M.; Diana, B.; Mantovani, F.; Realdon, O. The Benefits of emotion Regulation Interventions in Virtual Reality for the Improvement of Wellbeing in Adults and Older Adults: A Systematic Review. *J. Clin. Med.* **2020**, *9*, 500. [CrossRef] [PubMed]

91. Arcos-Carmona, I.M.; Castro-Sánchez, A.M.; Matarán-Peñarrocha, G.A.; Gutiérrez-Rubio, A.B.; Ramos-González, E.; Moreno-Lorenzo, C. Effects of aerobic exercise program and relaxation techniques on anxiety, quality of sleep, depression, and quality of life in patients with fibromyalgia: A randomized controlled trial. *Med. Clin.* **2011**, *137*, 398–401. [CrossRef]

92. Van Abbema, R.; Van Wilgen, C.P.; Van Der Schans, C.P.; Van Ittersum, M.W. Patients with more severe symptoms benefit the most from an intensive multimodal programme in patients with fibromyalgia. *Disabil. Rehabil.* **2010**, *33*, 743–750. [CrossRef]

93. Freeman, D.; Reeve, S.; Robinson, A.; Ehlers, A.; Clark, D.; Spanlang, B.; Slater, M. Virtual reality in the assessment, understanding, and treatment of mental health disorders. *Psychol. Med.* **2017**, *47*, 2393–2400. [CrossRef]

94. Fodor, L.A.; Coteț, C.D.; Cuijpers, P.; Szamoskozi, T.; David, D.; Cristea, I.A. The effectiveness of virtual reality based interventions for symptoms of anxiety and depression: A meta-analysis. *Sci. Rep.* **2018**, *8*, 10323. [CrossRef]

95. Masaoka, Y.; Homma, I. The source generator of respiratory-related anxiety potential in the human brain. *Neurosci. Lett.* **2000**, *283*, 21–24. [CrossRef]

96. Gormsen, L.; Rosenberg, R.; Bach, F.; Jensen, T.S. Depression, anxiety, health-related quality of life and pain in patients with chronic fibromyalgia and neuropathic pain. *Eur. J. Pain* **2010**, *14*, 127.e1–127.e8. [CrossRef]

97. Thieme, K.; Turk, D.C.; Flor, H. Comorbid Depression and Anxiety in Fibromyalgia Syndrome: Relationship to Somatic and Psychosocial Variables. *Psychosom. Med.* **2004**, *66*, 837–844. [CrossRef] [PubMed]

98. Montoro, C.I.; Duschek, S.; Schuepbach, D.; Gandarillas, M.; del Paso, G.A.R. Cerebral blood flow variability in fibromyalgia syndrome: Relationships with emotional, clinical and functional variables. *PLoS ONE* **2018**, *13*, e0204267. [CrossRef]

99. Rodriguez, A.; Tembl, J.; Mesa-Gresa, P.; Muñoz, M.; Montoya, P.; Rey, B. Altered cerebral blood flow velocity features in fibromyalgia patients in resting-state conditions. *PLoS ONE* **2017**, *12*, e0180253. [CrossRef]

100. Galvez-Sánchez, C.M.; del Paso, G.A.R.; Duschek, S. Cognitive Impairments in Fibromyalgia Syndrome: Associations with Positive and Negative Affect, Alexithymia, Pain Catastrophizing and Self-Esteem. *Front. Psychol.* **2018**, *9*, 377. [CrossRef] [PubMed]

101. Van Liew, C.; Leon, G.; Neese, M.; Cronan, T.A. You get used to it, or do you: Symptom length predicts less fibromyalgia physical impairment, but only for those with above-average self-efficacy. *Psychol. Health Med.* **2018**, *24*, 207–220. [CrossRef]

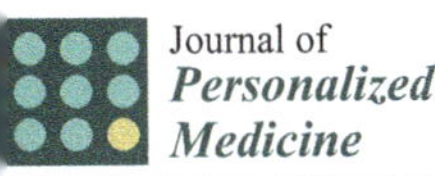

Journal of
Personalized
Medicine

MDPI

Review

Family Risk Factors That Jeopardize Child Development: Scoping Review

Aida Simões [1,2], Saudade Lopes [3], Maria dos Anjos Dixe [3] and Júlio Belo Fernandes [1,4,*]

1   Escola Superior de Saúde Egas Moniz, 2829-511 Almada, Portugal; aidasimoes@gmail.com
2   Centro de Investigação Interdisciplinar Egas Moniz (CiiEM), 2829-511 Almada, Portugal
3   Center for Innovative Care and Health Technology (ciTechcare), School of Health Sciences, Polytechnic of Leiria, 2411-901 Leiria, Portugal; saudade.lopes@ipleiria.pt (S.L.); maria.dixe@ipleiria.pt (M.d.A.D.)
4   Grupo de Patologia Médica, Nutrição e Exercício Clínico (PaMNEC)—Centro de Investigação Interdisciplinar Egas Moniz (CiiEM), 2829-511 Almada, Portugal
*   Correspondence: juliobelo01@gmail.com

Abstract: The obligation to protect children is defined by law. However, there is fragility in identifying actual or potential situations that jeopardize their development. This review aims to identify the family risk factors that jeopardize child development. A scoping review was conducted following the Joanna Briggs Institute for Evidence-Based Practice framework and the 2020 Preferred Reporting Items for Systematic Reviews and Meta-analyses (PRISMA) statement. The research was carried out on the electronic databases PubMed, CINAHL, Nursing & Allied Health Collection: Comprehensive, MEDLINE Complete, and MedicLatina, with a time limit of 2010 to 2021. The search was restricted to documents written in Portuguese, English, and French. A total of 3998 articles were initially identified. After selecting and analysing, 28 risk factors were extracted from 29 articles. Four categories of risk factors were identified—namely, patterns of social and economic interaction, family characteristics, caregiver's characteristics, and parenting. The results of this review allow the identification of family risk factors that jeopardize child development. This is significant for Child Protective Services workers as they carry out their risk assessments. This assessment is the first step in avoiding an accumulation of harm to at-risk children and allowing the development of interventions for minimising harm's impact on children's development.

Keywords: child; child abuse; maltreatment; neglect; risk factors; family; caregivers; child protective services

Citation: Simões, A.; Lopes, S.; dos Anjos Dixe, M.; Fernandes, J.B. Family Risk Factors That Jeopardize Child Development: Scoping Review. *J. Pers. Med.* **2022**, 12, 562. https://doi.org/10.3390/jpm12040562

Academic Editor: José Carmelo Adsuar Sala

Received: 6 January 2022
Accepted: 31 March 2022
Published: 1 April 2022

Publisher's Note: MDPI stays neutral with regard to jurisdictional claims in published maps and institutional affiliations.

1. Introduction

The family is a micro-system with an organization, both structural and functional. Each family member plays a socially defined role, referring us to a space of affection, harmony, and protection between its members. The family environment has been the subject of several studies on its implications for children's development and can be conceptualized as a resource or adversity [1].

Even though most children grow in desirable environments, a minority are victims of multiple types of maltreatment by their parents or caregivers [2].

When children are at risk of or are experiencing neglect or any other form of maltreatment, Child Protective Services (CPS) becomes involved in investigating the allegations. The CPS is a branch of the state's social services department that assesses, investigates, and intervenes in cases of an allegation of child abuse and neglect. The main focus is on promoting child's rights and safety and providing support for parents to strengthen families and promote a safe, nurturing environment for children [3]. While effective engagement is an essential component for helping children and their families, this process presents an ongoing challenge [4]. There is an underlying tension caused by the controlling function inherent to the CPS and the contribution to developing families' skills to produce better outcomes for children [5].

Dealing with the duality of this relationship can be challenging for families and CPS, given the expectations that CPS workers will engage in conflicting roles of supporting families on the one hand and ensuring the child's safety on the other. In addition, having the right to remove a child from their home causes a level of mistrust throughout the interaction [6].

For CPS to investigate any allegations of children who are at risk of or who are experiencing any type of abuse or neglect, the initial assessment is crucial. This assessment is performed by CPS workers and enables the collection of information that confirms or disproves the veracity of the allegations [7,8].

The CPS workers come from various professional areas, and in practice, it is verified that their assessments are based on criteria arising from their fields of training and expertise. This may lead to difficulty in gathering information, and consequently, it may hinder decision-making.

Previous research has revealed several risk factors frequently related to child maltreatment. For example, a study assessing the risk of child abuse showed a higher risk for mothers with lower education and social support [9]. Another study reviewed CPS reports from 2006 to 2008 for families in Connecticut's child abuse prevention program and identified several family risk factors—namely, histories of CPS, domestic violence, mental health, sexual abuse, substance abuse, and criminal involvement [10]. Children in families and environments exposed to these factors have an increased probability of experiencing neglect or any other type of abuse [11,12]. Although several studies approach the risk factors for child maltreatment and the improvements in risk assessment, recent research has not adequately looked at the factors related to the family.

A better understanding of family risk factors can support CPS workers in the identification of stressors and situations that put children at risk of neglect or abuse, allowing CPS workers to intervene before maltreatment occurs. Considering this gap in evidence, this review aims to identify the family risk factors that jeopardize child development.

2. Methods

This scoping review report was drawn based on the 2020 Preferred Reporting Items for Systematic Reviews and Meta-analyses (PRISMA) statement [13]. In addition, our methods followed the Joanna Briggs Institute for Evidence-Based Practice framework [14]. According to PCC, the following research question was defined: What are the family risk factors that jeopardize child development?

The PubMed, CINAHL, Nursing & Allied Health Collection: Comprehensive, MED-LINE Complete, and MedicLatina databases were searched using a combination of concepts in line with the DeCS/MeSH terms. The search equation was: ((Social service Or Social work OR Protection service) AND (Family OR Caregiver) AND (Neglect OR Abuse OR Maltreatment) AND (Child OR Child, preschool OR Adolescent)).

The selection criteria were: documents written in Portuguese, English, and French, published between 2010 and 2021, which addressed or referred to the family risk factors that jeopardize child development. All documents that did not meet the selection criteria were excluded from the review.

Two researchers independently carried out the search, selection, and extraction of data to increase consistency.

The article selection was performed in three phases. In the first phase, the title was analysed, followed by the abstract analysis, and, finally, the selected articles were read in full. When it was unclear whether an article fit this review, it went to the following analysis stage. Disagreements between reviewers were resolved through discussion. In occasional situations, if any doubt or inconsistency was present, the issues were discussed by all researchers.

Data were extracted using an instrument designed for data extraction, considering the defined research questions. Finally, all authors discussed the final extraction chart.

A data-driven thematic analysis adopted from Braun, Clarke, Hayfield, and Terry's guidelines [15] was undertaken. Two researchers reviewed data independently and manually coded using inductive analysis to identify common themes across the collected data. Data were separated into meaningful units of words or phrases on the same topic. Then, codes were assigned to the meaningful units, and categories were identified, reflecting differences and similarities in data. The two researchers compared their findings to finalize this analysis process, and discussion resolved any discrepancies. Finally, the whole research team reviewed the final findings.

From the analysis, the family risk factors were grouped under different categories.

3. Results

The study selection process is summarized below in the PRISMA flow chart (Figure 1). Initially, 3998 documents were identified in the different databases. Then, after analysing the complete texts, 29 articles (Table 1) presented knowledge that allowed answering the research question.

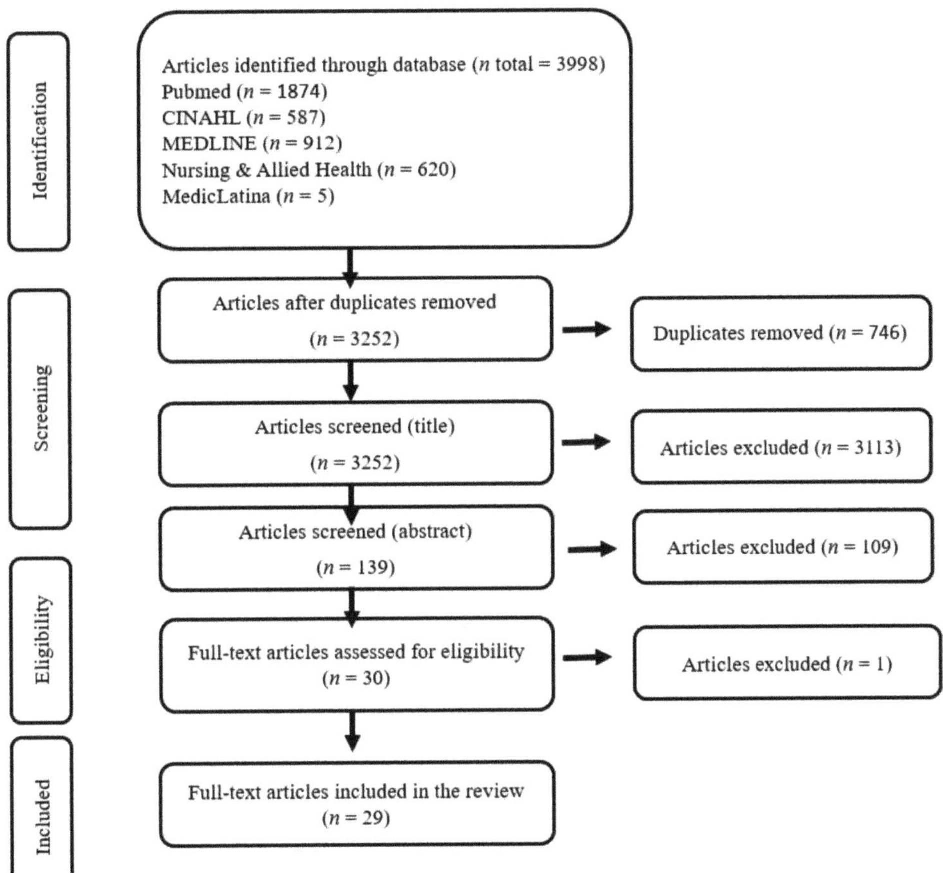

Figure 1. PRISMA flow chart.

Table 1. Selected articles.

Study (S)/Authors/Year	Title
S1—Donohue et al. (2016) [16]	Development and initial psychometric examination of the Home Safety and Beautification Assessment in mothers referred to treatment by child welfare agents.
S2—Gurwitch et al. (2016) [17]	Child-Adult Relationship Enhancement (CARE): An evidence-informed program for children with a history of trauma and other behavioural challenges.
S3—Casillas, Fauchier, Derkash, and Garrido (2016) [11]	Implementation of evidence-based home visiting programs aimed at reducing child maltreatment: A meta-analytic review.
S4—Peng et al. (2015) [18]	A systems approach to addressing child maltreatment in China: China needs a formalised child protection system.
S5—Loman and Siegel (2015) [4]	Effects of approach and services under differential response on long-term child safety and welfare.
S6—Winokur, Ellis, Drury, and Rogers (2015) [19]	Answering the big questions about differential response in Colorado: safety and cost outcomes from a randomised controlled trial.
S7—Jones (2015) [20]	Implementation of differential response: a racial equity analysis.
S8—Fuller, Paceley, and Schreiber (2015) [21]	Differential Response family assessments: listening to what parents say about service helpfulness.
S9—Duffy, Hughes, Asnes, and Leventhal (2015) [10]	Child maltreatment and risk patterns among participants in a child abuse prevention program.
S10—Goltz, Mena, and Swank (2014) [22]	Using growth curve analysis to examine challenges in instrumentation in longitudinal measurement in home visiting.
S11—Schneiderman, Hurlburt, Leslie, Zhang, and Horwitz (2012) [12]	Child, caregiver, and family characteristics associated with emergency department use by children who remain at home after a child protective services investigation.
S12—Benbenishty et al. (2015) [23]	Decision making in child protection: An international comparative study on maltreatment substantiation, risk assessment and interventions recommendations, and the role of professionals' child welfare attitudes.
S13—Macdonald et al. (2014) [24]	THE SAAF STUDY: evaluation of the Safeguarding Children Assessment and Analysis Framework (SAAF), compared with management as usual, for improving outcomes for children and young people who have experienced, or are at risk of, maltreatment.
S14—Glad, Jergeby, Gustafsson, and Sonnander (2014) [25]	Social worker and teacher apprehension of children's stimulation and support in the home environment and caregiver perception of the HOME Inventory in Sweden.
S15—Hirsch, Yang, Font, and Slack (2015) [26]	Physically hazardous housing and risk for child protective services involvement.
S16—Malo, Moreau, Lavergne, and Hélie (2016) [27]	Psychological maltreatment, the under-recognised violence against children: a new portrait from Quebec.
S17—Zimmermann et al. (2016) [28]	Growing up under adversity in Germany: Design and methods of a developmental study on risk and protective mechanisms in families with diverse psychosocial risk.
S18—Ben-David (2016) [29]	A Focus on Neglect: Comparing the Characteristics of Children and Parents in Cases of Neglect, Abuse, and Non-CAN (Child Abuse and Neglect) in Israeli Rulings on Termination of Parental Rights.
S19—Liel et al. (2020) [30]	Risk factors for child abuse, neglect and exposure to intimate partner violence in early childhood: Findings in a representative cross-sectional sample in Germany.
S20—Ajduković, Rajter, and Rezo (2018) [9]	Individual and contextual factors for the child abuse potential of Croatian mothers: The role of social support in times of economic hardship.
S21—Vial et al. (2020) [31]	Exploring the interrelatedness of risk factors for child maltreatment: A network approach.

Table 1. *Cont.*

Study (S)/Authors/Year	Title
S22—Laslett, Room, Dietze, and Ferris (2012) [32]	Alcohol's involvement in recurrent child abuse and neglect cases.
S23—Vincent and Petch (2017) [33]	Understanding child, family, environmental and agency risk factors: findings from an analysis of significant case reviews in Scotland.
S24—Logan-Greene and Jones (2018) [34]	Predicting chronic neglect: Understanding risk and protective factors for CPS-involved families.
S25—Gifford, Eldred, Sloan, and Evans, (2016) [35]	Parental Criminal Justice Involvement and Children's Involvement With Child Protective Services: Do Adult Drug Treatment Courts Prevent Child Maltreatment?
S26—Nilchian et al. (2012) [36]	Evaluation of factors influencing child abuse leading to oro-facial lesions in Isfahan, Iran: A qualitative approach.
S27—Palusci and Ilardi (2020) [8]	Risk Factors and Services to Reduce Child Sexual Abuse Recurrence.
S28—McConnell, Feldman, Aunos, and Prasad (2011) [37]	Parental cognitive impairment and child maltreatment in Canada.
S29—Sinanan (2011) [38]	The impact of child, family, and child protective services factors on reports of child sexual abuse recurrence.

A total of twenty-nine studies published between 2010 and 2021 were selected for final analysis. Regarding the country where studies were applied, we verified that the majority of studies were from the USA [4,8,10–12,16,17,19–22,26,29,34,35,38], eight were from Europe [9,23–25,28,30,31,33], two were from Canada [27,37], one was from China [18], one was from Australia [32], and another was from Iran [36].

The content analysis of the data in the articles allowed the identification of twenty-eight family risk factors that jeopardize child development, which were grouped into four categories. These results are presented in Table 2.

Table 2. Family risk factors.

Category	Risk Factors	Study
Patterns of social and economic interaction	Hazardous housing	S1, S8, S13, S15
	Low social support	S4, S9, S11, S12, S13, S16, S20, S28
	No means of transportation	S8
	Mismanaged finances	S2, S4, S5, S7, S9, S10, S11, S12, S14, S15, S17, S20, S26, S27, S29
	Violence in the community and neighbourhood	S8, S9, S23
Family characteristics	History of allegations	S8, S9, S10, S14, S15
	Domestic violence	S3, S5, S6, S8, S9, S11, S13, S16, S17, S19, S21, S24
	Family disagreements and conflicts	S4, S7, S8, S11, S12, S15, S16, S17, S19
	Single-parent families	S3, S4, S7, S9, S10, S14, S17
	Multi-child family	S15, S17, S19, S24
	Multiple caregivers	S9
	Existence of stepmothers and stepfathers	S4, S9, S15
	Being the firstborn	S3
	Poor communication between separated parents	S8, S16, S26

Table 2. *Cont.*

Category	Risk Factors	Study
Caregiver characteristics	Alcohol and/or drug abuse	S3, S5, S9, S10, S13, S14, S15, S17, S18, S22, S23, S26, S27
	Mental health problems	S5, S8, S9, S10, S11, S13, S14, S15, S17, S24, S26, S28
	History of inflicting maltreatment	S5, S26, S27
	Low level of education	S3, S9, S10, S12, S14, S15, S20
	Criminal record	S5, S9, S10, S11, S13, S14, S18, S25
	Lack of cooperation with CPS	S11, S12, S28
	Unintended pregnancy	S10, S14, S17
	History of having been maltreated	S3, S9, S10, S11, S13, S14, S21
	Age (under 18 years old)	S3, S6, S9, S10, S14, S15, S17, S19
Parenting	Unrealistic expectations towards the child	S11
	Negative attitudes towards the child	S10, S14, S16, S17
	Abusive and mistreating practices	S4, S5, S10, S11, S13, S14
	Multiple trips to children's emergency room	S9, S11
	Parents absent in childrearing	S4, S8, S16, S21

4. Discussion

Experiencing physical and emotional maltreatment in childhood can lead to the development of a broad range of long-term health conditions that can manifest as educational difficulties, anxiety, depression, trouble forming and maintaining relationships, drug use, and suicide attempts [39–42]. Therefore, it is essential to identify and, if possible, eliminate or mitigate factors that jeopardize child development.

This review helps to understand the family risk factors that jeopardize child development. Research in this area is crucial, especially as new data reveal the true impact of the cumulative harm of repeated abusive and neglect parenting practices on early brain development, emotional regulation, and cognitive and social development. The results from this review support prior research findings that when assessing families with chronic neglect and abusive practices, CPS deals with significant and multiple risk factors [43].

Multiple risk factors emerged from the review. The first category of risk factors demonstrates the relationship of social and economic interaction patterns in child development. The risk factors that encompass this category are hazardous housing, low social support, no means of transportation, mismanaged finances, and the presence of violence in the community and neighbourhood.

Problems in accessing basic needs, including income, employment, adequate housing, childcare, and transport, are risk factors. In addition, mismanaged finances are considered a risk factor that contributes to high family stress levels. In combination with other factors, low economic resources contribute to an increased propensity for child abuse and neglect [4,8,9,28,36,38].

The existence of means of transportation is significant for parents to have access to medical appointments, school activities, job interviews, and transport of essential goods for household activities [21].

Concerning family social exclusion, Macdonald et al. [24] concluded that, by itself, it is a risk factor for the situations of neglect and abusive practices by families.

We found that specific family characteristics such as a history of allegations, domestic violence, family disagreements and conflicts, single-parent families, multiple caregivers, the existence of stepmothers and stepfathers, multi-child families, being the firstborn, and poor communication between separated parents might also be risk factors during child development.

Previous studies found that family characteristics such as having a history of allegations, including a history of abuse and neglect, are risk factors for the child's development [10,21,22,25,26]. Furthermore, families with multiple allegations, either for different children or referring the same child several times, are also associated with child abuse and neglect [26]. In addition, children from single-parent families are more likely to be neglected than children from two-parent families [10,11,18,20,22,25,28]. Thus, there is broad agreement that child maltreatment should be analysed as a problem in the family system, although research focuses on the mother or father [44].

Ineffective communication is a barrier between the child's caregivers, especially when the parents are separated, with difficulties understanding care [21,27,36]. When the most consistent pattern in the parents' relationship involves violence, children exposed to it are more likely to abuse their partner physically. There is a risk of intergenerational transmission of partner violence, which increases when either parents or caregivers are violent [44].

The category caregiver's characteristics encompasses risk factors that include history of inflicting maltreatment, having been neglected, criminal record, alcohol and/or drug abuse, mental health problems, low level of education, lack of cooperation with CPS, being under 18 years old, and unintended pregnancy.

Several authors frame the use of alcohol or drugs in changes in family functioning [4,8,10,11,22,24–26,28,29,32,33,36]. These data are corroborated by a study by Felitti et al. [45], which assessed the adverse childhood experiences of 13,494 individuals. These researchers identified psychological, physical or sexual abuse, domestic violence, and living with substance-abusing and mentally ill family members as risk factors for the child's development.

Previous studies identified that physical illness and physical, intellectual, or cognitive impairments might be considered risk indicators. Laslett, Room, and Dietze [46] conclude that mental or physical illness and alcohol or drug abuse are caregiver characteristics that should be considered risk factors for the child's development.

The caregivers' low level of education is a predictor of abuse and neglect [9–11,22,23,25,26]. A study conducted by Hirsch et al. [26] found that a low level of education was a constant, with 79% of participants having no more than primary education, regardless of whether the associated issue was abuse, neglect, or other forms of maltreatment.

Another risk factor identified in this review was the caregiver's lack of cooperation with Child Protective Services. This lack of collaboration jeopardizes the child's well-being and increases the risk for abuse and neglect [9,12,23].

The last category shows the risk factors associated with parenting that may jeopardize the child's development—namely, not meeting the child's unique needs, unrealistic expectations towards the child, or negative attitudes towards the child, abusive and mistreating practices, multiple trips to children's emergency room, and parents absent in childrearing.

Negative attitudes towards the child are considered to be psychologically toxic parenting behaviours [27]. Along the same line, Zimmermann et al. [28] identified that one of the risk factors for abuse or neglect was perceiving the child as a burden.

There is a significant reduction in the parental skills and commitment of the caregiver's motivation for parenting when physical abuse and child neglect are involved, either due to lack of supervision, unmet basic needs, unsafe home environment, and lack of health care [4]. In addition, emotional sensitivity, parental guidance, the quality of the affective relationship, and the failure to promote the children's autonomy severely compromise cognitive development and reduce the affective sphere, translating into changes in the child's behaviour [28].

CPS assessment needs refinement to better identify cases of child abuse and neglect. This process can be accomplished by introducing an evaluation of family risk factors specific to child neglect and abusive practices [34]. Furthermore, the assessment should be holistic—not focusing on a single factor but considering the accumulation of harm perceived through the various interactions with CPS [43].

Current CPS practices focused on determining the risk of harm associated with the present allegations, not considering past patterns of abuse or neglect. A shift in thinking is necessary to minimize the harmful impact of recurrent neglect over time. CPS can achieve better results by adding a family risk factors assessment in its evaluation processes.

As critics have argued, the introduction of screening tools in CPS assessment processes needs to be followed by training and buy-in from frontline staff [47]. Therefore, training regarding family risk factors and their implications on the child's development should be mandatory for all CPS professionals who handle the allegations.

The results from this review can be helpful for CPS workers when assessing children and families to identify stressors that place a child at risk for child maltreatment. A comprehensive family assessment is essential for identifying children who have experienced or who are at risk of maltreatment. This assessment enables CPS workers to identify and prevent further abuse or neglect and support and improve parental abilities to guarantee a safe and nurturing environment that allows the child's development.

Our results can also be significant for future research, as they can be used as a foundation on which to develop screening tools for assessing family risk factors that jeopardize child development.

This research has several limitations. First, the researchers' choice to develop a scoping review combined with a data-driven thematic analysis instead of a meta-analysis may impact data reliability. Second, the databases' restrictions and imposed time limits may influence the results obtained. Third, we have to consider the exclusion of studies written in languages other than English, Spanish, or Portuguese. These methodological choices may have led to some relevant studies being excluded.

5. Conclusions

The result of this research intends to contribute to allow CPS to adequately assess the presence of risk factors that jeopardize child development. This initial assessment is a fundamental step that enables CPS to collect information that confirms or disproves an allegation's veracity and then act to minimize the impact of the risk factor on the child's development. This review addresses a critical evidence gap regarding the family risk factors that jeopardize child development. It allowed the identification of several articles from which family risk factors were extracted, falling into four categories: social and economic interaction patterns, family characteristics, caregiver's characteristics, and parenting. The identification of these four categories that comprise twenty-eight family risk factors can help CPS workers identify stressors and situations that put children at increased risk for maltreatment. However, despite the usefulness of these results, we must emphasize that although certain factors might be present in families where neglect and abuse occur, it should not be assumed that the presence of these factors causes child maltreatment.

Author Contributions: Conceptualization, A.S.; methodology, A.S. and J.B.F.; formal analysis, A.S., S.L., M.d.A.D. and J.B.F.; data curation, A.S.; writing—original draft preparation, A.S., S.L., M.d.A.D. and J.B.F.; writing—review and editing, A.S., S.L., M.d.A.D. and J.B.F.; supervision, A.S.; project administration, A.S. All authors have read and agreed to the published version of the manuscript.

Funding: This research received no external funding.

Institutional Review Board Statement: Not applicable.

Informed Consent Statement: Not applicable.

Data Availability Statement: The data presented in this study are available on request from the first author.

Acknowledgments: This publication was financed by national funds through the FCT—Foundation for Science and Technology, I.P., under the project UIDB/04585/2020. The researchers would like to thank the Centro de Investigação Interdisciplinar Egas Moniz (CiiEM) for the support provided for the publication of this article.

Conflicts of Interest: The authors declare no conflict of interest.

References

1. Horwitz, B.N.; Neiderhiser, J.M. Environment Interplay, Family Relationships, and Child Adjustment. *J. Marriage Fam.* **2011**, *73*, 804–816. [CrossRef] [PubMed]
2. World Health Organization. 2020. Available online: https://www.who.int/news-room/fact-sheets/detail/child-maltreatment (accessed on 28 November 2021).
3. Schreiber, J.C.; Fuller, T.; Paceley, M.S. Engagement in child protective services: Parent perceptions of worker skills. *Child. Youth Serv. Rev.* **2013**, *35*, 707–715. [CrossRef]
4. Loman, L.A.; Siegel, G.L. Effects of approach and services under differential response on long term child safety and welfare. *Child Abus. Negl.* **2015**, *39*, 86–97. [CrossRef] [PubMed]
5. Thrana, H.M.; Halvor, F. The emotional encounter with child welfare services: The importance of incorporating the emotional perspective in parents' encounters with child welfare workers. *Eur. J. Soc. Work* **2014**, *17*, 221–236. [CrossRef]
6. Toros, K.; LaSala, M.C. Estonian child protection workers' assessment perspectives: The need for competence and confidence. *Int. Soc. Work.* **2018**, *61*, 93–105. [CrossRef]
7. Pecora, P.J.; Whittaker, J.K.; Barth, R.P.; Vesneski, W.; Borja, S. *The Child Welfare Challenge: Policy, Practice and Research*, 4th ed.; Taylor and Francis: New York, NY, USA, 2019.
8. Palusci, V.J.; Ilardi, M. Risk Factors and Services to Reduce Child Sexual Abuse Recurrence. *Child Maltreat.* **2020**, *25*, 106–116. [CrossRef]
9. Ajduković, M.; Rajter, M.; Rezo, I. Individual and contextual factors for the child abuse potential of Croatian mothers: The role of social support in times of economic hardship. *Child Abuse Negl.* **2018**, *78*, 60–70. [CrossRef]
10. Duffy, J.Y.; Hughes, M.; Asnes, A.G.; Leventhal, J.M. Child maltreatment and risk patterns among participants in a child abuse prevention program. *Child Abus. Negl.* **2015**, *44*, 184–193. [CrossRef]
11. Casillas, K.L.; Fauchier, A.; Derkash, B.T.; Garrido, E.F. Implementation of evidence-based home visiting programs aimed at reducing child maltreatment: A meta-analytic review. *Child Abus. Negl.* **2016**, *53*, 64–80. [CrossRef]
12. Schneiderman, J.U.; Hurlburt, M.S.; Leslie, L.K.; Zhang, J.; Horwitz, S.M. Child, caregiver, and family characteristics associated with emergency department use by children who remain at home after a child protective services investigation. *Child Abus. Negl.* **2012**, *36*, 4–11. [CrossRef]
13. Page, M.J.; McKenzie, J.E.; Bossuyt, P.M.; Boutron, I.; Hoffmann, T.C.; Mulrow, C.D.; Shamseer, L.; Tetzlaff, J.F.; Akl, E.A.; Brennan, S.E.; et al. The PRISMA 2020 statement: An updated guideline for reporting systematic reviews. *BMJ* **2021**, *372*, n71. [CrossRef]
14. The Joanna Briggs Institute. *Joanna Briggs Institute Reviewers' Manual: 2015 Edition/Supplement*; The Joana Briggs Institute: Adelaide, South Australia, 2015. Available online: https://nursing.lsuhsc.edu/JBI/docs/ReviewersManuals/Scoping-.pdf (accessed on 5 November 2021).
15. Braun, V.; Clarke, V.; Hayfield, N.; Terry, G. Thematic analysis. In *Handbook of Research Methods in Health Social Sciences*; Liamputtong, P., Ed.; Springer: Singapore, 2019; pp. 843–860.
16. Donohue, B.; Pitts, M.; Chow, G.M.; Benning, S.D.; Soto-Nevarez, A.; Plant, C.P.; Allen, D.N. Development and initial psychometric examination of the Home Safety and Beautification Assessment in mothers referred to treatment by child welfare agents. *Psychol. Assess.* **2016**, *28*, 523–538. [CrossRef]
17. Gurwitch, R.H.; Messer, E.P.; Masse, J.; Olafson, E.; Boat, B.W.; Putnam, F.W. Child-Adult Relationship Enhancement (CARE): An evidence-informed program for children with a history of trauma and other behavioral challenges. *Child Abus. Negl.* **2016**, *53*, 138–145. [CrossRef]
18. Peng, J.; Shao, J.; Zhu, H.; Yu, C.; Yao, W.; Yao, H.; Shi, J.; Xiang, H. A systems approach to addressing child maltreatment in China: China needs a formalized child protection system. *Child Abus. Negl.* **2015**, *50*, 33–41. [CrossRef]
19. Winokur, M.; Ellis, R.; Drury, I.; Rogers, J. Answering the big questions about differential response in Colorado: Safety and cost outcomes from a randomized controlled trial. *Child Abus. Negl.* **2015**, *39*, 98–108. [CrossRef]
20. Jones, A. Implementation of differential response: A racial equity analysis. *Child Abus. Negl.* **2015**, *39*, 73–85. [CrossRef]
21. Fuller, T.L.; Paceley, M.S.; Schreiber, J.C. Differential Response family assessments: Listening to what parents say about service helpfulness. *Child Abus. Negl.* **2015**, *39*, 7–17. [CrossRef]
22. Goltz, H.H.; Mena, K.C.; Swank, P.R. Using growth curve analysis to examine challenges in instrumentation in longitudinal measurement in home visiting. *J. Evid. Based Soc. Work.* **2014**, *11*, 127–138. [CrossRef]
23. Benbenishty, R.; Davidson-Arad, B.; López, M.; Devaney, J.; Spratt, T.; Koopmans, C.; Knorth, E.J.; Witteman, C.L.; Del Valle, J.F.; Hayes, D. Decision making in child protection: An international comparative study on maltreatment substantiation, risk assessment and interventions recommendations, and the role of professionals' child welfare attitudes. *Child Abus. Negl.* **2015**, *49*, 63–75. [CrossRef]
24. Macdonald, G.; Lewis, J.; Macdonald, K.; Gardner, E.; Murphy, L.; Adams, C.; Ghate, D.; Cotmore, R.; Green, J. THE SAAF STUDY: Evaluation of the Safeguarding Children Assessment and Analysis Framework (SAAF), compared with management as usual, for improving outcomes for children and young people who have experienced, or are at risk of maltreatment. *Trials* **2014**, *15*, 453. [CrossRef]

25. Glad, J.; Jergeby, U.; Gustafsson, C.; Sonnander, K. Social worker and teacher apprehension of children's stimulation and support in the home environment and care-giver perception of the HOME Inventory in Sweden. *Br. J. Soc. Work.* **2014**, *44*, 2218–2236. [CrossRef]

26. Hirsch, B.K.; Yang, M.Y.; Font, S.; Slack, K.S. Physically Hazardous Housing and Risk for Child Protective Services Involvement. *Child Welf.* **2015**, *94*, 87–104.

27. Malo, C.; Moreau, J.; Lavergne, C.; Hélie, S. Psychological Maltreatment, the Under-Recognized Violence Against Children: A New Portrait from Quebec. *Child Welf.* **2016**, *95*, 77–99.

28. Zimmermann, P.; Vierhaus, M.; Eickhorst, A.; Sann, A.; Egger, C.; Förthner, J.; Gerlach, J.; Iwanski, A.; Liel, C.; Podewski, F.; et al. Growing up under adversity in Germany: Design and methods of a developmental study on risk and protective mechanisms in families with diverse psychosocial risk. *Bundesgesundheitsblatt Gesundh. Gesundheitsschutz.* **2016**, *59*, 1262–1270. [CrossRef]

29. Ben-David, V. A focus on neglect: Comparing the characteristics of children and parents in cases of neglect, abuse, and non-CAN (child abuse and neglect) in Israeli rulings on termination of parental rights. *J. Aggress. Maltreat. Trauma* **2016**, *25*, 721–740. [CrossRef]

30. Liel, C.; Ulrich, S.M.; Lorenz, S.; Eickhorst, A.; Fluke, J.; Walper, S. Risk factors for child abuse, neglect and exposure to intimate partner violence in early childhood: Findings in a representative cross-sectional sample in Germany. *Child Abus. Negl.* **2020**, *106*, 104487. [CrossRef]

31. Vial, A.; van der Put, C.; Stams, G.J.J.M.; Kossakowski, J.; Assink, M. Exploring the interrelatedness of risk factors for child maltreatment: A network approach. *Child Abus. Negl.* **2020**, *107*, 104622. [CrossRef]

32. Laslett, A.-M.; Room, R.; Dietze, P.; Ferris, J. Alcohol's involvement in recurrent child abuse and neglect cases. *Addiction* **2012**, *107*, 1786–1793. [CrossRef]

33. Vincent, S.; Petch, A. Understanding child, family, environmental and agency risk factors: Findings from an analysis of significant case reviews in Scotland. *Child Fam. Soc. Work* **2017**, *22*, 741–750. [CrossRef]

34. Logan-Greene, P.; Jones, A.S. Predicting chronic neglect: Understanding risk and protective factors for CPS-involved families. *Child Fam. Soc. Work* **2018**, *23*, 264–272. [CrossRef]

35. Gifford, E.J.; Eldred, L.M.; Sloan, F.A.; Evans, K.E. Parental Criminal Justice Involvement and Children's Involvement With Child Protective Services: Do Adult Drug Treatment Courts Prevent Child Maltreatment? *Subst. Use Misuse* **2016**, *51*, 179–192. [CrossRef] [PubMed]

36. Nilchian, F.; Jabbarifar, S.E.; Khalighinejad, N.; Sadri, L.; Saeidi, A.; Arbab, L. Evaluation of factors influencing child abuse leading to oro-facial lesions in Isfahan, Iran: A qualitative approach. *Dent. Res. J.* **2012**, *9*, 624–627. [CrossRef] [PubMed]

37. McConnell, D.; Feldman, M.; Aunos, M.; Prasad, N. Parental cognitive impairment and child maltreatment in Canada. *Child Abus. Negl.* **2011**, *35*, 621–632. [CrossRef] [PubMed]

38. Sinanan, A.N. The impact of child, family, and child protective services factors on reports of child sexual abuse recurrence. *J. Child Sex. Abus.* **2011**, *20*, 657–676. [CrossRef]

39. Hamilton, J.L.; Shapero, B.G.; Stange, J.P.; Hamlat, E.J.; Abramson, L.Y.; Alloy, L.B. Emotional maltreatment, peer victimization, and depressive versus anxiety symptoms during adolescence: Hopelessness as a mediator. *J. Clin. Child Adolesc. Psychol.* **2013**, *42*, 332–347. [CrossRef]

40. Rosenkranz, S.E.; Muller, R.T.; Henderson, J.L. Psychological maltreatment in relation to substance use problem severity among youth. *Child Abus. Negl.* **2012**, *36*, 438–448. [CrossRef]

41. Taillieu, T.L.; Brownridge, D.A. Aggressive parental discipline experienced in childhood and internalizing problems in early adulthood. *J. Fam. Violence* **2013**, *28*, 445–458. [CrossRef]

42. Taylor, J.; Bradbury-Jones, C.; Lazenbatt, A.; Soliman, F. Child maltreatment: Pathway to chronic and long-term conditions? *J. Public Health* **2016**, *38*, 426–431. [CrossRef]

43. Simões, A.C.; Lopes, S.; Dixe, M.A. Risk factors for the development of children and young people referred at a commission for the protection. *Referência* **2021**, *5*, e20046. [CrossRef]

44. Straus, M.A.; Douglas, E.M. Concordance Between Parents in Perpetration of Child Mistreatment: How Often Is It by Father-Only, Mother-Only, or by Both and What Difference Does It Make? *Trauma Violence Abus.* **2019**, *20*, 416–427. [CrossRef]

45. Felitti, V.J.; Anda, R.F.; Nordenberg, D.; Williamson, D.F.; Spitz, A.M.; Edwards, V.; Koss, M.P.; Marks, J.S. Relationship of Childhood Abuse and Household Dysfunction to Many of the Leading Causes of Death in Adults: The Adverse Childhood Experiences (ACE) Study. *Am. J. Prev. Med.* **2019**, *56*, 774–786. [CrossRef]

46. Laslett, A.M.; Room, R.; Dietze, P. Substance misuse, mental health problems and recurrent child maltreatment. *Adv. Dual Diagn.* **2014**, *7*, 15–23. [CrossRef]

47. Bunting, L.; Montgomery, L.; Mooney, S.; MacDonald, M.; Coulter, S.; Hayes, D.; Davidson, G. Trauma Informed Child Welfare Systems-A Rapid Evidence Review. *Int. J. Environ. Res. Public Health* **2019**, *16*, 2365. [CrossRef]

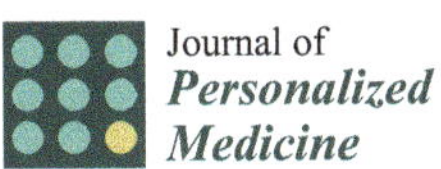

Journal of
Personalized
Medicine

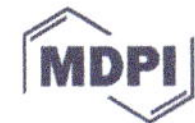

Review

Interventions to Promote a Healthy Sexuality among School Adolescents: A Scoping Review

Fernanda Loureiro *, Margarida Ferreira, Paula Sarreira-de-Oliveira and Vanessa Antunes

Centro de Investigação Interdisciplinar Egas Moniz (CiiEM), Escola Superior de Saúde Egas Moniz, 2829-511 Almada, Portugal; mferreira@egasmoniz.edu.pt (M.F.); psarreira@egasmoniz.edu.pt (P.S.-d.-O.); vantunes@egasmoniz.edu.pt (V.A.)
* Correspondence: floureiro@egasmoniz.edu.pt; Tel.: +351-212-946-807

Abstract: Schools are particularly suitable contexts for the implementation of interventions focused on adolescent sexual behavior. Sexual education and promotion have a multidisciplinary nature. Nurses' role and the spectrum of the carried-out interventions is not clear. We aimed to identify interventions that promote a healthy sexuality among school adolescents. Our review followed the Preferred Reporting Items for Systematic Reviews and Meta-Analyses extension for Scoping Reviews and was registered in the Open Science Framework. Published articles on sexuality in adolescents in school contexts were considered. The research limitations included primary studies; access in full text in English, Spanish, or Portuguese; and no data publication limitation. Research was carried out on the EBSCOhost, PubMed, SciELO, and Web of Science platforms; gray literature and the bibliographies of selected articles were also searched. A total of 56 studies were included in the sample. The studies used a broad range of research methods, and 10 types of interventions were identified. Multi-interventional programs and socio-emotional interventions showed a greater impact on long-term behavioral changes, and continuity seemed to be a key factor. Long-term studies are needed to reach a consensus on the effectiveness of interventions. Nurses' particular role on the multidisciplinary teams was found to be a gap in the research, and must be further explored.

Keywords: adolescent; nursing; review literature; sexuality

Citation: Loureiro, F.; Ferreira, M.; Sarreira-de-Oliveira, P.; Antunes, V. Interventions to Promote a Healthy Sexuality among School Adolescents: A Scoping Review. *J. Pers. Med.* **2021**, *11*, 1155. https://doi.org/10.3390/jpm11111155

Academic Editor: Ruslan Dorfman

Received: 7 September 2021
Accepted: 4 November 2021
Published: 7 November 2021

Publisher's Note: MDPI stays neutral with regard to jurisdictional claims in published maps and institutional affiliations.

1. Introduction

The World Health Organization [1] considers sexuality as a central aspect of human beings. It is influenced by psychological, social, biological, religious, spiritual, political, legal, economic, ethical, and historical issues.

Sexual development is considered a multidimensional process that is experienced more intensely by adolescents as they go through the changes of puberty, develop the capacity for intimacy, and experience sexual thoughts [2]. Adolescence is a complex stage of life that brings several challenges to health professionals. By traditional definition, it includes individuals from 10 to 19 years old. However, the definition has long posed a conundrum, and recently Sawyer at al. [3] suggested an extension to 10–24 years to correspond to a more current and updated concept. Regardless of age limits, it is a period of important biological growth, psychological development, and social role transitions.

The World Health Organization and other agencies consider sexual education as a priority within this age group due to sexual behavior implications, such as maternal mortality or sexually transmitted infections [4], and aspects such as gender-based violence and gender inequality. Since sexuality is an all-encompassing concept, there is no consensual definition of it. However, Goettsch [5] suggested a preliminary definition that includes: sexuality as an individual capacity, its experiential nature, body-oriented, and directed to genital excitation. The World Health Organization [1] gives a more comprehensive definition of sexuality that includes reproduction, sex, sexual orientation, gender identities and roles, pleasure, and intimacy, highlighting that not all of them are always experienced or expressed.

For many years now, schools have been considered privileged contexts for the implementation of health promotion and education, as they are built to foster personal and social development. Schools are the ideal place for building health-promoting communities, and are able to link children, families, and communities with other services (e.g., health services). The role of schools in health promotion is not a new phenomenon. In fact, historically, implementing health education interventions in schools has been recommended by several organizations and in several countries [6].

School-based education includes sexuality in its educational curricula, which is different from interventions, that can be implemented in a more/less structured way. Both approaches are used worldwide according to the context characteristics. School-based interventions are wildly recognized for their impact on adolescents' sexual health [6]. Many sex education programs, especially those centered on risks associated with sexual activity, focus on knowledge as a prerequisite for adopting preventive behaviors. However, results from surveys such as the Health Behavior in School-Aged Children showed a trend of systematic reduction in terms of knowledge and protective behaviors [7]. Simultaneously, scientific evidence has shown that existing knowledge is not directly expressed in preventive practices, and that programs that include an ecological and participatory approach are more effective [8]. Thus, the focus of intervention programs has been expanding at different levels: from risk prevention to well-being, from directed and specific to individual to comprehensive and structural, and from traditional knowledge transference to innovative tools [9].

Interventions such as school policy changes, parent involvement, and work with local communities have been identified as effective for promoting sexual health [10]. In addition, the influence of contextual factors such as peers, parents, siblings, and schools have been examined and established by researchers [11]. As the field of intervention has expanded, it became evident that sexual education and promotion has a multidisciplinary and cross-sectoral nature. Interventions are broad, and are implemented by different professionals such as teachers, social workers, or psychologists, among others.

In this context, nurses are often involved in schools' health promotion programs in general, but their role in these programs is not always clear or visible. Depending on the different realities, they can be in school-based health centers, or work in partnership with teachers or as part of multidisciplinary school health teams, and are often the only link between children and the health system [12]. They work directly with children and adolescents, but also collaborate in the training of teachers and other school personnel [13]. Additionally, annual preventive health examinations are seen as encounters in which screening adolescents for sexual and reproductive health is recommended [14]. Nurses work in a wide variety of settings (hospitals, health centers, schools), which gives them direct access to adolescent populations. In addition, nurses have an important role in promoting accessibility, inclusive communication, competent and guideline-based care, and confidentiality. Barriers to the implementation of health programs, identified by teachers, include lack of training and lack of time [8]. The integration of nurses in these programs represents an added value, and their unique combination of knowledge and specific skills [14] make them an essential and central element in these teams. A preliminary literature search revealed that the available studies on sexual education interventions are dispersed. Specific studies on nursing interventions in the school context also are scarce. The role of nursing and its unique contributions to this area remain less clear and less explored. Therefore, it is fundamental to firstly map the wide spectrum of interventions to promote adolescent sexuality, carried out in the school context. This can further contribute to a clearer identification of nursing's role, and to the planning of interventions that are scientifically accurate, sustainable, and age- and culturally appropriate.

A scoping review was conducted according to the steps defined by Tricco et al. [15] that aimed to identify interventions that promote a healthy sexuality among school adolescents. This methodology proved to be advantageous, as it allowed identifying gaps in the literature, mapping the available evidence [16] that will support the planning of interventions to promote a healthy sexuality among adolescents in schools. The following research question was defined, according to PICo: which are the interventions that promote a healthy sexuality among school adolescents? (Population: adolescents; Interest: interventions to promote a healthy sexuality; Context: school).

2. Materials and Methods

The steps defined by Tricco et al. [15] for the scoping review were followed as detailed below.

Protocol and Registration. The protocol was drawn according to the Preferred Reporting Items for Systematic Reviews and Meta-Analyses extension for Scoping Reviews (PRISMA-ScR) and registered prospectively with the Open Science Framework on 18 June 2021 (https://osf.io/v97ek/?view_only=).

Eligibility criteria. Considering the scarcity of studies on specific nursing interventions, and keeping in mind the multidisciplinary scope of health promotion, for the purposes of this study, we selected studies focused on multidisciplinary interventions. Published articles on nurses, teachers, psychologists, and social care professionals integrated in work groups on sexuality in adolescents from school context were considered for analysis. Empirical studies with quantitative, qualitative, and mixed methods were included to maximize the coverage of evidence available. Peer-reviewed papers available in open access and full text and written in English, Spanish, and Portuguese were included. As to the publication date, no time frame was established. Manuscripts were excluded if studies were performed in specific contexts and specific health conditions (for example, hospitalization or adolescents with mental disorders). Letters to the editor, editorials, literature reviews, theoretical studies, protocols, methodological studies (for example, instrument validation/construction), blog articles, advertising, and opinion articles were excluded. Studies in which subjects were family members or health professionals that did not identify or suggest any interventions were also excluded.

Information sources. A three-step approach was used, as recommended in the literature [17]. The search was initially performed in two databases: Medical Literature Analysis and Retrieval System Online (MEDLINE) and Cumulative Index to Nursing and Allied Health Literature (CINAHL). Then, an analysis of the words contained in the titles and summaries was performed to understand the best terms to be used in the review. The purpose was to identify the keywords to be included in search equation.

In step two, after identifying the MeSH keywords to be used, research was conducted on the electronic platform EBSCOhost in the following databases: Cumulative Index to Nursing and Allied Health Literature (CINAHL) (complete); MEDLINE (complete); Nursing & Allied Health Collection (comprehensive); Cochrane Central Register of Controlled Trials; Cochrane Database of Systematic Reviews; Cochrane Methodology Register; Library, Information Science & Technology Abstracts (LISTA); and MedicLatina. Additionally, PubMed, SciELO, ScienceDirect, and Web of Science were also searched. For grey literature, we used Open Grey, MedNar, and WorldWideScience.org—The Global Science Gateway.

In step three, the list of references from the articles selected in step two were systematically searched to find additional relevant literature for this review.

Search. The research equation, designed with keywords and Boolean operators, was: ((Adolescen *) AND (Sexuality) AND (Nurs *)). An asterisk operator (*) was used, so that the database could identify variants of the original word. Research was performed in March 2021 by all the authors, working in groups of two (F.L. and V.A.; P.O. and M.F.). Considering inclusion criteria and fields available in databases, the sample initially obtained was limited, as shown in Table A1 (Appendix A).

Selection of sources of evidence. Articles were selected initially by title, and when it was not clear if the article fitted this review, the abstract was read. Duplicates were removed, and inclusion/exclusion criteria were applied. Reviewers in groups of two

(F.L. and P.O.; V.A. and M.F.) screened the same publications to increase consistency. Any disagreements between reviewers were resolved through discussion with all reviewers until consensus was reached.

Data-charting process. The variables to be extracted were decided by all researchers, and a data-charting table was developed. The process was initially performed individually by each author. Then, working groups of two were formed (F.L. and P.O.; V.A. and M.F.) to compare the extracted data, resolve disagreements, and increase accuracy. In cases in which the articles contained insufficient information, the authors were contacted. The final extraction chart was discussed by all authors until reaching unanimity.

Data items. Data were extracted related to article characteristics such as reference, country, and methods (aim, population and sample, type of study). We also included the intervention implemented, as well as the main findings.

Critical appraisal of individual sources of evidence. To describe the quality of the selected articles ($n = 56$), studies were appraised by all authors. Divergent views regarding the critical appraisal were reviewed until consensus. The Hawker et al. [18] assessment tool, with a four-grade scale (1 = very poor; 2 = poor; 3 = fair; 4 = good) was used. The total score ranges between 9 and 36, and higher scores indicate higher quality. An article's quality appraisal was centered on the following items: 1—abstract and title; 2—introduction and aims; 3—method and data; 4—sampling; 5—data analysis; 6—ethics and bias; 7—results; 8—transferability or generalizability; and 9—implications and usefulness.

Synthesis of results. Results were synthetized in a table that included all information extracted individually and approved by all authors. The data collected summarized studies and interventions that were identified in this review. Information was collected related to article reference, country where the study was applied, methods, intervention, and findings.

3. Results

Selection of sources of evidence. A total of 149 articles were identified by title. From those, 93 were excluded by abstract. Articles excluded were mainly those that did not identify interventions. Manuscripts that presented only data concerning descriptive statistics for a diagnostic purpose in a particular context were also excluded. The process of study selection is summarized below in Figure 1 using a PRISMA flow chart.

Characteristics of sources of evidence. This review allowed the identification of a broad set of interventions to promote a healthy sexuality among adolescents in the school context. Through the International Classification of Health Interventions (ICHI), the World Health Organization [19] defines a health intervention as an act that has the purpose of assessing, improving, maintaining, promoting, or modifying health, functioning, or health conditions. These interventions can be performed for, with, or on behalf of a person or population. According to ICHI descriptors, interventions regarding sexuality can be mostly framed as interventions on body systems and function (ICHI code 1) or interventions on health-related behaviors (ICHI code 4). In this review, both types were retrieved from articles; however, interventions predominantly were oriented toward behaviors. On the other hand, it was not always clear which type of intervention was implemented; therefore, we categorized them as presented in Table A2 (Appendix A). The interventions were grouped by ascending order of frequency found in sample studies ($n = 56$).

Critical appraisal within sources of evidence. The results demonstrated that overall, the studies' quality was high. Quality appraisal ranged from 18 to 35. Sampling, ethics, and bias, as well as transferability, were the main limitations of the studies (Table A3—Appendix A).

Results of individual sources of evidence. The results from each study selected in this scoping review are synthetized in Table A4 (Appendix A).

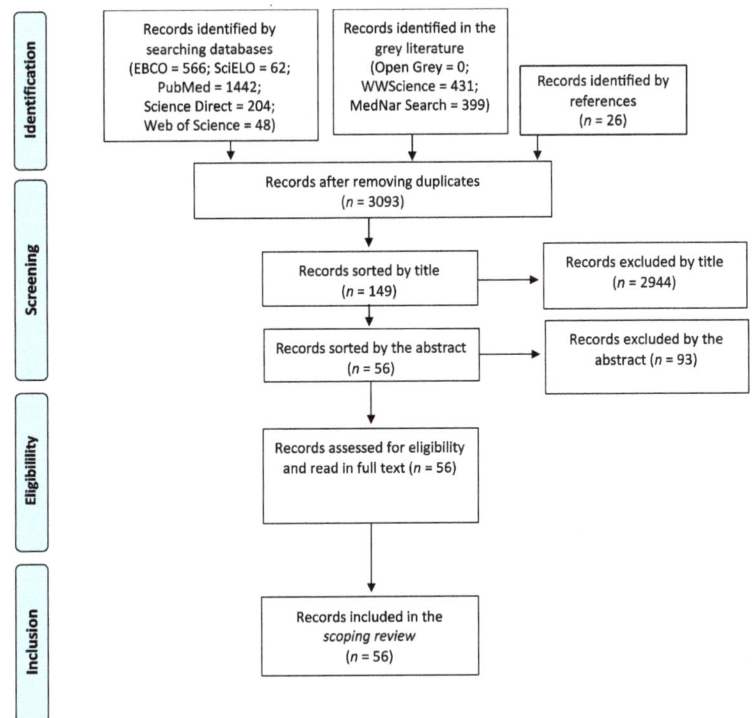

Figure 1. PRISMA flow chart of the study selection.

Synthesis of results. A total of 56 studies published between 1998 and 2021 were selected for final analysis. All studies had adolescents as subjects except for Barnes et al. [20], who studied nurses; and Valli and Cogo [21], whose study was related to school blogs on sexuality. Sample sizes ranged from 10 [22] to 11840 [23]. As to publication date, more than half of our article sample (*n* = 32) were published in the last 10 years. Regarding the country where studies were applied, we verified that there were studies from all around the world; however, three countries stood out: Brazil, with 16 articles; the USA, with 13 articles; and the UK, with 6 articles. Of the studies, 32 were of a quantitative nature, 18 used a qualitative approach, and 6 used mixed methods. Surveys were the most used form of collecting data (28), followed by combined techniques. These techniques included the use of surveys combined with interviews [24–26], focus groups [27,28], and an online environment [29]. A field diary and participating observation were also found as combined data collection techniques [22,30].

4. Discussion

Summary of evidence. The results indicated that adolescent sexuality is a relevant, current, and growing interest theme for health professionals, as we found articles from all around the world, and the great majority were recently published.

Evidence was mapped regarding the type of interventions performed in the school context, the factors that may influence their effectiveness, and a few considerations that were found on the multidisciplinary nature of school-based interventions.

Although studies that described an isolated intervention were found, mostly articles reported the findings of multiple interventional programs, such as SHARE [31–33] and Cuídate [34–36], or combined interventions, as stated above. The diversity of interventions found also reinforced the idea that adolescent health is still an evolving area [37] that requires a multidisciplinary approach.

Innovative approaches were also described, such as the use of blogs [21], Facebook [29], and online games [27,38], as they seemed to have greater acceptance by adolescents. As technologies continue to expand, online resources are becoming progressively relevant and used by adolescents, which raises concerns regarding vulnerability, but also presents opportunities for important impacts on healthy learning [39].

Interestingly, mobile phone intervention was found in six studies. Given the access and amount of time spent by adolescents with these devices, this intervention seems particularly suitable for the adolescent population. As an intervention that uses existing resources, mobile phone intervention is cost effective and sustainable, with the ability to reach many adolescents even in low-income countries. Furthermore, there is evidence that the use of mobile text messages may lead to improved adolescent sexual and reproductive health [40].

Interventions delivered through school-based health centers (SBHCs) are described in two studies. The existence of SBHCs has proven to have an impact on adolescents regarding satisfaction with their health and adherence to health-promoting behaviors [41]. Not all countries have SBHCs, since they are not part of their health and education systems. Nevertheless, policy makers should consider including this strategy in their agendas, as it is a more comprehensive and integrated approach. It has proven to raise adolescents' access to health care services, overcoming identified barriers such as charges, transportation, accessibility, availability, and privacy concerns [23].

Sex education sessions, group discussions, and workshops can be framed as the more traditional interventions. They can be implemented alone, simultaneously, integrated in a broader program, or used combined with other interventions. The studies that addressed them were mostly descriptive, with few considerations of their effectiveness as isolated interventions. With respect to sex education sessions, nurses often have a prominent role, particularly school nurses, as they have a broader knowledge of health-related issues. Brewin et al. [42] reported barriers related to privacy, time, confidentiality, and fear of conflict.

Peer education was only mentioned in four studies. This is an intervention that creates greater expectations around its impact on adolescent sexual behavior because, when performed and conveyed by peers with a similar age or status, it becomes more appealing and credible [43]. However, no study could demonstrate peer education effectiveness by itself. Stephenson et al. [43] argued that it should be considered as part of a broader program.

Concerning interventions' effectiveness, some studies did not assess interventions' impact on adolescent behavior or knowledge, only describing the implementation experience in the school context. Even so, a more comprehensive approach that includes multiple types of interventions seems to be more effective in promoting positive changes in sexual behavior [44]. These findings were aligned with the multidimensional scope of adolescent sexuality.

In general, the articles evaluating the effectiveness of programs demonstrated a very low sustainability in the modification of risk behaviors [31,36,43,45,46] of young people and adolescents. Of the articles included, only one showed maintenance of the positive effects in terms of reduced pregnancies, delayed sexual debut, and intentions to use condoms. Again, it described a more comprehensive approach: a training intervention for children's social competence, classroom management and instruction, and parenting practices without interventions specifically aimed at sexuality [47].

In addition, interventions focused on psycho-affective and socio-emotional skills showed a greater impact on long-term behavioral changes. These findings were in line with the growing interest in socio-emotional skills learning (SEL) that, especially since the beginning of this century, has shown a positive impact on school success, well-being, and health of the participants [48], and which are at the base of health-promotion programs in schools such as the Collaborative for Academic, Social, and Emotional Learning

(CASEL) (Chicago, IL, USA) or the Schools for Health in Europe Network Foundation (SHE) (Haderslev, Denmark).

Furthermore, we believe that the fact that programs are mostly implemented in local and regional contexts and only in a specific period of time limits their long-term effectiveness. Continuity seems to be a key factor in maintaining the change in adolescent behavior with regard to their sexuality.

The fact that so many studies and so many different interventions were found, with little evidence of their effectiveness, may also signify a difficulty in officially instituting and operationalizing them in the long term.

It is worth noting the difficulties in categorizing the domains of sexuality and standardizing the language regarding interventions. Despite the evident effort of the scientific community, there is still no universal consensus on them. Thus, there seems to be agreement on the multidisciplinary nature of interventions that promote adolescent sexuality.

As to limitations, we must consider the possibility of having excluded or missed some relevant studies due to the databases used, and the exclusion of studies written in languages other than English, Spanish, or Portuguese.

5. Conclusions

As previously mentioned, nurses are often involved in schools' health-promotion programs in general, but their role in these programs is not always clear or visible. This research did not allow us to draw conclusions about this topic. Nonetheless, it is interesting to note that most studies had nurses or nursing professors as their first author, although they did not focus exclusively on the role of nurses/nursing care. Again, this can be explained by the multidisciplinary nature of the interventions.

Finding which interventions worked best to promote a healthy sexuality among school adolescents was challenging. As the studies were carried out in very different contexts, and there are few long-term evaluations of the implemented interventions, it was not possible to make considerations about their effectiveness.

This review allowed the identification of interventions implemented in schools to promote adolescents' healthy sexuality; namely, event history calendar, group discussion, interventions delivered through SBHC, peer education, online intervention, mobile phone intervention, combined interventions, workshops, sex education sessions, and multiple interventional programs. These findings were in line with the multidimensional scope of adolescent sexuality. The studies found were recent and were published all around the world, which sustained the idea that this is a relevant and evolving theme.

Although most authors were nursing professionals or nursing students, the particular role of nurses on the multidisciplinary team was not explored. This is clearly a gap in the evidence that requires further investigation. However, this review gave a clear picture of the interventions that can be implemented to promote adolescent sexuality. The effectiveness of those strategies should be further explored. Decision makers should integrate these strategies in their agendas and use them as collaboration measures between the health and education sectors.

Author Contributions: Conceptualization, F.L., M.F., P.S.-d.-O. and V.A.; methodology, F.L., M.F., P.S.-d.-O. and V.A.; software, F.L., M.F., P.S.-d.-O. and V.A.; validation, F.L., M.F., P.S.-d.-O. and V.A.; formal analysis, F.L., M.F., P.S.-d.-O. and V.A.; investigation, F.L., M.F., P.S.-d.-O. and V.A.; resources, F.L., M.F., P.S.-d.-O. and V.A.; data curation, F.L., M.F., P.S.-d.-O. and V.A; writing—original draft preparation, F.L.; writing—review and editing, M.F., P.S.-d.-O. and V.A.; visualization, F.L., M.F., P.S.-d.-O. and V.A.; supervision, F.L., M.F., P.S.-d.-O. and V.A.; project administration, F.L., M.F., P.S.-d.-O. and V.A.; funding acquisition, F.L., M.F., P.S.-d.-O. and V.A. All authors have read and agreed to the published version of the manuscript.

Funding: This work was financed by national funds through the FCT—Foundation for Science and Technology, I.P., under the project UIDB/04585/2020. The researchers would like to thank the Centro de Investigação Interdisciplinar Egas Moniz (CiiEM) for the support provided for the publication of this article.

Institutional Review Board Statement: The study was conducted according to the guidelines of the Declaration of Helsinki, and registered prospectively with the Open Science Framework on 18 June 2021 (https://osf.io/v97ek/?view_only=).

Conflicts of Interest: The authors declare no conflict of interest.

Appendix A

Table A1. Platforms and limiters used in search strategy.

Platform	Limiters
EBSCOhost	Adolescen * AND Sexuality AND Nurs * Portuguese, Spanish, or English language full text available
PubMed	Adolescen * AND Sexuality AND nurs * Portuguese, Spanish, or English language Full text available
SciELO	Adolescente OR adolescência AND sexualidade AND enfermagem
ScienceDirect	(Adolescent OR Adolescence) AND Sexuality AND (nursing OR nurse) Open access
Web of Science	Adolescen * AND Sexuality AND nurs * Portuguese, Spanish, or English language Full text available
Open Grey	Adolescen * AND Sexuality AND nurs *
MedNar	Adolescen * AND Sexuality AND nurs * Full text available
WorldWideScience	(Adolescent OR Adolescence) AND Sexuality AND (nursing OR nurse) Full text available

* Placing an asterisk is a strategy used in serach so that all variants of words are considered.

Table A2. Synthesis of interventions retrieved from studies.

Type of Intervention	Author, Year [49–82]
Event history calendar	(Martyn et al., 2012)
Group discussion	(Beserra et al., 2008; Fonseca et al., 2010)
Interventions delivered through School-Based Health Centers	(Bersamin et al., 2018; Denny et al., 2012)
Peer education	(Hatami et al., 2015; Okanlawon and Asuzu, 2013; Stephenson et al., 2008, 2004)
Online intervention	(Aragão et al., 2018; Castillo-Arcos et al., 2016; Enah et al., 2015; Souza et al., 2017; Valli and Cogo, 2013)
Mobile phone intervention	(Alhassan et al., 2019; Cornelius et al., 2019, 2012; French et al., 2016; Hickman and Schaar, 2018; Rokicki et al., 2017) [49]
Combined interventions	(Aventin et al., 2015; Barnes et al., 2004; Beserra et al., 2017; Gallegos et al., 2008; Hirvonen et al., 2021; Madeni et al., 2011; Oliveira et al., 2016)
Workshops	(Amaral and Fonseca, 2006; Beserra et al., 2006; Camargo and Ferrari, 2009; Carvalho et al., 2005; Freitas and Dias, 2010; Gubert et al., 2009; Levandowski and Schmidt, 2010; Santos et al., 2017; Soares et al., 2008) [50]
Sex education sessions	(Dunn et al., 1998; Elliott et al., 2013; Golbasi and Taskin, 2009; Grandahl et al., 2016; Lieberman et al., 2000; Moodi et al., 2013; Rani et al., 2016; Serowoky et al., 2015; Walker et al., 2006; Yakubu et al., 2019)
Multiple interventions program	(Henderson et al., 2007; Jemmott III et al., 1998; Jemmott et al., 2015; Lonczak et al., 2002; Richards et al., 2019; Siegel et al., 1998; Tucker et al., 2007; Villarruel et al., 2010, 2006; Wight et al., 2002)

Table A3. Critical appraisal of studies included in the scoping review.

Study	Abstract and Title	Introduction and Aims	Method and Data	Sampling	Data Analysis	Ethics and Bias	Results	Transferability or Generalizability	Implications and Usefulness	TOTAL
[58]	4	3	4	4	4	4	4	4	4	35
[59]	4	4	4	4	4	3	4	4	4	35
[24]	4	4	4	4	4	3	4	4	4	35
[49]	4	3	4	4	4	3	4	4	4	34
[47]	4	4	4	4	4	3	4	4	3	34
[74]	4	3	4	4	4	3	4	4	4	34
[43]	4	3	4	4	4	3	4	4	4	34
[51]	4	4	4	3	4	2	4	4	4	33
[23]	4	4	3	4	4	2	4	4	4	33
[27]	4	3	4	4	4	2	4	4	4	33
[45]	4	3	4	4	4	2	4	4	4	33
[70]	4	3	4	4	4	3	4	4	3	33
[80]	4	3	4	4	4	3	4	4	3	33
[33]	4	4	4	4	4	1	4	4	4	33
[82]	4	3	4	4	4	3	4	4	3	33
[64]	4	4	4	3	3	3	4	3	4	32
[65]	4	4	4	4	4	3	4	3	2	32
[31]	4	2	4	4	4	2	4	4	4	32
[72]	4	4	4	3	4	3	4	3	3	32
[77]	4	4	3	3	4	3	4	3	4	32
[54]	4	3	4	3	4	3	4	3	3	31
[57]	4	3	4	3	4	3	4	3	3	31
[46]	4	3	4	3	4	1	4	4	4	31
[34]	4	4	4	3	4	1	4	3	4	31
[79]	4	3	4	3	4	3	4	3	3	31
[21]	4	3	4	3	4	3	3	4	3	31
[35]	4	3	4	3	4	3	4	3	3	31
[81]	4	2	3	4	4	2	4	4	4	31
[61]	4	3	3	3	4	2	4	3	4	30
[68]	4	3	4	3	4	3	4	3	2	30
[69]	3	3	4	3	4	3	4	3	3	30
[25]	4	3	4	3	4	2	4	3	3	30
[30]	3	3	4	2	4	3	4	3	4	30
[32]	4	3	3	3	4	2	4	3	4	30

Table A3. *Cont.*

Study	Abstract and Title	Introduction and Aims	Method and Data	Sampling	Data Analysis	Ethics and Bias	Results	Transferability or Generalizability	Implications and Usefulness	TOTAL
[29]	4	3	4	2	4	3	4	2	3	29
[22]	3	3	4	2	4	3	4	3	3	29
[56]	4	3	3	3	4	3	3	3	3	29
[36]	4	2	3	3	4	3	4	3	3	29
[26]	4	3	4	3	4	3	4	3	4	28
[75]	4	3	4	2	3	3	3	3	3	28
[53]	4	2	3	2	3	3	4	2	4	27
[66]	4	4	3	2	3	2	4	2	3	27
[38]	4	4	3	2	3	3	3	2	3	27
[20]	3	3	4	3	3	2	3	3	2	26
[76]	3	3	3	3	4	2	4	2	2	26
[55]	3	3	3	3	3	2	3	3	2	25
[62]	4	3	3	2	3	2	3	3	2	25
[73]	3	3	3	3	3	1	3	3	3	25
[28]	4	3	2	2	3	2	4	2	3	25
[63]	3	3	3	2	3	3	3	2	2	24
[67]	3	2	3	2	4	2	4	2	2	24
[50]	3	3	3	2	2	3	3	2	2	23
[52]	3	3	3	2	2	2	3	2	3	23
[60]	3	3	2	3	2	1	4	3	2	23
[71]	2	3	3	2	2	2	3	2	2	21
[78]	3	3	1	2	2	1	2	2	2	18

4 = Good, 3 = Fair, 2 = Poor, 1 = Very poor.

Table A4. Study characteristics.

Study	Country	Aim	Type of Study	Population and Sample	Interventions	Key Findings
(Hirvonen et al., 2021)	UK	To understand the perceptions of adolescent students regarding the use of Facebook social media in sexual and reproductive health learning.	Mixed methods	1413 teenagers (14 to 16 years)	Combined interventions: peers' intervention and use of private Facebook groups	Social media groups formed around peer supporters' existing friendship networks hold potential for diffusing messages in peer-based sexual health interventions.
(Alhassan et al., 2019)	Ghana	To assess mobile phone usage among adolescents and young adult populations pursuing tertiary education and their use of these technologies in the education and prevention of STI.	Quantitative	250 teenagers (18 to 24 years)	Mobile phone interventions	Future mobile phone programs should be considered for STI education and prevention, as they were found to be more comfortable than traditional messaging or phone calls.
(Cornelius et al., 2019)	USA	To examine adolescents in the USA and Botswana, their mobile phone and social media usage, and their perceptions of safer-sex interventions delivered via social media.	Qualitative	28 teenagers (13 to 18 years)	Mobile phone interventions	Findings provided a starting point for researchers interested in developing a social media intervention with global implications for sexual health promotion.
(Golbasi and Taskin, 2009)	Turkey	To evaluate the effectiveness of school-based reproductive health education for adolescent girls on the reproductive knowledge level of the girls.	Quasi-experimental	189 adolescents (age not mentioned)	Sex education sessions	The school-based program was conducted by nursing educators, and the program was effective in increasing the students' levels of knowledge on reproductive health.
(Richards et al., 2019)	Dominican Republic	To evaluate the effectiveness of MAMI's CSEP in changing knowledge of STIs and pregnancy.	Mixed methods	600 students aged 11–25 years old	Multiple interventional program (comprehensive sexual education program: education sessions, interactive activities, visual aids)	The MAMI's CSEP improved knowledge of STIs and pregnancy and attitudes toward risky sexual behavior among program recipients.
(Yakubu et al., 2019)	Ghana	To assess an educational intervention program on knowledge, attitude, and behavior toward pregnancy prevention based on the HBM amongst adolescent girls in Northern Ghana.	RCT	363 adolescents (13 to 19 years).	Sex education sessions	Educational intervention, which was guided by HBM, significantly improved sexual abstinence and the knowledge of adolescents on pregnancy prevention.
(Aragão et al., 2018)	Brazil	To understand the perceptions of adolescent students regarding the use of Facebook social media in sexual and reproductive health learning.	Qualitative	96 adolescents (mean age 15 years)	Online interventions (Facebook)	Virtual spaces on the Internet offer potential for the production of health care, especially among adolescents, as it contributes to the sexual and reproductive health education in an interactive, playful, and practical way.

Table A4. *Cont.*

Study	Country	Aim	Type of Study	Population and Sample	Interventions	Key Findings
(Bersamin et al., 2018)	USA	To investigate the associations between SBHCs and sexual behavior and contraceptive use among 11th graders.	Quantitative	11840 adolescents (average age 16.6)	Interventions delivered through SBHCs	Exposure to SBHCs in general, and availability of specific reproductive health services, may be an effective strategy to support healthy sexual behaviors among youth.
(Hickman and Schaar, 2018)	USA	To develop and evaluate adolescent satisfaction with a text-messaging educational intervention to promote healthy behaviors, reduce the incidence of unhealthy behaviors, and prevent high-risk behaviors.	Mixed methods	202 adolescents (14 to 18 years)	Mobile phone interventions	Text messaging is a good way to educate adolescents and promote healthy habits, as it shows a high rate of intended behavioral change by adolescents.
(Beserra et al., 2017)	Brazil	To analyze the perception of adolescents about the life activity "express sexuality".	Qualitative	25 teenagers (15 to 18 years)	Combined interventions: video projection followed by discussion and clarification of doubts	The use of videos followed by discussion is a valid and useful strategy to help adolescents in expressing their sexuality.
(Rokicki et al., 2017)	Ghana	To evaluate whether text-messaging programs can improve reproductive health among adolescent girls in low- and middle-income countries.	RCT	756 adolescents (14 to 24 years)	Mobile phone interventions	Text-messaging programs can lead to large improvements in reproductive health knowledge, and have the potential to lower pregnancy risk for sexually active adolescent girls.
(Santos et al., 2017)	Brazil	To report the experience of conducting a workshop with teenagers about STIs.	Qualitative	34 adolescents (average age, 18 years old)	Workshops	Group educational experiences provide adolescents with the opportunity to build shared knowledge, and professionals learn about adolescents' doubts, and therefore plan new health education meetings.
(Souza et al., 2017)	Brazil	To describe the online game and reflect on its theoretical–methodological basis.	Qualitative	60 adolescents aged 15–18 years	Online game (Straight Talk)	Conceived as a pedagogic device, the online game has the capacity to implicate the adolescent in problem-based situations and allows the invention of other forms to deal with sexuality without the demand of support from a teacher.
(Castillo-Arcos et al., 2016)	Mexico	To evaluate the effect of an internet-based intervention to reduce sexual risk behaviors and increase resilience to sexual risk behaviors among Mexican adolescents.	Quasi-experimental	193 adolescents (14 to 17 years)	Online interventions (sex education sessions)	The intervention improved self-reported resilience to risky sexual behaviors, though not with a reduction in those behaviors.

Table A4. *Cont.*

Study	Country	Aim	Type of Study	Population and Sample	Interventions	Key Findings
(French et al., 2016)	UK	To explore young people's views of and experiences with a mobile phone text-messaging intervention to promote safer-sex behavior.	Qualitative	20 adolescents (16 to 24 years)	Mobile phone interventions	The intervention increased knowledge, confidence, and safer-sex behaviors.
(Grandahl et al., 2016)	Sweden	To improve primary prevention of HPV by promoting vaccination and increased condom use among upper secondary schools.	RCT	741 adolescents (aged 16 years)	Sex education sessions (face-to-face structured interventions)	Face-to-face education delivery by health care providers, such as school nurses, is a highly feasible and effective way to increase adolescents' beliefs and behavior toward primary prevention of HPV, regardless of socioeconomic status, ethnicity, or cultural background.
(Oliveira et al., 2016)	Brazil	To analyze the limits and the potentialities of the Papo Reto game, for construction of knowledge in the field of sexuality with adolescents.	Qualitative	23 adolescents (15 to 18 years)	Combined interventions (virtual game, workshops)	The game can be used as a pedagogic device for dealing with the subject of sexuality in adolescents. The results confirmed the potentiality of the contents for dealing with the complexity of reality from the point of view of gender.
(Rani et al., 2016)	India	To compare the knowledge and attitude regarding pubertal changes among pre-adolescent girls before and after the pubertal preparedness program	Quasi-experimental	104 pre-adolescent (12–14 years)	Sex education sessions	Pubertal preparedness programs and FAQs reinforcement sessions are effective in enhancing knowledge and developing a favorable attitude among pre-adolescent girls.
(Aventin et al., 2015)	Ireland	To design, develop, and optimize an educational intervention about young men and unintended teenage pregnancy based around an interactive film.	Mixed methods	360 adolescents (14 to 17 years)	Combined interventions: interactive film-based interventions (If I were Jack) with group discussion	The model of intervention reported in this paper was presented not as an ideal, but as an exemplar that other researchers might utilize, modify, and improve.
(Enah et al., 2015)	USA	To assess the acceptability and relevance of a web-based HIV prevention game for African American rural adolescents.	Mixed methods	42 adolescents (12 to 16 years)	Online interventions (game: Fast Car)	Using games for HIV prevention was found to be appealing and acceptable, but it was not found to be the best approach to HIV prevention with the target population.

Table A4. *Cont.*

Study	Country	Aim	Type of Study	Population and Sample	Interventions	Key Findings
(Hatami et al., 2015)	Iran	To evaluate the effect of organizing interactions using peer education in schools on the knowledge and attitude toward sexual health.	Quantitative	282 teenagers (14 to 18 years)	Peer education	The use of peer education in schools informally could enhance the knowledge and approach toward aspects of physical health, sexual behaviors, and social and mental changes among female adolescents.
(Jemmott et al., 2015)	2015 South Africa	To test the effect of an HIV/STI risk-reduction intervention.	RCT	1057 adolescents 9–18 years old	Sex education sessions	The HIV/STI risk-reduction intervention reduced unprotected intercourse and caused positive changes on theoretical constructs. Theory-based behavioral interventions with early adolescents can have long-lived effects in the context of a generalized severe HIV epidemic.
(Serowoky et al., 2015)	USA	To plan, implement, and evaluate a sustainable model of sexual health group programming (Cuídate) in a high school with a large Latino student population.	Quasi-experimental	24 adolescents (13 to 18 years)	Multiple interventional program (Cuídate)	The intervention showed significant increases in STI or HIV knowledge, self-efficacy, and intention to use condoms. It can be sustained in a school-based health center with results of efficacy.
(Elliott et al., 2013)	UK	To assess the effectiveness of the Scottish government's National Sexual Health Demonstration Project (HR2).	Quasi-experimental	5283 pupils aged 15–16 years	Sex education sessions	Combining sex education and sexual health services has a limited impact on young people's sexual health.
(Moodi et al., 2013)	Iran	To evaluate the effect of an educational program for puberty health on improving intermediate and high school female students' knowledge in Birjand, Iran.	Quasi-experimental	302 female students (mean age 12.9)	Sex education sessions	Performing educational programs during puberty has a crucial role in young girls' knowledge increase.
(Okanlawon and Asuzu, 2013)	Nigeria	To involve adolescents in school-based health-promotion activities that would improve their perception of risk in sexual behavior.	Quasi-experimental	519 adolescents	Peer education	Adolescents' active participation in health-promotion activities should be encouraged, as it improves the perception of risk in sexual behavior among adolescents.
(Valli and Cogo, 2013)	Brazil	To analyze the structure of school blogs on sexuality and their utilization by adolescents.	Quantitative	11 blogs about sexuality	Online interventions (blog)	The blog is a virtual interaction tool common among adolescents that allows the adolescent to establish relationships with other teens interested in the topic, decreasing feelings of doubt, isolation, and shyness.

Table A4. *Cont.*

Study	Country	Aim	Type of Study	Population and Sample	Interventions	Key Findings
(Cornelius et al., 2012)	USA	To understand adolescents' perceptions of mobile cell phone text-messaging-enhanced and mobile cell phone-based HIV-prevention interventions.	Qualitative	11 teenagers (13 to 18 years)	Mobile phone interventions	The messages increased participants' HIV awareness and knowledge.
(Denny et al., 2012)	New Zealand	To determine the association between availability and quality of school health services and reproductive health outcomes among sexually active students.	Quantitative	2745 adolescents (13 to 17 years)	Interventions delivered through SBHCs	Health services may be able to lower the incidence of pregnancy by providing access to comprehensive health services, including contraceptive care that is easily available and appropriate for the student population.
(Martyn et al., 2012)	USA	To explore the effects of an event history calendar approach on adolescent sexual risk communication and sexual activity.	Mixed methods	30 adolescents (15 to 19 years)	Event history calendar	School nurses could use the event history calendar approach to improve adolescent communication on sexual risks and tailoring of interventions.
(Madeni et al., 2011)	Tanzania	To evaluate a reproductive health awareness program for the improvement of reproductive health for unmarried adolescent girls and boys in urban Tanzania.	Quasi-experimental	305 adolescents (11 to 16 years)	Combined interventions (sex education sessions and group discussions)	The reproductive health program improved the students' knowledge and behavior about sexuality and decision making after the program for both girls and boys. Their attitudes were not likely to change based on the educational intervention.
(Fonseca et al., 2010)	Brazil	To find the perception of adolescents on the sexual orientation actions in a public school and to identify the actions' fragilities and potentials.	Qualitative	15 adolescents (15 to 17 years)	Group discussions	Participative methodology promotes a welcoming and productive work climate and provides larger involvement and learning.
(Freitas and Dias, 2010)	Brazil	To understand teenagers' perceptions about the development of their sexuality.	Qualitative	12 teenagers (11 to 19 years)	Workshops	Teenagers' perceptions about their sexuality emerged from the debates and shared knowledge during the workshops.
(Levandowski and Schmidt, 2010)	Brazil	To enable the exchange of experiences and reflection about sexuality-related actions and choices.	Qualitative	270 adolescents (12 to 15 years)	Workshops	The intervention reduced psychosocial risk factors, providing a healthy development.

Table A4. *Cont.*

Study	Country	Aim	Type of Study	Population and Sample	Interventions	Key Findings
(Villarruel et al., 2010)	Mexico	To examine the effectiveness of a safer-sex program (Cuídate) on sexual behavior, use of condoms, and use of other contraceptives among Mexican youth 48 months after the intervention.	RCT	708 adolescents (mean age 19.22)	Multiple interventional program (Cuídate)	Results demonstrated the efficacy of Cuídate among Mexican adolescents. Future research, policy, and practice efforts should be directed at sustaining safe-sex practices across adolescents' developmental and relationship trajectories.
(Camargo and Ferrari, 2009)	Brazil	To analyze the knowledge of adolescents on sexuality, contraceptive methods, pregnancy, and STDs/AIDS before and after prevention workshops.	Qualitative	117 adolescents (14 to 16 years)	Workshops	There is a need for systematic work, in the medium and long term, in schools regarding adolescent sexuality, as there was no increase in knowledge about STD transmission methods.
(Gubert et al., 2009)	Brazil	To address the use of educational technology as a strategy for health education among the teenagers in the school.	Qualitative	30 teenagers (14 to 18 years)	Workshops	Nursing professionals should produce/readjust new technologies that support the educational process in health education, valuing the skills and aspirations of adolescents, going beyond traditional health education activities based on specific actions and that do not recognize the real needs.
(Beserra et al., 2008)	Brazil	To investigate the adolescents' sexuality from the educative action of a nurse in the prevention of STDs.	Qualitative	10 adolescents (14 to 16 years)	Group discussions	The intervention allowed adolescents to explore and discuss many subjects that involved their sexuality, and it was also a moment to take actions on health education with the objective to prevent risks.
(Gallegos et al., 2008)	Mexico	To test the efficacy of a behavioral intervention designed to decrease risk of sexual behaviors for HIV/AIDS and unplanned pregnancies in Mexican adolescents.	RCT	832 adolescents, age 14–17	Combined interventions: sex education sessions and interactive games	The behavioral intervention represented an important effort, and was effective in promoting safe sexual behaviors among Mexican adolescents.
(Soares et al., 2008)	Brazil	To understand how adolescents live and exercise their sexuality.	Qualitative	350 adolescents (15 to 19 years)	Workshops	The workshops favored the discussion of attitude changes in the adolescents through the information, reflection, and expression of ideas and feelings, representing a process to be complemented by the family, school, and local social politics.

Table A4. *Cont.*

Study	Country	Aim	Type of Study	Population and Sample	Interventions	Key Findings
(Henderson et al., 2007)	Scotland	To assess the impact of a theoretically based sex education program (SHARE) delivered by teachers compared with conventional education in terms of conceptions and terminations registered by the NHS.	RCT	4196 female (mean age 20)	Multiple intervention program (SHARE)	Enhanced teacher-led school sex education (SHARE) improved knowledge and reduced regret, but did not reduce conceptions or terminations compared with conventional sex education.
(Tucker et al., 2007)	2006 UK-Lothian	To test for improved outcomes for the new Lothian Healthy Respect's SHARE on teenage sexual behavior outcomes in the Lothian region.	Quasi-experimental	4381 secondary school pupils (average age 14.6 years)	Multiple intervention program (SHARE)	The findings demonstrated limited impact on sexual health behavior outcomes and raised questions about the likely and achievable sexual health gains for teenagers from school-based interventions.
(Amaral and Fonseca, 2006)	Brazil	To understand adolescents' social representations on sexual initiation concerning gender.	Qualitative	16 adolescents (11 to 16 years)	Workshops	The strategy allowed the understanding of the social representations of teenagers about sexual initiation, being of great importance for planning the work developed with teenagers, supporting debates and reflections on the experience of healthy and responsible sexuality by young people.
(Beserra et al., 2006)	Brazil	To describe an experience to promote health and prevent STDs among teenagers.	Qualitative	28 adolescents (13 to 16 years)	Workshops	The strategy was effective at promoting teenagers' adoption of preventative measures.
(Villarruel et al., 2006)	USA	To test the efficacy of a prevention intervention to reduce sexual risk behavior among Latino adolescents.	RCT	553 adolescents, aged 13 to 18 years	Multiple interventional program (Cuídate)	Results provided evidence for efficacy for HIV prevention in decreasing sexual activity and increasing condom use among Latino adolescents.
(Walker et al., 2006)	Mexico	To assess effects on condom use and other sexual behavior of an HIV prevention program at school that promotes the use of condoms with and without emergency contraception.	RCT	First-year high school students ($n = 10954$) (16–17 years)	Sex education sessions	A rigorously designed, implemented, and evaluated HIV education course based in public high schools did not reduce risk behavior, so such courses need to be redesigned and evaluated.

Table A4. *Cont.*

Study	Country	Aim	Type of Study	Population and Sample	Interventions	Key Findings
(Carvalho et al., 2005)	Brazil	To determine how the intervention in sexual guidance was experienced by adolescents.	Qualitative	13 adolescents (13 to 15 years)	Workshops	The analysis demonstrated a reconstruction / redefinition of meaning for the ideas related to sexuality, to gender, and to the wider social context.
(Barnes et al., 2004)	Australia	To evaluate the impact of changes in the health system and services on the roles and responsibilities of child health nurses and to identify professional development needs.	Qualitative	10 nurses	Combined interventions: health education and health information displays.	The school-based youth health nurse program provides nurses with a new, challenging, autonomous role within the school environment, and the opportunity to expand their role to incorporate all aspects of the health-promoting schools' framework.
(Stephenson et al., 2004)	UK	To examine the effectiveness of one form of peer-led sex education.	RCT	8000 students (13 to 14 years)	Peer education	Peer-led sex education was effective in some ways, but broader strategies are needed to improve young people's sexual health. The role of single-sex sessions should be further investigated.
(Lonczak et al., 2002)	USA	To examine the long-term effects of the full SSDP intervention on sexual behavior and associated outcomes assessed at age 21 years.	Non-randomized controlled trial	349 former fifth-grade students (aged 21 years)	Multiple interventional program (SSDP)	A theory-based social development program that promotes academic success, social competence, and bonding to school during the elementary grades can prevent risky sexual practices and adverse health consequences in early adulthood.
(Wight et al., 2002)	Scotland	To determine whether a theoretically based sex education program for adolescents (SHARE) delivered by teachers reduced unsafe sexual intercourse compared with current practice.	RCT	8430 pupils aged 13–15 years	Multiple intervention program (SHARE)	Compared with conventional sex education, this specially designed intervention did not reduce sexual risk-taking in adolescents.
(Lieberman et al., 2000)	USA	To assess the impact of an abstinence-based model for sexual education.	Quantitative	312 students (mean age 12.9)	Multiple intervention program (IMPPACT)	A small-group abstinence-based intervention can have some impact on adolescents' attitudes and relationships (particularly with their parents).
(Dunn et al., 1998)	Canada	To evaluate a school-based HIV prevention intervention in adolescents.	Quasi-experimental	160 adolescents (14 to 15 years)	Sex education sessions	School-based interventions can improve adolescents' short-term HIV/AIDS prevention knowledge, attitudes, self-efficacy, and behavioral intentions.

Table A4. *Cont.*

Study	Country	Aim	Type of Study	Population and Sample	Interventions	Key Findings
(Jemmott III et al., 1998)	USA	To evaluate the effects of abstinence and safer-sex HIV risk-reduction interventions on young inner-city African American adolescent's HIV sexual risk behaviors when implemented by adult facilitators as compared with peer cofacilitators.	RCT	659 adolescents (mean age 11.8)	Sex education sessions	Both abstinence and safer-sex interventions can reduce HIV sexual risk behaviors, but safer-sex interventions may have longer-lasting effects, and may be especially effective with sexually experienced adolescents.
(Siegel et al., 1998)	USA	To determine the short-term effect of a middle and high school–based AIDS and sexuality intervention (RAPP) on knowledge, self-efficacy, and behavior intention.	Non-randomized controlled trial	Middle and high school students ($n = 3635$)	Multiple interventional program (RAPP): games, role playing, take-home exercises	At short-term follow-up, the RAPP intervention had a powerful effect on knowledge for all students and a moderate effect on sexual self-efficacy and safe behavior intention, particularly for high school students.
(Stephenson et al., 2008)	UK	To assess the long-term effects of a peer-led sex education program.	RCT	9000 students (13–14 years)	Peer education	Compared with conventional school sex education at age 13–14 y, this form of peer-led sex education was not associated with a change in teenage abortions, but may have led to fewer teenage births, and was popular with pupils. It merits consideration within broader teenage-pregnancy-prevention strategies.

References

1. World Health Organization. Implementing the global reprodutive health strategy. *Policy Br. World Health Organ. Dept. Reprod. Health Res.* **2006**, *2*, 7.
2. Holland-Hall, C.; Quint, E.H. Sexuality and disability in adolescents. *Pediatr. Clin. N. Am.* **2017**, *64*, 435–449. [CrossRef]
3. Sawyer, S.M.; Azzopardi, P.S.; Wickremarathne, D.; Patton, G.C. The age of adolescence. *Lancet Child Adolesc. Health* **2018**, *2*, 223–228. [CrossRef]
4. Mullinax, M.; Mathur, S.; Santelli, J. *Adolescent Sexual Health and Sexuality Education*; Cherry, A.L., Baltag, V., Dillon, M.E., Eds.; Springer International Publishing: Berlin/Heidelberg, Germany, 2017. [CrossRef]
5. Goettsch, S.L. Clarifying basic concepts: Conceptualizing sexuality. *J. Sex Res.* **1989**, *26*, 249–255. [CrossRef]
6. Young, I. Health promotion in schools—A historical perspective. *Promot. Educ.* **2005**, *12*, 112–117. [CrossRef] [PubMed]
7. Inchley, J.; Currie, D.; Budisavljevic, S.; Torsheim, T.; Jåstad, A.; Cosma, A.; Kelly, C.; Már Arnarsson, Á. *Spotlight on Adolescent Health and Well-Being Survey in Europe and Canada International Report Volume 1. Key Findings*; HBSC: Glasgow, UK, 2018.
8. Leung, H.; Shek, D.; Leung, E.; Shek, E. Development of contextually-relevant sexuality education: Lessons from a comprehensive review of adolescent sexuality education across cultures. *Int. J. Environ. Res. Public Health* **2019**, *16*, 621. [CrossRef] [PubMed]
9. Michielsen, K.; De Meyer, S.; Ivanova, O.; Anderson, R.; Decat, P.; Herbiet, C.; Kabiru, C.W.; Ketting, E.; Lees, J.; Moreau, C.; et al. Reorienting adolescent sexual and reproductive health research: Reflections from an international conference. *Reprod. Health* **2015**, *13*, 3. [CrossRef] [PubMed]
10. Shackleton, N.; Jamal, F.; Viner, R.M.; Dickson, K.; Patton, G.; Bonell, C. School-based interventions going beyond health education to promote adolescent health: Systematic review of reviews. *J. Adolesc. Health* **2016**, *58*, 382–396. [CrossRef] [PubMed]
11. Mmari, K.; Sabherwal, S. A review of risk and protective factors for adolescent sexual and reproductive health in developing countries: An Update. *J. Adolesc. Health* **2013**, *53*, 562–572. [CrossRef] [PubMed]
12. Willgerodt, M.A.; Brock, D.M.; Maughan, E.D. Public school nursing practice in the United States. *J. Sch. Nurs.* **2018**, *34*, 232–244. [CrossRef] [PubMed]
13. Leroy, Z.C.; Wallin, R.; Lee, S. The role of school health services in addressing the needs of students with chronic health conditions. *J. Sch. Nurs.* **2017**, *33*, 64–72. [CrossRef] [PubMed]
14. Santa Maria, D.; Guilamo-Ramos, V.; Jemmott, L.S.; Derouin, A.; Villarruel, A. Nurses on the front lines. *AJN Am. J. Nurs.* **2017**, *117*, 42–51. [CrossRef] [PubMed]
15. Tricco, A.C.; Lillie, E.; Zarin, W.; O'Brien, K.K.; Colquhoun, H.; Levac, D.; Moher, D.; Peters, M.D.J.; Horsley, T.; Weeks, L.; et al. PRISMA Extension for Scoping Reviews (PRISMA-ScR): Checklist and explanation. *Ann. Intern. Med.* **2018**, *169*, 467. [CrossRef]
16. Munn, Z.; Peters, M.D.J.; Stern, C.; Tufanaru, C.; McArthur, A.; Aromataris, E. Systematic review or scoping review? Guidance for authors when choosing between a systematic or scoping review approach. *BMC Med. Res. Methodol.* **2018**, *18*, 143. [CrossRef] [PubMed]
17. Peters, M.; Godfrey, C.M.; Mcinerney, P.; Baldini Soares, C.; Khalil, H.; Parker, D. Guidance for the Conduct of JBI Scoping Reviews. In *Joana Briggs Institute Reviewer's Manual*; Aromataris, E., Munn, Z., Eds.; The Joanna Briggs Institute: Adelaide, Australia, 2017; pp. 141–146.
18. Hawker, S.; Payne, S.; Kerr, C.; Hardey, M.; Powell, J. Appraising the evidence: Reviewing disparate data systematically. *Qual. Health Res.* **2002**, *12*, 1284–1299. [CrossRef]
19. World Health Organization. International Classification of Health Interventions. Available online: https://www.who.int/standards/classifications/international-classification-of-health-interventions (accessed on 7 September 2021).
20. Barnes, M.; Courtney, M.D.; Pratt, J.; Walsh, A.M. School-based youth health nurses: Roles, responsibilities, challenges, and rewards. *Public Health Nurs.* **2004**, *21*, 316–322. [CrossRef]
21. Valli, G.P.; Cogo, A.L.P. School blogs about sexuality: An exploratory documentary study. *Rev. Gaúcha Enferm.* **2013**, *34*, 31–37. [CrossRef]
22. Beserra, E.P.; da Pinheiro, P.N.C.; Barroso, M.G.T. Educative action of nurse in the prevention of sexually transmitted diseases: An investigation with the adolescents. *Esc. Anna Nery* **2008**, *12*, 522–528. [CrossRef]
23. Bersamin, M.; Paschall, M.J.; Fisher, D.A. Oregon school-based health centers and sexual and contraceptive behaviors among adolescents. *J. Sch. Nurs.* **2018**, *34*, 359–366. [CrossRef] [PubMed]
24. Grandahl, M.; Rosenblad, A.; Stenhammar, C.; Tydén, T.; Westerling, R.; Larsson, M.; Oscarsson, M.; Andrae, B.; Dalianis, T.; Nevéus, T. School-based intervention for the prevention of HPV among adolescents: A cluster randomised controlled study. *BMJ Open* **2016**, *6*, e009875. [CrossRef]
25. Hirvonen, M.; Purcell, C.; Elliott, L.; Bailey, J.V.; Simpson, S.A.; McDaid, L.; Moore, L.; Mitchell, K.R. Peer-to-peer sharing of social media messages on sexual health in a school-based intervention: Opportunities and challenges identified in the STASH feasibility trial. *J. Med. Internet Res.* **2021**, *23*, e20898. [CrossRef]
26. Martyn, K.K.; Darling-Fisher, C.; Pardee, M.; Ronis, D.L.; Felicetti, I.L.; Saftner, M.A. Improving sexual risk communication with adolescents using event history calendars. *J. Sch. Nurs.* **2012**, *28*, 108–115. [CrossRef]
27. Enah, C.; Piper, K.; Moneyham, L. Qualitative evaluation of the relevance and acceptability of a web-based HIV prevention game for rural adolescents. *J. Pediatr. Nurs.* **2015**, *30*, 321–328. [CrossRef] [PubMed]

28. Richards, S.D.; Mendelson, E.; Flynn, G.; Messina, L.; Bushley, D.; Halpern, M.; Amesty, S.; Stonbraker, S. Evaluation of a comprehensive sexuality education program in La Romana, Dominican Republic. *Int. J. Adolesc. Med. Health* **2019**, 1–18. [CrossRef] [PubMed]

29. Aragão, J.M.N.; do Gubert, F.A.; Torres, R.A.M.; da Silva, A.S.R.; Vieira, N.F.C. The use of facebook in health education: Perceptions of adolescent students. *Rev. Bras. Enferm.* **2018**, *71*, 265–271. [CrossRef] [PubMed]

30. Soares, S.M.; Amaral, M.A.; Silva, L.B.; Silva, P.A.B. Workshops on sexuality in adolescence: Revealing voices, unveiling views student's of the medium teaching glances. *Esc. Anna Nery* **2008**, *12*, 485–491. [CrossRef]

31. Henderson, M.; Wight, D.; Raab, G.M.; Abraham, C.; Parkes, A.; Scott, S.; Hart, G. Impact of a Theoretically Based Sex Education Programme (SHARE) delivered by teachers on NHS registered conceptions and terminations: Final results of cluster randomised trial. *BMJ* **2007**, *334*, 133. [CrossRef]

32. Tucker, J.S.; Fitzmaurice, A.E.; Imamura, M.; Penfold, S.; Penney, G.C.; Van Teijlingen, E.; Shucksmith, J.; Philip, K.L. The effect of the national demonstration project healthy respect on teenage sexual health behaviour. *Eur. J. Public Health* **2007**, *17*, 33–41. [CrossRef]

33. Wight, D.; Raab, G.M.; Henderson, M.; Abraham, C.; Buston, K.; Hart, G.; Scott, S. Limits of teacher delivered sex education: Interim behavioural outcomes from randomised trial. *BMJ* **2002**, *324*, 1430. [CrossRef]

34. Serowoky, M.L.; George, N.; Yarandi, H. Using the program logic model to evaluate ¡Cuídate!: A sexual health program for latino adolescents in a school-based health center. *Worldviews Evid.-Based Nurs.* **2015**, *12*, 297–305. [CrossRef] [PubMed]

35. Villarruel, A.M.; Jemmott, J.B.; Jemmott, L.S. A randomized controlled trial testing an HIV Prevention Intervention for Latino Youth. *Arch. Pediatr. Adolesc. Med.* **2006**, *160*, 772. [CrossRef] [PubMed]

36. Villarruel, A.M.; Zhou, Y.; Gallegos, E.C.; Ronis, D.L. Examining long-term effects of cuídate-a sexual risk reduction program in Mexican Youth. *Rev. Panam. Salud Pública* **2010**, *27*, 345–351. [CrossRef]

37. Salam, R.A.; Das, J.K.; Lassi, Z.S.; Bhutta, Z.A. Adolescent health interventions: Conclusions, evidence gaps, and research priorities. *J. Adolesc. Health* **2016**, *59*, S88–S92. [CrossRef] [PubMed]

38. De Souza, V.; Gazzinelli, M.F.; Soares, A.N.; Fernandes, M.M.; de Oliveira, R.N.G.; da Fonseca, R.M.G.S. The game as strategy for approach to sexuality with adolescents: Theoretical-methodological reflections. *Rev. Bras. Enferm.* **2017**, *70*, 376–383. [CrossRef]

39. Giovanelli, A.; Ozer, E.M.; Dahl, R.E. Leveraging technology to improve health in adolescence: A developmental science perspective. *J. Adolesc. Health* **2020**, *67*, S7–S13. [CrossRef] [PubMed]

40. L'Engle, K.L.; Mangone, E.R.; Parcesepe, A.M.; Agarwal, S.; Ippoliti, N.B. Mobile phone interventions for adolescent sexual and reproductive health: A systematic review. *Pediatrics* **2016**, *138*, e20160884. [CrossRef] [PubMed]

41. McNall, M.A.; Lichty, L.F.; Mavis, B. The impact of school-based health centers on the health outcomes of middle school and high school students. *Am. J. Public Health* **2010**, *100*, 1604–1610. [CrossRef]

42. Brewin, D.; Koren, A.; Morgan, B.; Shipley, S.; Hardy, R.L. Behind closed doors. *J. Sch. Nurs.* **2014**, *30*, 31–41. [CrossRef]

43. Stephenson, J.; Strange, V.; Allen, E.; Copas, A.; Johnson, A.; Bonell, C.; Babiker, A.; Oakley, A. The Long-Term Effects of a Peer-Led Sex Education Programme (RIPPLE): A cluster randomised trial in schools in England. *PLoS Med.* **2008**, *5*, e224. [CrossRef] [PubMed]

44. Denford, S.; Abraham, C.; Campbell, R.; Busse, H. A Comprehensive review of reviews of school-based interventions to improve sexual-health. *Health Psychol. Rev.* **2017**, *11*, 33–52. [CrossRef] [PubMed]

45. Jemmott, J.B.; Jemmott, L.S.; O'Leary, A.; Ngwane, Z.; Lewis, D.A.; Bellamy, S.L.; Icard, L.D.; Carty, C.; Heeren, G.A.; Tyler, J.C.; et al. HIV/STI risk-reduction intervention efficacy with South African adolescents over 54 months. *Health Psychol.* **2015**, *34*, 610–621. [CrossRef] [PubMed]

46. Lieberman, L.D.; Gray, H.; Wier, M.; Fiorentino, R.; Maloney, P. Long-term outcomes of an abstinence-based, small-group pregnancy prevention program in New York City Schools. *Fam. Plann. Perspect.* **2000**, *32*, 237–245. [CrossRef]

47. Lonczak, H.S.; Abbott, R.D.; Hawkins, J.D.; Kosterman, R.; Catalano, R.F. Effects of the seattle social development project on sexual behavior, pregnancy, birth, and sexually transmitted disease outcomes by age 21 Years. *Arch. Pediatr. Adolesc. Med.* **2002**, *156*, 438. [CrossRef] [PubMed]

48. Domitrovich, C.E.; Durlak, J.A.; Staley, K.C.; Weissberg, R.P. Social-emotional competence: An essential factor for promoting positive adjustment and reducing risk in school children. *Child Dev.* **2017**, *88*, 408–416. [CrossRef] [PubMed]

49. Alhassan, R.K.; Abdul-Fatawu, A.; Adzimah-Yeboah, B.; Nyaledzigbor, W.; Agana, S.; Mwini-Nyaledzigbor, P.P. Determinants of Use of Mobile Phones for Sexually Transmitted Infections (STIs) education and prevention among adolescents and young adult population in Ghana: Implications of public health policy and interventions design. *Reprod. Health* **2019**, *16*, 120. [CrossRef]

50. Amaral, M.A.; da Fonseca, R.M.G.S. Between desire and fear: Female adolescents' social representation on sexual initiation. *Rev. Esc. Enferm. USP* **2006**, *40*, 469–476. [CrossRef] [PubMed]

51. Aventin, Á.; Lohan, M.; O'Halloran, P.; Henderson, M. Design and development of a film-based intervention about teenage men and unintended pregnancy: Applying the medical research council framework in practice. *Eval. Program Plann.* **2015**, *49*, 19–30. [CrossRef]

52. Beserra, E.P.; Sousa, L.B.; Cardoso, V.P.; Alves, M.D.S. Perception of adolescents about the life activity "express sexuality". *Rev. Pesqui. Cuid. Fundam. Online* **2017**, *9*, 340–346. [CrossRef]

53. Beserra, E.P.; de Araújo, M.F.M.; Barroso, M.G.T. Health promotion in transmissible diseases—An investigation among teenagers. *ACTA Paul. Enferm.* **2006**, *19*, 402–407. [CrossRef]

54. Camargo, E.Á.I.; Ferrari, R.A.P. Adolescents: Knowledge about sexuality before and after participating in prevention workshops. *Cien. Saude Colet.* **2009**, *14*, 937–946. [CrossRef]

55. Carvalho, A.M.; Rodrigues, C.S.; Medrado, K.S. Workshop in human sexuality with adolescents. *Estud. Psicol.* **2005**, *10*, 377–384. [CrossRef]

56. Castillo-Arcos, L.D.C.; Benavides-Torres, R.A.; López-Rosales, F.; Onofre-Rodríguez, D.J.; Valdez-Montero, C.; Maas-Góngora, L. The effect of an internet-based intervention designed to reduce HIV/AIDS sexual risk among mexican adolescents. *AIDS Care* **2016**, *28*, 191–196. [CrossRef]

57. Cornelius, J.B.; Whitaker-Brown, C.; Neely, T.; Kennedy, A.; Okoro, F. Mobile phone, social media usage, and perceptions of delivering a social media safer sex intervention for adolescents: Results from two countries. *Adolesc. Health Med. Ther.* **2019**, *10*, 29–37. [CrossRef]

58. Cornelius, J.B.; St. Lawrence, J.S.; Howard, J.C.; Shah, D.; Poka, A.; McDonald, D.; White, A.C. Adolescents' perceptions of a mobile cell phone text messaging-enhanced intervention and development of a mobile cell phone-based HIV prevention intervention. *J. Spec. Pediatr. Nurs.* **2012**, *17*, 61–69. [CrossRef] [PubMed]

59. Denny, S.; Robinson, E.; Lawler, C.; Bagshaw, S.; Farrant, B.; Bell, F.; Dawson, D.; Nicholson, D.; Hart, M.; Fleming, T.; et al. Association between availability and quality of health services in schools and reproductive health outcomes among students: A multilevel observational study. *Am. J. Public Health* **2012**, *102*, e14–e20. [CrossRef]

60. Dunn, L.; Ross, B.; Caines, T.; Howorth, P. A School-Based HIV/AIDS prevention education program: Outcomes of peer-led versus community health nurse-led interventions. *J. Pract. Nurs.* **1998**, *42*, 49.

61. Elliott, L.; Henderson, M.; Nixon, C.; Wight, D. Has untargeted sexual health promotion for young people reached its limit? A quasi-experimental study. *J. Epidemiol. Commun. Health* **2013**, *67*, 398–404. [CrossRef] [PubMed]

62. Da Fonseca, A.D.; Gomes, V.L.D.O.; Teixeira, K.C. Perception of adolescents about an educative action in sexual orientation conducted by nursing academics'. *Esc. Anna Nery* **2010**, *14*, 330–337. [CrossRef]

63. De Freitas, K.R.; Dias, S.M.Z. Teenagers' perceptions regarding their sexuality. *Texto Context. Enferm.* **2010**, *19*, 351–357. [CrossRef]

64. French, R.S.; McCarthy, O.; Baraitser, P.; Wellings, K.; Bailey, J.V.; Free, C. Young people's views and experiences of a mobile phone texting intervention to promote safer sex behavior. *JMIR mHealth uHealth* **2016**, *4*, e26. [CrossRef]

65. Gallegos, E.C.; Villarruel, A.M.; Loveland-Cherry, C.; Ronis, D.L.; Yan Zhou, M. Intervención para reducir riesgo en conductas sexuales de adolescentes: Un ensayo aleatorizado y controlado. *Salud Publica Mex.* **2008**, *50*, 59–66. [CrossRef]

66. Golbasi, Z.; Taskin, L. Evaluation of school-based reproductive health education program for adolescent girls. *Int. J. Adolesc. Med. Health* **2009**, *21*, 395–404. [CrossRef] [PubMed]

67. Gubert, F.A.; dos Santos, A.C.L.; Aragão, K.A.; Pereira, D.C.R.; Vieira, N.F.C.; Pinheiro, P.N.C. Educational technology in the school context: Strategy for health education in a public school in fortaleza-CE. *Rev. Eletronica Enferm.* **2009**, *11*, 165–172.

68. Hatami, M.; Kazemi, A.; Mehrabi, T. Effect of peer education in school on sexual health knowledge and attitude in girl adolescents. *J. Educ. Health Promot.* **2015**, *4*, 78. [CrossRef] [PubMed]

69. Hickman, N.E.; Schaar, G. Impact of an educational text message intervention on adolescents' knowledge and high-risk behaviors. *Compr. Child. Adolesc. Nurs.* **2018**, *41*, 71–82. [CrossRef] [PubMed]

70. Jemmott, J.B., III; Sweet Jemmott, L.; Fong, G.T. Abstinence and safer sex HIV risk-reduction interventions for African American Adolescents. *JAMA* **1998**, *279*, 1529. [CrossRef]

71. Levandowski, D.C.; Schmidt, M.M. Workshop addressing sexuality and dating directed to adolescents. *Paid* **2010**, *20*, 431–436. [CrossRef]

72. Madeni, F.; Horiuchi, S.; Iida, M. Evaluation of a reproductive health awareness program for adolescence in urban Tanzania-A quasi-experimental pre-test post-test research. *Reprod. Health* **2011**, *8*, 21. [CrossRef] [PubMed]

73. Moodi, M.; Shahnazi, H.; Sharifirad, G.-R.; Zamanipour, N. Evaluating puberty health program effect on knowledge increase among female intermediate and high school students in Birjand, Iran. *J. Educ. Health Promot.* **2013**, *2*, 57. [CrossRef] [PubMed]

74. Okanlawon, F.A.; Asuzu, M.C. Secondary school adolescents' perception of risk in sexual behaviour in rural community of Oyo State, Nigeria. *J. Community Med. Prim. Health Care* **2013**, *24*, 21–28.

75. De Oliveira, R.N.G.; Gessner, R.; de Souza, V.; da Fonseca, R.M.G.S. Limits and possibilities of an online game for building adolescents' knowledge of sexuality. *Cien. Saude Colet.* **2016**, *21*, 2383–2392. [CrossRef]

76. Rani, M.; Sheoran, P.; Kumar, Y.; Singh, N. Evaluating the effectiveness of pubertal preparedness program in terms of knowledge and attitude regarding pubertal changes among pre-adolescent girls. *J. Fam. Reprod. Health* **2016**, *10*, 122–128.

77. Rokicki, S.; Cohen, J.; Salomon, J.A.; Fink, G. Impact of a text-messaging program on adolescent reproductive health: A cluster–randomized trial in Ghana. *Am. J. Public Health* **2017**, *107*, 298–305. [CrossRef] [PubMed]

78. Santos, M.P.; de Alencar, A.B.; Lima, S.V.M.A.; Silva, G.M.; Carvalho, C.M.D.L.; da Farre, A.G.M.C.; de Sousa, L.B. Educational pre-carnival on sexually transmitted infections with school adolescents. *Rev. Enferm. UFPE Line* **2017**, *11*, 5116. [CrossRef]

79. Siegel, D.M.; Aten, M.J.; Roghmann, K.J.; Enaharo, M. Early effects of a school-based human immunodeficiency virus infection and sexual risk prevention intervention. *Arch. Pediatr. Adolesc. Med.* **1998**, *152*, 961–970. [CrossRef]

80. Stephenson, J.; Strange, V.; Forrest, S.; Oakley, A.; Copas, A.; Allen, E.; Babiker, A.; Black, S.; Ali, M.; Monteiro, H.; et al. Pupil-Led Sex Education in England (RIPPLE Study): Cluster-randomised intervention trial. *Lancet* **2004**, *364*, 338–346. [CrossRef]

81. Walker, D.; Gutierrez, J.P.; Torres, P.; Bertozzi, S.M. HIV prevention in Mexican schools: Prospective randomised evaluation of intervention. *BMJ* **2006**, *332*, 1189–1194. [CrossRef]
82. Yakubu, I.; Garmaroudi, G.; Sadeghi, R.; Tol, A.; Yekaninejad, M.S.; Yidana, A. Assessing the impact of an educational intervention program on sexual abstinence based on the health belief model amongst adolescent girls in Northern Ghana, a cluster randomised control trial. *Reprod. Health* **2019**, *16*, 124. [CrossRef] [PubMed]

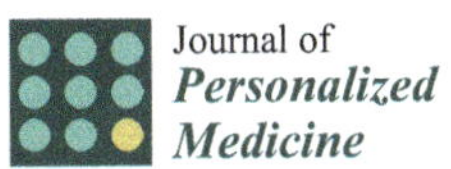

Journal of
Personalized
Medicine

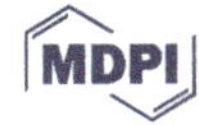

Review

The SGLT-2 Inhibitors in Personalized Therapy of Diabetes Mellitus Patients

Mariana Cornelia Tilinca, Robert Aurelian Tiuca *, Ioan Tilea and Andreea Varga

"G. E. Palade" University of Medicine, Pharmacy, Science and Technology of Targu Mures, 540142 Targu Mures, Romania; mariana.tilinca@umfst.ro (M.C.T.); ioan.tilea@umfst.ro (I.T.); andreea.varga@umfst.ro (A.V.)
* Correspondence: tiuca.robert@gmail.com

Abstract: Diabetes mellitus (DM) represents a major public health problem, with yearly increasing prevalence. DM is considered a progressive vascular disease that develops macro and microvascular complications, with a great impact on the quality of life of diabetic patients. Over time, DM has become one of the most studied diseases; indeed, finding new pharmacological ways to control it is the main purpose of the research involved in this issue. Sodium–glucose cotransporter 2 inhibitors (SGLT-2i) are a modern drug class of glucose-lowering agents, whose use in DM patients has increased in the past few years. Besides the positive outcomes regarding glycemic control and cardiovascular protection in DM patients, SGLT-2i have also been associated with metabolic benefits, blood pressure reduction, and improved kidney function. The recent perception and understanding of SGLT-2i pathophysiological pathways place this class of drugs towards a particularized patient-centered approach, moving away from the well-known glycemic control strategy. SGLT-2i have been shown not only to reduce death from cardiovascular causes, but also to reduce the risk of stroke and heart failure hospitalization. This article aims to review and highlight the existing literature on the effects of SGLT-2i, emphasizing their role as oral antihyperglycemic agents in type 2 DM, with important cardiovascular and metabolic benefits.

Keywords: diabetes mellitus; SGLT-2 inhibitors; antidiabetic agents; cardiovascular outcomes; personalized therapy

Citation: Tilinca, M.C.; Tiuca, R.A.; Tilea, I.; Varga, A. The SGLT-2 Inhibitors in Personalized Therapy of Diabetes Mellitus Patients. *J. Pers. Med.* **2021**, *11*, 1249. https://doi.org/10.3390/jpm11121249

Academic Editors: Fábio G. Teixeira, Catarina Godinho and Júlio Belo Fernandes

Received: 29 October 2021
Accepted: 23 November 2021
Published: 25 November 2021

Publisher's Note: MDPI stays neutral with regard to jurisdictional claims in published maps and institutional affiliations.

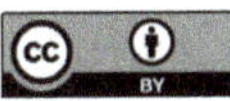

1. Introduction

Diabetes mellitus (DM) is a major public health problem, with yearly increasing prevalence. Worldwide, more than 460 million people have DM, with estimations stating that there will be over 700 million cases in the next 20 years [1]. DM is an important risk factor for cardiovascular disease (CVD). Once present, CVD is the main cause of morbidity and mortality in diabetic patients [2,3]. Hence, when managing DM, physicians should be paying attention not only to the proper control of blood glucose, but also to the obtainment of cardiovascular protection. Several glucose-lowering agents, such as metformin or glucagon-like peptide 1 receptor agonists (GLP-1 RAs), have proven important cardiovascular benefits [4–8].

Sodium–glucose cotransporter 2 inhibitors (SGLT-2i) are a modern drug class of glucose-lowering agents, whose use in DM patients has increased in recent years. Currently, the American Diabetes Association (ADA) recommends SGLT-2i as a second-line drug option, after metformin, for managing type 2 DM patients with established CVD [9]. Besides the positive outcomes regarding glycemic control and cardiovascular protection in DM, SGLT-2i have also been associated with metabolic benefits (such as weight loss), blood pressure reduction, and improved kidney function [10–13]. The positive effects of SGLT-2i have been demonstrated in individuals with and without type 2 DM [14,15].

This article aims to review and highlight the existing literature on the effects of SGLT-2i, emphasizing their role as oral antihyperglycemic agents in type 2 DM, with important cardiovascular and metabolic benefits.

2. Mechanism of Action of SGLT-2i and Clinical Effects—A Brief Overview

2.1. Mechanism of Action of SGLT-2i

In healthy persons, almost all filtered glucose is reabsorbed ($\approx$180 g daily) and almost no glucose is found in the urine as a consequence of SGLT-2 and SGLT-1 action benefits. SGLT-2 proteins are mainly found in the proximal renal convoluted tubule segment 1, and are responsible for up to 90% of filtered glucose reabsorption, while, in humans, SGLT-1 acts on segment 3 of the proximal tubule and in the intestine, where it reabsorbs the remaining 10% of glucose [16–19]. The Na^+/K^+ ATP pump located on the membrane of the tubular cells provides the energy for glucose reabsorption, which is an active transport mechanism [18]. SGLT-2 can also be found in the brain, liver, thyroid, heart, and skeletal muscle, although in much lower amounts [20]. The physiological renal threshold for glucose reabsorption corresponds to a blood glucose concentration of 180 mg/dL. Patients with DM type 1 and 2 have an increased renal threshold, and, consequently, the expression of SGLT-2 can be up-regulated in diabetic patients, worsening preexisting hyperglycemia [21]. The mechanism of action of SGLT-2i consists of blocking glucose reabsorption at the proximal renal tubule, resulting in glucosuria, osmotic diuresis, and natriuresis, thus reducing blood glucose without stimulating insulin release [22,23]. Currently, in the United States and Europe, there are five SGLT-2i widely used in type 1 and 2 DM patients, which are as follows: canagliflozin (INVOKANA), dapagliflozin (FORXIGA, FARXIGA), empagliflozin (JARDIANCE), ertugliflozin (STEGLATRO), and sotagliflozin (ZYNQUISTA) (Table 1) [18,21,24].

Table 1. List of the currently most used SGLT-2i in the United States and Europe.

Name	Available Doses (Milligrams)	Route of Administration
Canagliflozin (INVOKANA®)	100, 300	Oral, q.a.m
Dapagliflozin (FORXIGA™, FARXIGA™)	5, 10	Oral, q.a.m
Empagliflozin (JARDIANCE®)	10, 25	Oral, q.a.m
Ertugliflozin (STEGLATRO®)	5, 15	Oral, q.a.m
Sotagliflozin (ZYNQUISTA™)	200	Oral, q.a.m
Abbreviations	q.a.m, every morning	

2.2. Clinical Effects of SGLT-2i

By suppressing glucose reabsorption and increasing glucosuria ($\approx$75 g glucose/day, which corresponds to almost 300 kcal/day), as well as promoting osmotic diuresis ($\approx$400 mL/day), SGLT-2i reduce blood glucose and promote weight loss [18]. The reduction in fasting and postprandial glucose caused by SGLT-2i is associated with decreased insulin secretion and increased plasma glucagon concentration [25]. Furthermore, by reducing glucotoxicity, SGLT-2i may improve beta-cell function [26,27].

Taking into consideration the fact that the glucose-lowering effect depends on kidney function, dysfunction of the renal system may alter this effect. Therefore, regarding the glucose-lowering efficacy, therapy with SGLT-2i is not recommended in patients with an estimated glomerular filtration rate (eGFR) <45 mL/min. On the other hand, given that SGLT-2i are associated with positive renal outcomes, therapy with this drug class may be considered in diabetic patients with renal impairment, to improve kidney function [28–30]. Decreased insulin secretion results in lipolysis and increased circulating free fatty acids [18]. Glucagon elevation also contributes to lipolysis, and reduces visceral fat [31]. SGLT-2i can reduce the levels of uric acid in a dose-dependent manner [32]. A summary of the mechanism of action and the clinical effects associated with SGLT-2i is illustrated in Figure 1.

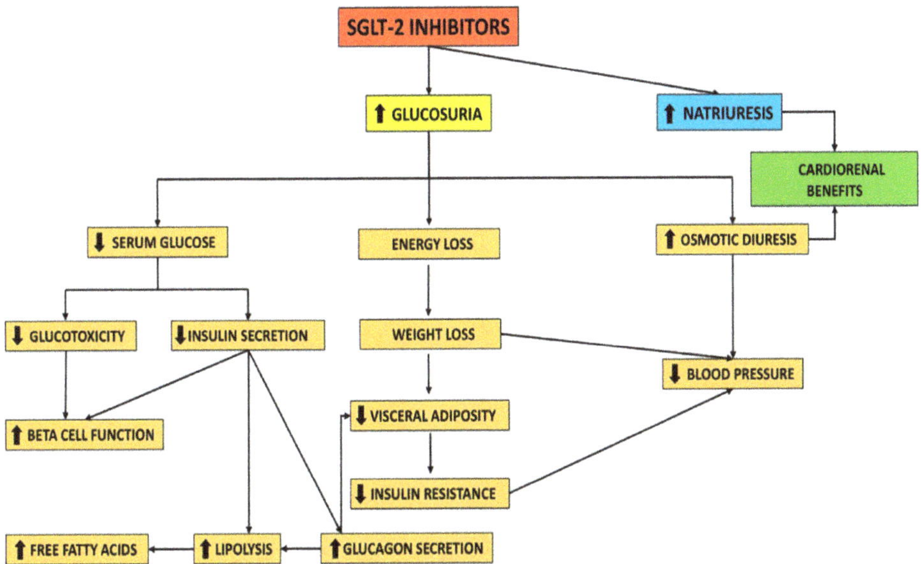

Figure 1. Mechanism of action of SGLT-2 inhibitors.

3. SGLT-2i as Antidiabetic Agents

Diabetes mellitus is a complex metabolic disorder frequently associated with excess weight, hypertension, dyslipidemia, and non-alcoholic fatty liver disease (NAFLD) [33,34]. Moreover, diabetic patients have an increased risk of cardiovascular and renal complications [3,35]. Therefore, an optimal antidiabetic drug should not only possess a good glucose-lowering capacity, but should also exhibit benefits on body weight, blood pressure, lipid profile, NAFLD, cardiovascular function, and renal function. SGLT-2i have been shown to meet many of these criteria. Besides SGLT-2i, glucagon-like peptide 1 (GLP-1) receptor agonists, another modern drug class, exhibit similar benefits in diabetic patients [36,37].

3.1. Improving Glycemic Control

SGLT-2i have consistently proven their efficacy in improving glycemic control in patients with type 2 DM in numerous studies, reducing the levels of glycated hemoglobin (HbA1c), and improving the fasting and postprandial glycemic values [38].

Bailey et al. assessed the efficacy and safety of dapagliflozin in patients with type 2 DM poorly controlled with metformin, in a phase 3, double-blind, placebo-controlled trial. A total of 546 patients were randomized to dapagliflozin 2.5, 5, or 10 mg, or a placebo, once daily. It was noted that treatment with dapagliflozin produced greater HbA1c reduction vs. the placebo (−0.67% with dapagliflozin 2.5 mg, −0.70% with dapagliflozin 5 mg, and −0.84% with dapagliflozin 10 mg vs. −0.30% with the placebo; P for all three doses of dapagliflozin vs. placebo: <0.0001) [39]. A meta-analysis of 45 clinical trials, published in 2013 by Vasilakou et al., showed that HbA1c was reduced by 0.79% (95% confidence interval (CI): −0.96% to −0.62%) with SGLT-2i in monotherapy, and by 0.61% (95% CI: −0.69% to −0.53%) with SGLT-2 as an add-on therapy to other antidiabetic agents [40].

In a 26-week, randomized, double-blind, placebo-controlled study, canagliflozin was assessed regarding its safety and efficacy in subjects with type 2 DM and poor glycemic control, uncontrolled with diet and exercise. Canagliflozin (100 and 300 mg) significantly reduced HbA1c compared to the placebo (−0.77% vs. −1.03% vs. −0.14%, respectively; $p < 0.001$ for both doses of canagliflozin) [41]. In a 24-week, randomized, controlled trial, the efficacy and safety of empagliflozin were evaluated when added to linagliptin and metformin in patients with inadequately controlled type 2 DM [42]. Empagliflozin (10 and 25 mg) significantly reduced HbA1c by −0.79% and −0.70%, respectively, versus the placebo. Fasting plasma glucose (FPG) was also significantly reduced by empagliflozin vs. placebo ($p < 0.001$) [40]. A phase 3 study evaluated the efficacy and safety of ertugliflozin plus sitagliptin in patients with type 2 DM inadequately controlled by diet and exercise [43]. After 26 weeks, it was noted that HbA1c was reduced by 1.7%, 1.6%, and 0.4% with ertugliflozin 15 mg plus sitagliptin 100 mg, ertugliflozin 5 mg plus sitagliptin 100 mg, and the placebo, respectively. FPG and postprandial glucose were also significantly reduced in both the ertugliflozin plus sitagliptin groups compared to the placebo group [43].

Shyangdan et al. published a meta-analysis in 2016, which had the objective to indirectly compare SGLT-2i in diabetes treatment. Few differences between SGLT-2i were noted. In monotherapy, canagliflozin 300 mg achieved a greater HbA1c reduction vs. canagliflozin 100 mg (risk ratio (RR): 0.72%) and dapagliflozin 10 mg (RR: 0.63%), without significant differences when compared to empagliflozin [44]. Goring et al. conducted a meta-analysis that assessed the change in HbA1c when adding thiazolidinediones (TZD), sulphonylureas (SU), dipeptidyl peptidase inhibitors (DDP4-i), or dapagliflozin to the treatment of diabetic patients who were uncontrolled with metformin in monotherapy. Dapagliflozin had a treatment effect on HbA1c of −0.08%, relative to DDP4-i, and −0.02%, relative to TZD, with similar HbA1c reduction when compared with SU [45]. Canagliflozin 100 and 300 mg reduced HbA1c by 0.59% and 0.75%, respectively, in a meta-analysis of six randomized controlled trials, which assessed the efficacy and tolerability of canagliflozin as an add-on therapy to metformin in patients with type 2 DM. Moreover, FPG was reduced by 1.49 mmol/L (canagliflozin 100 mg) and 1.80 mmol/L (canagliflozin 300 mg) [46].

According to a meta-analysis of randomized controlled trials, published in 2014, when added to other antidiabetic drugs, dapagliflozin reduced HbA1c and FPG by 0.52% and 20 mg/dL, respectively [47]. A meta-analysis that included 38 trials and 23,997 participants showed that SGLT-2i improved glucose control, achieving a decrease in HbA1c between 0.6–0.9% and a decrease in FPG between 1.1–1.9 mmol/L [48]. The efficacy of ertugliflozin was assessed when given to patients with type 2 DM, who were treated with metformin [49]. After 26 weeks, ertugliflozin 5 and 15 mg reduced HbA1c by 0.7% and 0.9%, respectively [49]. A randomized, double-blind, placebo-controlled 4-week study compared dapagliflozin 10 mg/day with a placebo in adult patients with type 2 DM, monitoring a 24 h glycemic profile using continuous glucose monitoring. After 4 weeks, dapagliflozin 10 mg/day achieved a mean glucose reduction of 18.2 mg/dL vs. 5.8 mg/dL increase with a placebo ($p < 0.001$) [50].

In a 24-week, randomized, controlled trial, empagliflozin 10 or 25 mg was added to pioglitazone in patients with type 2 DM, with or without metformin. Empagliflozin achieved a HbA1c reduction of −0.6% (10 mg) and −0.7% (25 mg) vs. −0.1% with a placebo (P for both doses of empagliflozin < 0.001) [51]. FPG was reduced by −0.94 mmol/L (10 mg) and −1.22 mmol/L (25 mg) vs. +0.36 mmol/L with a placebo (P for both doses of empagliflozin < 0.001) [51]. Empagliflozin 10 and 25 mg was evaluated regarding its efficacy when added to liraglutide 0.9 mg/day in a 52-week, randomized, phase 4 trial [52]. After 52 weeks, empagliflozin 10 and 25 mg improved HbA1c by 0.55% and 0.77%, respectively. FPG was also reduced by 32.5 mg/dL and 36 mg/dL, respectively [52]. Terra et al. investigated the efficacy of ertugliflozin 5 and 15 mg in patients with diabetes that was were inadequately controlled with diet and exercise [53]. After 26 weeks, the treatment with ertugliflozin significantly reduced HbA1c from the baseline by 0.99% (5 mg) and 1.16% (15 mg), improving FPG and postprandial glucose as well [53].

A summary of the presented studies, regarding the effects of SGLT-2i on improving glycemic control, is illustrated in Supplementary Table S1.

3.2. Body Weight Reduction Benefits and Effects on Blood Pressure

SGLT-2i also have weight reduction benefits in diabetic patients, which may help in diminishing insulin resistance, reducing complications, and improving quality of life.

Body weight loss was observed in patients with type 2 DM who were taking SGLT-2i as a monotherapy or in combination with other antidiabetic agents.

Regarding body composition, Bolinder et al. showed, through dual-energy X-ray absorptiometry, that dapagliflozin reduced total body weight by mostly reducing fat mass [54]. Moreover, dapagliflozin reduced visceral and subcutaneous adiposity, according to a magnetic resonance imaging sub-study [54]. On the other hand, Fadini et al. found that, compared to a placebo, dapagliflozin did not affect fat mass when the body composition was analyzed by bio-impedenzometry [55].

Ferrannini et al. observed that, even though glucosuria is persistent over time, body weight loss reaches a plateau, given that chronic glucosuria may induce an adaptive increase in energy intake. Therefore, SGLT-2i may induce greater weight loss if combined with reduced caloric intake [56]. Ji et al. noted a dose-dependent weight loss effect for dapagliflozin 5 mg and 10 mg compared with a placebo (−1.64 kg vs. −2.25 kg vs. −0.27 kg, respectively) [57]. Kaku et al. reported similar results, regarding body weight reduction effects, for dapagliflozin 5 mg and 10 mg compared with a placebo (−2.13 kg vs. −2.22 kg vs. −0.84 kg, respectively) [58]. Combining SGLT-2i with other agents that possess weight reduction benefits via different mechanisms may lead to major weight loss [11]. The co-administration of dapagliflozin once daily (10 mg) and exenatide, a member of the GLP-1 RAs family, once weekly (2 mg) resulted in a greater mean bodyweight loss in patients with type 2 DM than that achieved with monotherapies alone. The change in baseline weight was −3.41 kg for the exenatide plus dapagliflozin group, −1.54 kg for the exenatide group, and −2.19 kg for the dapagliflozin group [59]. Strojek et al. observed that adding dapagliflozin to glimepiride, a member of the sulphonylureas family, improved body weight compared with a placebo. Dapagliflozin 2.5, 5, and 10 mg/day added to glimepiride 4 mg/day produced a weight loss of −1.36, −1.54, and −2.41 kg, respectively, vs. −0.77 kg with a placebo [60].

Canagliflozin exhibits positive and dose-dependent effects on body weight, HbA1c, and systolic blood pressure reduction. Patients who achieved greater weight loss also achieved greater reductions in HbA1c and systolic blood pressure. A weight loss of 1% was associated with a 0.045% reduction in HbA1c and a 0.62 mmHg reduction in systolic blood pressure [61]. In the same direction, in a recent meta-analysis, SGLT-2i was were proven to have a mean reduction, both in systolic and diastolic blood pressure, assessed by 24 h ambulatory blood pressure monitoring. Independent of the SGLT-2i dose, this effect is comparable with a low dose of hydrochlorothiazide [62]. According to the results of a the Systolic Blood Pressure Intervention trial (SPRINT trial), in hypertensive patients without diabetes, who have increased cardiovascular risk, targeting a systolic blood pressure of ≤120 mmHg (intensive strategy), rather than ≤140 mmHg (standard strategy), was associated with lower incidence of major adverse cardiovascular events and all-cause mortality [63,64]. Buckley et al. conducted a study to determine the effects of intensive blood pressure on cardiovascular outcomes in subjects with type 2 DM and additional risk factors for cardiovascular disease. Intensive blood pressure treatment reduced the incidence of cardiovascular death, nonfatal myocardial infarction, revascularization, and heart failure (HF) [65]. In a review conducted by Oliva et al., SGLT-2i (dapagliflozin and canagliflozin) were associated with a reduction of 4–10 mmHg in systolic blood pressure in both hypertensive and normotensive patients with type 2 DM [66]. Tikkanen et al. demonstrated that empagliflozin produced a significant reduction in 24 h systolic and diastolic blood pressure in patients with type 2 DM [67]. Moreover, empagliflozin also produced a significant reduction in 24 h systolic (−5.1 mmHg) and diastolic (−2.0 mmHg) blood pressure in non-diabetic patients, without acute changes regarding renal oxygenation [68]. Therefore, although this modern drug class is not approved as an antihypertensive agent, by reducing body weight and high blood pressure, SGLT-2i have a positive impact on reducing both cardiovascular and renal risk, regardless of the presence or absence of diabetes.

3.3. SGLT-2i and Cardiorenal Continuum

Diabetic patients are prone to developing atherosclerotic cardiovascular disease (AS-CVD), HF, and renal disease. The pathophysiological chain of the cardiorenal continuum illustrates a continuous progression up to the end stage of heart disease; with a focus on a diabetic subgroup, such as type 2 DM, this is the cardinal point in the cardiorenal continuum, as is shown in Figure 2 [69]. Cardioprotective outcomes in type 2 DM patients mediated by SGLT-2i are related to systemic and direct myocardial effects. In cardiac homeostasis, the main effects address decreasing myocardial fibrosis/steatosis, reducing cardiac and vascular inflammation, and improving systolic and diastolic myocardial function [70]. SGLT-2i have moderate benefits in patients with baseline ASCVD, decreasing the major adverse cardiovascular events (MACE) by 14% [14].

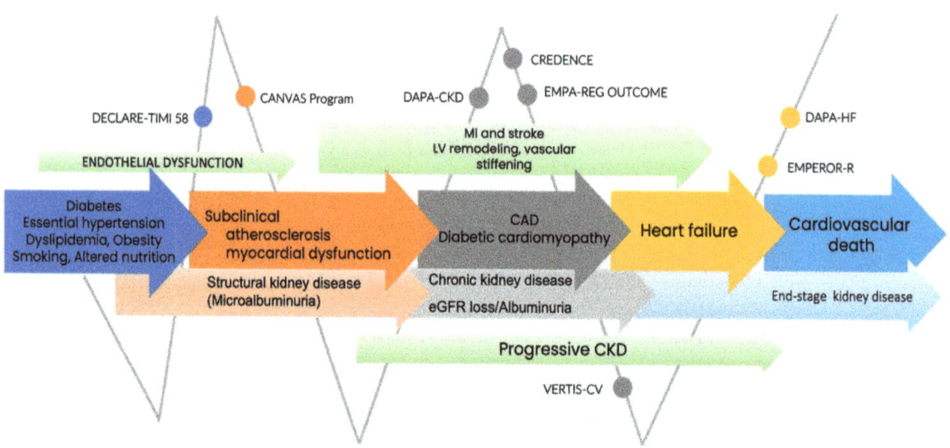

Figure 2. SGLT-2 randomized studies in cardiorenal continuum. Abbreviations: CAD, coronary artery disease; CKD, chronic kidney disease; eGFR, estimated glomerular filtration rate; LV, left ventricle; MI, myocardial infarction.

Referring to the effects of empagliflozin in type 2 DM patients with coronary artery disease, Bilgin et al. stated, in the SUPER GATE study, that the use of this SGLT-2i significantly reduced the anthropometric indices (body weight and mass index, and waist and hip circumferences) associated with type 2 DM. In this subset of patients, the metabolic parameters, including low-density lipoprotein cholesterol levels, were improved, along with targeted blood pressure values and heart rate. The kidney function, assessed by serum creatinine levels and eGFR, was not significantly modified [71].

The multicenter, double-blind, randomized controlled VERTIS-CV trial tested the effect of ertugliflozin on patients with type 2 DM and established ASCVD, and showed the non-inferiority of this SGLT-2i compared to a placebo, in terms of MACE and reduction in risk of the first hospitalization for HF, but not for known HF patients [72]. The cardioprotection mechanisms of SGLT-2i use were conclusively proved in in vivo models by dapagliflozin, which decreases myocardial fibrosis through the inhibition of fibroblast multiplication in the endothelial-to-mesenchymal transition (EndMT) via AMPKα-mediated inhibition of TGF-β/Smad signaling [73]. In ischemic myocardial injury in nondiabetic HF, with reduced ejection fraction (HFrEF) porcine models, empagliflozin showed improved diastolic dysfunction, alleviating left ventricle and cardiomyocyte stiffness [74].

Chronic kidney disease (CKD) is recognized in 30% of patients with type 1 DM and 40% of patients with type 2 DM [75]. Initially, empagliflozin, canagliflozin, and dapagliflozin demonstrated nephroprotection in DM patients without advanced CKD [76–78]. Clinical trials and real-world clinical practice data of SGLT-2i use in patients with type 2 DM, evaluating renal outcome, showed both a reduction in the loss of eGFR and end-stage kidney disease [79]. In patients with CKD in different stages, independent of diabetes condition, DAPA-CKD (Dapagliflozin and Prevention of Adverse Outcomes in Chronic Kidney Disease) and CREDENCE (Canagliflozin and Renal Events in Diabetes with Established Nephropathy Clinical Evaluation) trials walk one through renal protection. The CREDENCE trial confirmed the use of canagliflozin down to an eGFR of 30 mL/min/1.73 m^2. Nonetheless, it remains to be clarified whether this beneficial effect can be attributed to the drug itself, or whether it is an SGLT-2 class effect [80–82]. Ertugliflozin reduced renal risk by 19%, but still did not prove significant benefits in composite renal outcomes, including renal death, need for dialysis or kidney transplantation, or a two-fold increase in serum creatinine, in the VERTIS CV study [72].

3.3.1. The Era of SGLT-2i Benefits in Heart Failure

The risk of developing HF in DM patients is at least two times higher compared to non-diabetic patients [83]. The potential mechanism by which SGLT-2i intervene in both the preserved and reduced HF risk of type 2 DM patients is related to multiple pathophysiological processes addressing three major directions, which are as follows:

1. Decreased preload (increased osmotic diuresis and natriuresis);

2. Decreased afterload (lowered blood pressure, reduced arterial stiffness, and vascular resistance);

3. Strengthening of myocardial contractility (inhibition of cardiomyocyte Na$^+$/H exchanger; increased myocardial energetics, systolic and diastolic function, cardiac output, heart rate, O^2 consumption, and mediated coronary blood flow; reduction in myocardial Ca^{2+}/calmodulin-dependent protein kinase II activity and left ventricular mass) [70,84].

SGLT-2i demonstrated positive effects on the scaling down of admission rates in HF patients, and the lowering of CV (cardiovascular) and all-cause mortality in diabetic patients [72,78,85–87]. The use of three SGLT-2i (empagliflozin, canagliflozin, and dapagliflozin) have a Class 1 level of evidence A, in that they lower the risk of HF hospitalization in DM patients by 35%, 33%, and 27%, respectively, as stated in the 2019 European Society of Cardiology Guidelines on diabetes, pre-diabetes, and cardiovascular diseases [88].

The first clinical trial exploring the effectiveness of SGTL-2i on cardiovascular outcomes in HFrEF patients, EMPA-REG OUTCOME (Empagliflozin Cardiovascular Outcome Event Trial in Type 2 Diabetes Mellitus Patients), met the primary outcome in lowering the deaths from cardiovascular causes, nonfatal myocardial infarction or stroke, and the secondary outcome for hospitalization for HF (hHF) [70]. The 10 mg, once daily dose efficacy of empagliflozin, as an add-on to the optimal HF therapy, was explored in patients with HFrEF, New York Heart Association (NYHA) functional class II–IV, in the EMPEROR Reduced trial [89]. Empagliflozin reduced the risk of death due to CV events and acute HF episodes by 5.3% compared to a placebo, $p < 0.001$, at a 16-month follow-up. No significant differences were observed between empagliflozin-treated patients and patients treated with a placebo, in terms of hypoglycemic episodes, amputation of the lower limb, and bone fractures [89]. Empagliflozin effects in patients with HF with preserved ejection fraction (HFpEF), with or without type 2 DM, were investigated in EMPEROR—Preserved (Empagliflozin Outcome Trial in Patients with Chronic Heart Failure with Preserved Ejection Fraction). The novelty of the results consists of demonstrating the reduction in the combined risk of cardiovascular death or hHF [90].

The CANVAS study program (Canagliflozin Cardiovascular Assessment Study and Canagliflozin Cardiovascular Assessment Study—Renal) also confirmed the reduction in hHF in patients with type 2 DM and ASCVD, or patients at high risk for CV occurrence, and also confirmed the reduction in hospitalization of patients with no past events of HF. Canagliflozin diminished the risk of death from cardiovascular causes, nonfatal myocardial infarction, or stroke; however, an increased risk of amputation was recorded compared to a placebo [82].

For dapagliflozin, the DAPA-HF (Dapagliflozin and Prevention of Adverse Outcomes in Heart Failure) study showed a reduction in hospitalization for HF and death from cardiovascular causes compared to a placebo, though this favored patients with NYHA II functional class compared to those with NYHA III or IV functional class [91]. Positive results and a beneficial protection profile of dapagliflozin were also observed in non-diabetic patients with HF and CKD [92].

A summary of the presented clinical trials in Sections 3.3 and 3.3.1 is illustrated in Supplementary Table S2.

The results of the following ongoing trials will offer evidence-based data on the role of dapagliflozin in selected outcomes: Dapagliflozin Evaluation to Improve the LIVEs of Patients With Preserved Ejection Fraction Heart Failure (DELIVER), DAPA ACT HF-TIMI 68, Efficacy and Safety of Dapagliflozin in Acute Heart Failure (DICTATE-AHF), Dapagliflozin Heart Failure Readmission Study, DAPA MI Study, and Effectiveness of Dapagliflozin for Weight Loss [93–98].

4. Conclusions

The recent understanding of the pathophysiological pathways of SGLT-2i places this class of drugs towards a particularized, patient-centered approach, moving away from the well-known glycemic control strategy. SGLT-2i exhibit beneficial outcomes regarding glycemic control in type 2 DM, while also exhibiting weight loss benefits; the latter effect is especially observed when combined with other weight-reduction agents. SGLT-2i, by promoting weight loss and positively impacting high blood pressure, may have an additional cardiorenal protective role. Moreover, SGLT-2i have been shown not only to reduce death from cardiovascular causes, but also to reduce the risk of stroke and hospitalization due to heart failure. As a result of the positive cardiovascular and renal outcomes reported by numerous studies, SGLT-2i might be considered as one of the most reliable and efficient treatment options in diabetic patients nowadays, given that one of the main goals in treating type 2 DM is to preservee and improve cardiorenal function. Relying on the results of SGLT-2i studies, with beneficial effects on cardiovascular outcomes and mortality in patients with type 2 DM, as well as in non-diabetic patients, prescribing this class of drugs in medical practice is becoming a priority in personalized medicine.

Supplementary Materials: The following are available online at https://www.mdpi.com/article/10.3390/jpm11121249/s1, Table S1: summary of SGLT-2i effects on glycemic control as found in several studies. Table S2: summary of SGLT-2i cardiorenal outcomes as reported in randomized clinical trials.

Author Contributions: Conceptualization, M.C.T. and A.V.; writing—original draft preparation, R.A.T. and A.V.; writing—review and editing, M.C.T., R.A.T., I.T. and A.V.; visualization, M.C.T. and I.T., supervision, M.C.T. and A.V. All authors have read and agreed to the published version of the manuscript.

Funding: This research received no external funding.

Institutional Review Board Statement: Not applicable.

Informed Consent Statement: Not applicable.

Data Availability Statement: Not applicable.

Conflicts of Interest: The authors declare no conflict of interest.

References

1. International Diabetes Federation. IDF Diabetes Atlas—9th Edition. 2019. Available online: http://www.diabetesatlas.org/ (accessed on 4 September 2021).
2. Raghavan, S.; Vassy, J.L.; Ho, Y.L.; Song, R.J.; Gagnon, D.R.; Cho, K.; Wilson, P.W.F.; Phillips, L.S. Diabetes mellitus-related all-cause and cardiovascular mortality in a national cohort of adults. *J. Am. Heart Assoc.* **2019**, *8*, e011295. [CrossRef]
3. Schmidt, A.M. Diabetes mellitus and cardiovascular disease. *Arterioscler. Thromb. Vasc. Biol.* **2019**, *39*, 558–568. [CrossRef] [PubMed]

4. Han, Y.; Xie, H.; Liu, Y.; Gao, P.; Yang, X.; Shen, Z. Effect of metformin on all-cause and cardiovascular mortality in patients with coronary artery diseases: A systematic review and an updated meta-analysis. *Cardiovasc. Diabetol.* **2019**, *18*, 96. [CrossRef]
5. Griffin, S.J.; Leaver, J.K.; Irving, G.J. Impact of metformin on cardiovascular disease: A meta-analysis of randomised trials among people with type 2 diabetes. *Diabetologia* **2017**, *60*, 1620–1629. [CrossRef]
6. Marso, S.P.; Daniels, G.H.; Brown-Frandsen, K.; Kristensen, P.; Mann, J.F.; Nauck, M.A.; Nissen, S.E.; Pocock, S.; Poulter, N.R.; Ravn, L.S.; et al. Liraglutide and cardiovascular outcomes in type 2 diabetes. *N. Engl. J. Med.* **2016**, *375*, 311–322. [CrossRef]
7. Marso, S.P.; Bain, S.C.; Consoli, A.; Eliaschewitz, F.G.; Jódar, E.; Leiter, L.A.; Lingvay, I.; Rosenstock, J.; Seufert, J.; Warren, M.L.; et al. Semaglutide and cardiovascular outcomes in patients with type 2 diabetes. *N. Engl. J. Med.* **2016**, *375*, 1834–1844. [CrossRef]
8. Holman, R.R.; Bethel, M.A.; Mentz, R.J.; Thompson, V.P.; Lokhnygina, Y.; Buse, J.B.; Chan, J.C.; Choi, J.; Gustavson, S.M.; Iqbal, N.; et al. Effects of once-weekly exenatide on cardiovascular outcomes in type 2 diabetes. *N. Engl. J. Med.* **2017**, *377*, 1228–1239. [CrossRef] [PubMed]
9. American Diabetes Association. 9. Pharmacologic approaches to glycemic treatment: Standards of Medical Care in Diabetes— 2021. *Diabetes Care* **2021**, *44* (Suppl. S1), S111–S124. [CrossRef] [PubMed]
10. Guthrie, R. Canagliflozin and cardiovascular and renal events in type 2 diabetes. *Postgrad. Med.* **2018**, *130*, 149–153. [CrossRef]
11. Pereira, M.J.; Eriksson, J.W. Emerging role of SGLT-2 inhibitors for the treatment of obesity. *Drugs* **2019**, *79*, 219–230. [CrossRef]
12. Briasoulis, A.; Al Dhaybi, O.; Bakris, G.L. SGLT2 inhibitors and mechanisms of hypertension. *Curr. Cardiol. Rep.* **2018**, *20*, 1. [CrossRef]
13. Davidson, J.A. SGLT2 inhibitors in patients with type 2 diabetes and renal disease: Overview of current evidence. *Postgrad. Med.* **2019**, *131*, 251–260. [CrossRef]
14. Zelniker, T.A.; Wiviott, S.D.; Raz, I.; Im, K.; Goodrich, E.L.; Bonaca, M.P.; Mosenzon, O.; Kato, E.T.; Cahn, A.; Furtado, R.H.M.; et al. SGLT2 inhibitors for primary and secondary prevention of cardiovascular and renal outcomes in type 2 diabetes: A systematic review and meta-analysis of cardiovascular outcome trials. *Lancet* **2019**, *393*, 31–39. [CrossRef]
15. McMurray, J.J.V.; Solomon, S.D.; Inzucchi, S.E.; Køber, L.; Kosiborod, M.N.; Martinez, F.A.; Ponikowski, P.; Sabatine, M.S.; Anand, I.S.; Bělohlávek, J.; et al. Dapagliflozin in patients with heart failure and reduced ejection fraction. *N. Engl. J. Med.* **2019**, *381*, 1995–2008. [CrossRef] [PubMed]
16. Scheen, A.J. Pharmacodynamics, efficacy and safety of sodium-glucose co-transporter type 2 (SGLT2) inhibitors for the treatment of type 2 diabetes mellitus. *Drugs* **2015**, *75*, 33–59. [CrossRef] [PubMed]
17. Ghezzi, C.; Loo, D.D.F.; Wright, E.M. Physiology of renal glucose handling via SGLT1, SGLT2 and GLUT2. *Diabetologia* **2018**, *61*, 2087–2097. [CrossRef] [PubMed]
18. Brown, E.; Rajeev, S.P.; Cuthbertson, D.J.; Wilding, J.P.H. A review of the mechanism of action, metabolic profile and haemodynamic effects of sodium-glucose co-transporter-2 inhibitors. *Diabetes Obes. Metab.* **2019**, *21* (Suppl. S2), 9–18. [CrossRef]
19. Hummel, C.S.; Lu, C.; Loo, D.D.; Hirayama, B.A.; Voss, A.A.; Wright, E.M. Glucose transport by human renal Na+/D-glucose cotransporters SGLT1 and SGLT2. *Am. J. Physiol. Cell Physiol.* **2011**, *300*, C14–C21. [CrossRef]
20. Wright, E.M.; Loo, D.D.; Hirayama, B.A. Biology of human sodium glucose transporters. *Physiol. Rev.* **2011**, *91*, 733–794. [CrossRef]
21. Moses, R.G.; Colagiuri, S.; Pollock, C. SGLT2 inhibitors: New medicines for addressing unmet needs in type 2 diabetes. *Australas. Med. J.* **2014**, *7*, 405–415. [CrossRef]
22. Hsia, D.S.; Grove, O.; Cefalu, W.T. An update on sodium-glucose co-transporter-2 inhibitors for the treatment of diabetes mellitus. *Curr. Opin. Endocrinol. Diabetes Obes.* **2017**, *24*, 73–79. [CrossRef]
23. Giugliano, D.; Longo, M.; Scappaticcio, L.; Caruso, P.; Esposito, K. Sodium-glucose transporter-2 inhibitors for prevention and treatment of cardiorenal complications of type 2 diabetes. *Cardiovasc. Diabetol.* **2021**, *20*, 17. [CrossRef] [PubMed]
24. Bhatt, D.L.; Szarek, M.; Steg, P.G.; Cannon, C.P.; Leiter, L.A.; McGuire, D.K.; Lewis, J.B.; Riddle, M.C.; Voors, A.A.; Metra, M.; et al. Sotagliflozin in patients with diabetes and recent worsening heart failure. *N. Engl. J. Med.* **2021**, *384*, 117–128. [CrossRef] [PubMed]
25. Ferrannini, E. Sodium-glucose co-transporters and their inhibition: Clinical physiology. *Cell Metab.* **2017**, *26*, 27–38. [CrossRef] [PubMed]
26. Takahara, M.; Shiraiwa, T.; Matsuoka, T.A.; Katakami, N.; Shimomura, I. Ameliorated pancreatic β cell dysfunction in type 2 diabetic patients treated with a sodium-glucose cotransporter 2 inhibitor ipragliflozin. *Endocr. J.* **2015**, *62*, 77–86. [CrossRef]
27. Polidori, D.; Mari, A.; Ferrannini, E. Canagliflozin, a sodium glucose co-transporter 2 inhibitor, improves model-based indices of beta cell function in patients with type 2 diabetes. *Diabetologia* **2014**, *57*, 891–901. [CrossRef]
28. Saisho, Y. SGLT2 inhibitors: The star in the treatment of type 2 diabetes? *Diseases* **2020**, *8*, 14. [CrossRef]
29. Neuen, B.L.; Young, T.; Heerspink, H.J.L.; Neal, B.; Perkovic, V.; Billot, L.; Mahaffey, K.W.; Charytan, D.M.; Wheeler, D.C.; Arnott, C.; et al. SGLT2 inhibitors for the prevention of kidney failure in patients with type 2 diabetes: A systematic review and meta-analysis. *Lancet Diabetes Endocrinol.* **2019**, *7*, 845–854. [CrossRef]
30. Jardine, M.J.; Zhou, Z.; Mahaffey, K.W.; Oshima, M.; Agarwal, R.; Bakris, G.; Bajaj, H.S.; Bull, S.; Cannon, C.P.; Charytan, D.M.; et al. Renal, cardiovascular, and safety outcomes of canagliflozin by baseline kidney function: A secondary analysis of the CREDENCE randomized trial. *J. Am. Soc. Nephrol.* **2020**, *31*, 1128–1139. [CrossRef]

31. Sheu, W.H.H.; Chan, S.P.; Matawaran, B.J.; Deerochanawong, C.; Mithal, A.; Chan, J.; Suastika, K.; Khoo, C.M.; Nguyen, H.M.; Linong, J.; et al. Use of SGLT-2 inhibitors in patients with type 2 diabetes mellitus and abdominal obesity: An Asian perspective and expert recommendations. *Diabetes Metab. J.* **2020**, *44*, 11–32. [CrossRef]

32. DeFronzo, R.A.; Norton, L.; Abdul-Ghani, M. Renal, metabolic and cardiovascular considerations of SGLT2 inhibition. *Nat. Rev. Nephrol.* **2017**, *13*, 11–26. [CrossRef]

33. American Diabetes Association. 2. Classification and diagnosis of diabetes: Standards of medical care in diabetes—2021. *Diabetes Care* **2021**, *44* (Suppl. S1), S15–S33. [CrossRef]

34. American Diabetes Association. 4. Comprehensive medical evaluation and assessment of comorbidities: Standards of medical care in diabetes—2021. *Diabetes Care* **2021**, *44* (Suppl. S1), S40–S52. [CrossRef]

35. Koye, D.N.; Magliano, D.J.; Nelson, R.G.; Pavkov, M.E. The global epidemiology of diabetes and kidney disease. *Adv. Chronic Kidney Dis.* **2018**, *25*, 121–132. [CrossRef]

36. Tilinca, M.C.; Tiuca, R.A.; Burlacu, A.; Varga, A. 2021 update on the use of liraglutide in the modern treatment of 'diabesity': A narrative review. *Medicina* **2021**, *57*, 669. [CrossRef] [PubMed]

37. Tilinca, M.C.; Tiuca, R.A.; Niculas, C.; Varga, A.; Tilea, I. Future perspectives in diabesity treatment: Semaglutide, a glucagon-like peptide 1 receptor agonist (Review). *Exp. Ther. Med.* **2021**, *22*, 1167. [CrossRef] [PubMed]

38. Monami, M.; Nardini, C.; Mannucci, E. Efficacy and safety of sodium glucose co-transport-2 inhibitors in type 2 diabetes: A meta-analysis of randomized clinical trials. *Diabetes Obes. Metab.* **2014**, *16*, 457–466. [CrossRef] [PubMed]

39. Bailey, C.J.; Gross, J.L.; Pieters, A.; Bastien, A.; List, J.F. Effect of dapagliflozin in patients with type 2 diabetes who have inadequate glycaemic control with metformin: A randomised, double-blind, placebo-controlled trial. *Lancet* **2010**, *375*, 2223–2233. [CrossRef]

40. Vasilakou, D.; Karagiannis, T.; Athanasiadou, E.; Mainou, M.; Liakos, A.; Bekiari, E.; Sarigianni, M.; Matthews, D.R.; Tsapas, A. Sodium-glucose cotransporter 2 inhibitors for type 2 diabetes: A systematic review and meta-analysis. *Ann. Intern. Med.* **2013**, *159*, 262–274. [CrossRef] [PubMed]

41. Stenlöf, K.; Cefalu, W.T.; Kim, K.A.; Alba, M.; Usiskin, K.; Tong, C.; Canovatchel, W.; Meininger, G. Efficacy and safety of canagliflozin monotherapy in subjects with type 2 diabetes mellitus inadequately controlled with diet and exercise. *Diabetes Obes. Metab.* **2013**, *15*, 372–382. [CrossRef]

42. Søfteland, E.; Meier, J.J.; Vangen, B.; Toorawa, R.; Maldonado-Lutomirsky, M.; Broedl, U.C. Empagliflozin as Add-on Therapy in Patients with Type 2 Diabetes Inadequately Controlled with Linagliptin and Metformin: A 24-Week Randomized, Double-Blind, Parallel-Group Trial. *Diabetes Care* **2017**, *40*, 201–209. [CrossRef]

43. Miller, S.; Krumins, T.; Zhou, H.; Huyck, S.; Johnson, J.; Golm, G.; Terra, S.G.; Mancuso, J.P.; Engel, S.S.; Lauring, B. Ertugliflozin and Sitagliptin Co-initiation in Patients with Type 2 Diabetes: The VERTIS SITA Randomized Study. *Diabetes Ther.* **2018**, *9*, 253–268. [CrossRef]

44. Shyangdan, D.S.; Uthman, O.A.; Waugh, N. SGLT-2 receptor inhibitors for treating patients with type 2 diabetes mellitus: A systematic review and network meta-analysis. *BMJ Open* **2016**, *6*, e009417. [CrossRef]

45. Goring, S.; Hawkins, N.; Wygant, G.; Roudaut, M.; Townsend, R.; Wood, I.; Barnett, A.H. Dapagliflozin compared with other oral anti-diabetes treatments when added to metformin monotherapy: A systematic review and network meta-analysis. *Diabetes Obes. Metab.* **2014**, *16*, 433–442. [CrossRef] [PubMed]

46. Yang, T.; Lu, M.; Ma, L.; Zhou, Y.; Cui, Y. Efficacy and tolerability of canagliflozin as add-on to metformin in the treatment of type 2 diabetes mellitus: A meta-analysis. *Eur. J. Clin. Pharmacol.* **2015**, *71*, 1325–1332. [CrossRef] [PubMed]

47. Sun, Y.N.; Zhou, Y.; Chen, X.; Che, W.S.; Leung, S.W. The efficacy of dapagliflozin combined with hypoglycaemic drugs in treating type 2 diabetes mellitus: Meta-analysis of randomised controlled trials. *BMJ Open* **2014**, *4*, e004619. [CrossRef] [PubMed]

48. Zaccardi, F.; Webb, D.R.; Htike, Z.Z.; Youssef, D.; Khunti, K.; Davies, M.J. Efficacy and safety of sodium-glucose co-transporter-2 inhibitors in type 2 diabetes mellitus: Systematic review and network meta-analysis. *Diabetes Obes. Metab.* **2016**, *18*, 783–794. [CrossRef]

49. Rosenstock, J.; Frias, J.; Páll, D.; Charbonnel, B.; Pascu, R.; Saur, D.; Darekar, A.; Huyck, S.; Shi, H.; Lauring, B.; et al. Effect of ertugliflozin on glucose control, body weight, blood pressure and bone density in type 2 diabetes mellitus inadequately controlled on metformin monotherapy (VERTIS MET). *Diabetes Obes. Metab.* **2018**, *20*, 520–529. [CrossRef]

50. Henry, R.R.; Strange, P.; Zhou, R.; Pettus, J.; Shi, L.; Zhuplatov, S.B.; Mansfield, T.; Klein, D.; Katz, A. Effects of dapagliflozin on 24-hour glycemic control in patients with type 2 diabetes: A randomized controlled trial. *Diabetes Technol. Ther.* **2018**, *20*, 715–724. [CrossRef]

51. Kovacs, C.S.; Seshiah, V.; Swallow, R.; Jones, R.; Rattunde, H.; Woerle, H.J.; Broedl, U.C.; EMPA-REG PIO™ Trial Investigators. Empagliflozin improves glycaemic and weight control as add-on therapy to pioglitazone or pioglitazone plus metformin in patients with type 2 diabetes: A 24-week, randomized, placebo-controlled trial. *Diabetes Obes. Metab.* **2014**, *16*, 147–158. [CrossRef]

52. Terauchi, Y.; Utsunomiya, K.; Yasui, A.; Seki, T.; Cheng, G.; Shiki, K.; Lee, J. Safety and efficacy of empagliflozin as add-on therapy to GLP-1 receptor agonist (Liraglutide) in japanese patients with type 2 diabetes mellitus: A randomised, double-blind, parallel-group phase 4 study. *Diabetes Ther.* **2019**, *10*, 951–963. [CrossRef]

53. Terra, S.G.; Focht, K.; Davies, M.; Frias, J.; Derosa, G.; Darekar, A.; Golm, G.; Johnson, J.; Saur, D.; Lauring, B.; et al. Phase III, efficacy and safety study of ertugliflozin monotherapy in people with type 2 diabetes mellitus inadequately controlled with diet and exercise alone. *Diabetes Obes. Metab.* **2017**, *19*, 721–728. [CrossRef] [PubMed]

54. Bolinder, J.; Ljunggren, Ö.; Kullberg, J.; Johansson, L.; Wilding, J.; Langkilde, A.M.; Sugg, J.; Parikh, S. Effects of dapagliflozin on body weight, total fat mass, and regional adipose tissue distribution in patients with type 2 diabetes mellitus with inadequate glycemic control on metformin. *J. Clin. Endocrinol. Metab.* **2012**, *97*, 1020–1031. [CrossRef] [PubMed]

55. Fadini, G.P.; Bonora, B.M.; Zatti, G.; Vitturi, N.; Iori, E.; Marescotti, M.C.; Albiero, M.; Avogaro, A. Effects of the SGLT2 inhibitor dapagliflozin on HDL cholesterol, particle size, and cholesterol efflux capacity in patients with type 2 diabetes: A randomized placebo-controlled trial. *Cardiovasc. Diabetol.* **2017**, *16*, 42. [CrossRef]

56. Ferrannini, G.; Hach, T.; Crowe, S.; Sanghvi, A.; Hall, K.D.; Ferrannini, E. Energy balance after sodium-glucose cotransporter 2 inhibition. *Diabetes Care* **2015**, *38*, 1730–1735. [CrossRef]

57. Ji, L.; Ma, J.; Li, H.; Mansfield, T.A.; T'joen, C.L.; Iqbal, N.; Ptaszynska, A.; List, J.F. Dapagliflozin as monotherapy in drug-naive Asian patients with type 2 diabetes mellitus: A randomized, blinded, prospective phase III study. *Clin. Ther.* **2014**, *36*, 84–100.e9. [CrossRef]

58. Kaku, K.; Kiyosue, A.; Inoue, S.; Ueda, N.; Tokudome, T.; Yang, J.; Langkilde, A.M. Efficacy and safety of dapagliflozin monotherapy in Japanese patients with type 2 diabetes inadequately controlled by diet and exercise. *Diabetes Obes. Metab.* **2014**, *16*, 1102–1110. [CrossRef]

59. Frías, J.P.; Guja, C.; Hardy, E.; Ahmed, A.; Dong, F.; Öhman, P.; Jabbour, S.A. Exenatide once weekly plus dapagliflozin once daily versus exenatide or dapagliflozin alone in patients with type 2 diabetes inadequately controlled with metformin monotherapy (DURATION-8): A 28 week, multicentre, double-blind, phase 3, randomised controlled trial. *Lancet Diabetes Endocrinol.* **2016**, *4*, 1004–1016. [PubMed]

60. Strojek, K.; Yoon, K.H.; Hruba, V.; Sugg, J.; Langkilde, A.M.; Parikh, S. Dapagliflozin added to glimepiride in patients with type 2 diabetes mellitus sustains glycemic control and weight loss over 48 weeks: A randomized, double-blind, parallel-group, placebo-controlled trial. *Diabetes Ther.* **2014**, *5*, 267–283. [CrossRef]

61. Cefalu, W.T.; Stenlöf, K.; Leiter, L.A.; Wilding, J.P.; Blonde, L.; Polidori, D.; Xie, J.; Sullivan, D.; Usiskin, K.; Canovatchel, W.; et al. Effects of canagliflozin on body weight and relationship to HbA1c and blood pressure changes in patients with type 2 diabetes. *Diabetologia* **2015**, *58*, 1183–1187. [CrossRef]

62. Georgianos, P.I.; Agarwal, R. Ambulatory Blood Pressure Reduction With SGLT-2 Inhibitors: Dose-Response Meta-analysis and Comparative Evaluation with Low-Dose Hydrochlorothiazide. *Diabetes Care* **2019**, *42*, 693–700. [CrossRef]

63. Wright, J.T., Jr.; Williamson, J.D.; Whelton, P.K.; Snyder, J.K.; Sink, K.M.; Rocco, M.V.; Reboussin, D.M.; Rahman, M.; Oparil, S.; Lewis, C.E.; et al. A Randomized Trial of Intensive versus Standard Blood-Pressure Control. *N. Engl. J. Med.* **2015**, *373*, 2103–2116.

64. Lewis, C.E.; Fine, L.J.; Beddhu, S.; Cheung, A.K.; Cushman, W.C.; Cutler, J.A.; Evans, G.W.; Johnson, K.C.; Kitzman, D.W.; Oparil, S.; et al. Final Report of a Trial of Intensive versus Standard Blood-Pressure Control. *N. Engl. J. Med.* **2021**, *384*, 1921–1930. [PubMed]

65. Buckley, L.F.; Dixon, D.L.; Wohlford, G.F., IV; Wijesinghe, D.S.; Baker, W.L.; Van Tassell, B.W. Intensive Versus Standard Blood Pressure Control in SPRINT-Eligible Participants of ACCORD-BP. *Diabetes Care* **2017**, *40*, 1733–1738. [CrossRef]

66. Oliva, R.V.; Bakris, G.L. Blood pressure effects of sodium-glucose co-transport 2 (SGLT2) inhibitors. *J. Am. Soc. Hypertens.* **2014**, *8*, 330–339. [CrossRef]

67. Tikkanen, I.; Narko, K.; Zeller, C.; Green, A.; Salsali, A.; Broedl, U.C.; Woerle, H.J. EMPA-REG BP Investigators. Empagliflozin reduces blood pressure in patients with type 2 diabetes and hypertension. *Diabetes Care* **2015**, *38*, 420–428. [CrossRef]

68. Zanchi, A.; Burnier, M.; Muller, M.E.; Ghajarzadeh-Wurzner, A.; Maillard, M.; Loncle, N.; Milani, B.; Dufour, N.; Bonny, O.; Pruijm, M. Acute and Chronic Effects of SGLT2 Inhibitor Empagliflozin on Renal Oxygenation and Blood Pressure Control in Nondiabetic Normotensive Subjects: A Randomized, Placebo-Controlled Trial. *J. Am. Heart Assoc.* **2020**, *9*, e016173. [CrossRef] [PubMed]

69. Fontes-Carvalho, R.; Santos-Ferreira, D.; Raz, I.; Marx, N.; Ruschitzka, F.; Cosentino, F. Protective effects of SGLT-2 inhibitors across the cardiorenal continuum: Two faces of the same coin. *Eur. J. Prev. Cardiol.* **2021**, zwab034. [CrossRef]

70. Kaplan, A.; Abidi, E.; El-Yazbi, A.; Eid, A.; Booz, G.W.; Zouein, F.A. Direct cardiovascular impact of SGLT2 inhibitors: Mechanisms and effects. *Heart Fail. Rev.* **2018**, *23*, 419–437. [CrossRef] [PubMed]

71. Bilgin, S.; Kurtkulagi, O.; Duman, T.T.; Tel, B.M.A.; Kahveci, G.; Kiran, M.; Erge, E.; Aktas, G. Sodium glucose co-transporter-2 inhibitor, Empagliflozin, is associated with significant reduction in weight, body mass index, fasting glucose, and A1c levels in Type 2 diabetic patients with established coronary heart disease: The SUPER GATE study. *Ir. J. Med. Sci.* **2021**, 1–6. [CrossRef] [PubMed]

72. Cannon, C.P.; Pratley, R.; Dagogo-Jack, S.; Mancuso, J.; Huyck, S.; Masiukiewicz, U.; Charbonnel, B.; Frederich, R.; Gallo, S.; Cosentino, F.; et al. Cardiovascular outcomes with ertugliflozin in type 2 diabetes. *N. Engl. J. Med.* **2020**, *383*, 1425–1435. [CrossRef] [PubMed]

73. Tian, J.; Zhang, M.; Suo, M.; Liu, D.; Wang, X.; Liu, M.; Pan, J.; Jin, T.; An, F. Dapagliflozin alleviates cardiac fibrosis through suppressing EndMT and fibroblast activation via AMPKα/TGF-β/Smad signalling in type 2 diabetic rats. *J. Cell. Mol. Med.* **2021**, *25*, 7642–7659. [CrossRef]

74. Santos-Gallego, C.G.; Requena-Ibanez, J.A.; San Antonio, R.; Garcia-Ropero, A.; Ishikawa, K.; Watanabe, S.; Picatoste, B.; Vargas-Delgado, A.P.; Flores-Umanzor, E.J.; Sanz, J.; et al. Empagliflozin ameliorates diastolic dysfunction and left ventricular fibrosis/stiffness in nondiabetic heart failure: A multimodality study. *JACC Cardiovasc. Imaging* **2021**, *14*, 393–407. [CrossRef]

75. Saran, R.; Li, Y.; Robinson, B.; Abbot, K.C.; Agodoa, L.Y.C.; Ayanian, J.; Bragg-Gresham, J.; Balkrishnan, R.; Chen, J.L.; Cope, E.; et al. US Renal Data System 2015 Annual Data Report: Epidemiology of kidney disease in the United States. *Am. J. Kidney Dis.* **2016**, *67*, S1–S305. [CrossRef] [PubMed]

76. Wanner, C.; Inzucchi, S.E.; Zinman, B.; EMPA-REG OUTCOME Investigators. Empagliflozin and progression of kidney disease in type 2 diabetes. *N. Engl. J. Med.* **2016**, *375*, 1801–1802. [CrossRef] [PubMed]

77. Neal, B.; Perkovic, V.; Mahaffey, K.W.; de Zeeuw, D.; Fulcher, G.; Erondu, N.; Shaw, W.; Law, G.; Desai, M.; Matthews, D.R. Canagliflozin and cardiovascular and renal events in type 2 diabetes. *N. Engl. J. Med.* **2017**, *377*, 644–657. [CrossRef]

78. Wiviott, S.D.; Raz, I.; Bonaca, M.P.; Mosenzon, O.; Kato, E.T.; Cahn, A.; Silverman, M.G.; Zelniker, T.A.; Kuder, J.F.; Murphy, S.A.; et al. Dapagliflozin and cardiovascular outcomes in type 2 diabetes. *N. Engl. J. Med.* **2019**, *380*, 347–357. [CrossRef]

79. Heerspink, H.J.L.; Karasik, A.; Thuresson, M.; Melzer-Cohen, C.; Chodick, G.; Khunti, K.; Wilding, J.P.H.; Garcia Rodriguez, L.A.; Cea-Soriano, L.; Kohsaka, S.; et al. Kidney outcomes associated with use of SGLT2 inhibitors in real-world clinical practice (CVD-REAL 3): A multinational observational cohort study. *Lancet Diabetes Endocrinol.* **2020**, *8*, 27–35. [CrossRef]

80. Heerspink, H.J.L.; Stefánsson, B.V.; Correa-Rotter, R.; Chertow, G.M.; Greene, T.; Hou, F.F.; Mann, J.F.E.; McMurray, J.J.V.; Lindberg, M.; Rossing, P.; et al. Dapagliflozin in patients with chronic kidney disease. *N. Engl. J. Med.* **2020**, *383*, 1436–1446. [CrossRef]

81. Perkovic, V.; Jardine, M.J.; Neal, B.; Bompoint, S.; Heerspink, H.J.L.; Charytan, D.M.; Edwards, R.; Agarwal, R.; Bakris, G.; Bull, S.; et al. Canagliflozin and renal outcomes in type 2 diabetes and nephropathy. *N. Engl. J. Med.* **2019**, *380*, 2295–2306. [CrossRef]

82. Mahaffey, K.W.; Neal, B.; Perkovic, V.; de Zeeuw, D.; Fulcher, G.; Erondu, N.; Shaw, W.; Fabbrini, E.; Sun, T.; Li, Q.; et al. Canagliflozin for primary and secondary prevention of cardiovascular events: Results from the CANVAS program (Canagliflozin Cardiovascular Assessment Study). *Circulation* **2018**, *137*, 323–334. [CrossRef]

83. Kenny, H.C.; Abel, E.D. Heart Failure in type 2 diabetes mellitus. *Circ. Res.* **2019**, *124*, 121–141. [CrossRef] [PubMed]

84. Lam, C.S.P.; Chandramouli, C.; Ahooja, V.; Verma, S. SGLT-2 Inhibitors in heart failure: Current management, unmet needs, and therapeutic prospects. *J. Am. Heart Assoc.* **2019**, *8*, e013389. [CrossRef] [PubMed]

85. Zinman, B.; Wanner, C.; Lachin, J.M.; Fitchett, D.; Bluhmki, E.; Hantel, S.; Mattheus, M.; Devins, T.; Johansen, O.E.; Woerle, H.J.; et al. Empagliflozin, cardiovascular outcomes, and mortality in type 2 diabetes. *N. Engl. J. Med.* **2015**, *373*, 2117–2128. [CrossRef] [PubMed]

86. Fitchett, D.; Zinman, B.; Wanner, C.; Lachin, J.M.; Hantel, S.; Salsali, A.; Johansen, O.E.; Woerle, H.J.; Broedl, U.C.; Inzucchi, S.E.; et al. Heart failure outcomes with empagliflozin in patients with type 2 diabetes at high cardiovascular risk: Results of the EMPA-REG OUTCOME® trial. *Eur. Heart J.* **2016**, *37*, 1526–1534. [CrossRef] [PubMed]

87. Neal, B.; Perkovic, V.; Matthews, D.R. Canagliflozin and cardiovascular and renal events in type 2 diabetes. *N. Engl. J. Med.* **2017**, *377*, 2099. [CrossRef] [PubMed]

88. Cosentino, F.; Grant, P.J.; Aboyans, V.; Bailey, C.J.; Ceriello, A.; Delgado, V.; Federici, M.; Filippatos, G.; Grobbee, D.E.; Hansen, T.B.; et al. 2019 ESC Guidelines on diabetes, pre-diabetes, and cardiovascular diseases developed in collaboration with the EASD. *Eur. Heart J.* **2020**, *41*, 255–323. [CrossRef]

89. Packer, M.; Anker, S.D.; Butler, J.; Filippatos, G.; Pocock, S.J.; Carson, P.; Januzzi, J.; Verma, S.; Tsutsui, H.; Brueckmann, M.; et al. Cardiovascular and renal outcomes with empagliflozin in heart failure. *N. Engl. J. Med.* **2020**, *383*, 1413–1424. [CrossRef] [PubMed]

90. Anker, S.D.; Butler, J.; Filippatos, G.; Ferreira, J.P.; Bocchi, E.; Böhm, M.; Brunner-La Rocca, H.P.; Choi, D.J.; Chopra, V.; Chuquiure-Valenzuela, E.; et al. Empagliflozin in Heart Failure with a Preserved Ejection Fraction. *N. Engl. J. Med.* **2021**, *385*, 1451–1461. [CrossRef]

91. Bragagni, A.; Piani, F.; Borghi, C. Surprises in cardiology: Efficacy of gliflozines in heart failure even in the absence of diabetes. *Eur. Heart J. Suppl.* **2021**, *23* (Suppl. E), E40–E44. [CrossRef]

92. Zargar, A.H.; Trailokya, A.A.; Ghag, S.; Pawar, R.; Aiwale, A.; Zalke, A. Current role of dapagliflozin in clinical practice. *J. Assoc. Phys. India* **2021**, *69*, 11–12.

93. Solomon, S.D.; de Boer, R.A.; DeMets, D.; Hernandez, A.F.; Inzucchi, S.E.; Kosiborod, M.N.; Lam, C.S.P.; Martinez, F.; Shah, S.J.; Lindholm, D.; et al. Dapagliflozin in heart failure with preserved and mildly reduced ejection fraction: Rationale and design of the DELIVER trial. *Eur. J. Heart Fail.* **2021**, *23*, 1217–1225. [CrossRef] [PubMed]

94. Dapagliflozin and Effect on Cardiovascular Events in Acute Heart Failure -Thrombolysis in Myocardial Infarction 68 (DAPA ACT HF-TIMI 68). Available online: https://clinicaltrials.gov/ct2/show/NCT04363697 (accessed on 6 September 2021).

95. Cox, Z.L.; Collins, S.P.; Aaron, M.; Hernandez, G.A.; Iii, A.T.M.; Davidson, B.T.; Fowler, M.; Lindsell, C.J.; Harrel, F.E., Jr.; Jenkins, C.A.; et al. Efficacy and safety of dapagliflozin in acute heart failure: Rationale and design of the DICTATE-AHF trial. *Am. Heart J.* **2021**, *232*, 116–124. [CrossRef] [PubMed]

96. Dapagliflozin Heart Failure Readmission. Available online: https://www.clinicaltrials.gov/ct2/show/NCT04249778 (accessed on 6 September 2021).

97. Dapagliflozin Effects on Cardiovascular Events in Patients with an Acute Heart Attack (DAPA-MI). Available online: https://www.clinicaltrials.gov/ct2/show/NCT04564742 (accessed on 6 September 2021).

98. Effectiveness of Dapagliflozin for Weight Loss. Available online: https://clinicaltrials.gov/ct2/show/NCT03968224 (accessed on 6 September 2021).

Journal of
*Personalized
Medicine*

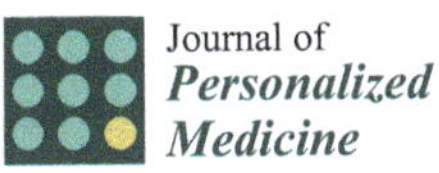

Review

Adherence to Therapy in Glaucoma Treatment—A Review

Alexandra-Cătălina Zaharia *, Otilia-Maria Dumitrescu, Mădălina Radu and Roxana-Elena Rogoz

Department of Ophthalmology, "Dr. Carol Davila" Central Military Emergency Hospital,
010825 Bucharest, Romania; otiliamariadumitrescu@gmail.com (O.-M.D.); madalina.rd@yahoo.com (M.R.);
rogozroxana@yahoo.com (R.-E.R.)
* Correspondence: alexandra.zahariac@gmail.com; Tel.: +40-723007817

Abstract: Glaucoma is a chronic disease and the second leading cause of irreversible vision loss worldwide, whose initial treatment consists of self-administered topical ocular hypotensive eyedrops. Adherence with glaucoma medications is a fundamental problem in the care of glaucoma patients as up to 50% of patients fail to receive the intended benefits of the treatment. The literature has identified many barriers to patients' compliance, from factors depending on the type of medication administered, communication between physician and patients, to factors dependent on patients' behaviour and lifestyle. Failure to take medication as prescribed increases the risk that patients will not receive the desired benefit, which often leads to a worsening of the disease. Our aim is to synthesize the methods used for measuring adherence of patients to glaucoma therapy and the interventions used for addressing adherence, laying emphasis on a patient-centred approach, taking time to educate patients about their chronic disease and to assess their views on treatment.

Keywords: patient adherence; glaucoma; personalized care; patient compliance

Citation: Zaharia, A.-C.; Dumitrescu, O.-M.; Radu, M.; Rogoz, R.-E. Adherence to Therapy in Glaucoma Treatment—A Review. *J. Pers. Med.* **2022**, *12*, 514. https://doi.org/10.3390/jpm12040514

Academic Editors: Fábio G. Teixeira, Catarina Godinho and Júlio Belo Fernandes

Received: 18 February 2022
Accepted: 21 March 2022
Published: 22 March 2022

Publisher's Note: MDPI stays neutral with regard to jurisdictional claims in published maps and institutional affiliations.

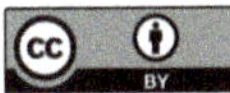

1. Introduction

Glaucoma is an optic neuropathy that poses a significant public health problem, affecting approximatively sixty million people worldwide. The goal of the currently available glaucoma medication is to preserve visual function by lowering intraocular pressure to a level that is likely to prevent further optic nerve damage, but patients are unlikely to experience the clinical benefits of their therapy if they do not adhere to their medication regimen [1,2].

Poor adherence to medical treatment is a common issue in medicine, especially with chronic diseases such as arterial hypertension and diabetes, where omission of medication can result in clinically significant symptoms [3]. Nonadherence to therapy has also been described in many chronic eye conditions that require frequent or long term eyedrop administration, including in the treatment of corneal ulcers [4,5] and dry eye syndrome secondary to chronic ocular surface diseases or to refractive surgery [6,7] in infants, who may be uncooperative [8]. Furthermore, there is literature that indicates that another recognized barrier to the patient's compliance is the cost of medication, as in the case of intravitreal injections, which are used for a variety of retinal conditions [9]. Given the asymptomatic nature of glaucoma and the lifelong therapeutic regimen without apparent subjective improvement, glaucoma patients are at risk of non-compliance with their treatment [10].

An ideal treatment regimen should achieve glaucoma control with the lowest risk and fewest adverse effects, whilst preserving the patient's visual function and quality of life. Visual impairment due to glaucoma has a negative effect on physical and mental health. It seems that the simple knowledge of having a chronic, irreversible, and potentially blinding disease can have a negative impact on the quality of life of patients. The Collaborative Initial Glaucoma Treatment Study assessed the fear of blindness in patients with glaucoma through questionnaires. At the baseline, after being told about their glaucoma diagnosis, 34% of patients reported either a moderate or high degree of worry regarding blindness, which decreased to 17% by 6 months and to 11% over a 5-year period. The decrease noted over time was probably due to the reassurance associated with receiving treatment, regular clinical follow-up, adaptation to the diagnosis, and a good adherence to treatment [11]. Many studies found that glaucoma therapy adherence was associated with an increased quality of life. Although the quality of life may be a highly subjective concept, it should be regarded as a central aspect of therapeutic decisions in glaucoma as it can allow clinicians to understand patients' perspective better and promote adherence to the treatment regimen [12].

Ophthalmologists are beginning to discover that nonadherence is more prevalent than previously realized and to understand the burden of glaucoma patients. Several studies of adherence with glaucoma therapy regimens point out that adherence on average is suboptimal, but research is still needed regarding how to detect and address nonadherence. The aim of this review is to provide an overview of patients' compliance with glaucoma treatments. Perhaps physicians should consider patient-centred approaches such as empowering patients in their own treatment through education and support, which could be regarded as important first steps in reinforcing adherence or correcting nonadherence [13].

2. Materials and Methods

We conducted a literature search for this review using the MEDLINE database. The following search terms were included: "adherence to glaucoma medication", "methods of measuring adherence", "nonadherence", "barriers to adherence with glaucoma medication", "electronic medication monitoring", "self-tonometry", "topical treatment in glaucoma" and "questionnaires for glaucoma adherence". The articles retrieved were reviewed for their title, abstract, and language (non-English articles were excluded). Inclusion criteria consisted of manuscripts written in English that had appeared before February 2022. We concentrated on the studies that best described patient adherence to a medication regimen, evaluated efficacy and/or compared methods regarding measuring adherence and new studies addressing adherence in glaucoma. After relevant articles were retrieved using these keywords, a search was conducted through the reference lists of the chosen studies and additional papers were selected.

3. Literature Review

3.1. Definition of Adherence and Compliance

Before discussing methods and barriers of adherence to glaucoma therapy, it is essential to first define compliance and adherence as the terms are often used synonymously. Adherence refers to the prevalence of use of the initial medication at various time points and is founded upon patients' understanding of their illness severity, their belief in the efficacy of a treatment, and in their ability to control their symptoms by using this treatment [12]. On the other hand, the term "compliance" has been defined as the extent to which the patient is passively following the physician's orders or recommendations and suggests that the therapy is not based on a therapeutic alliance between the patient and the physician. Both terms imperfectly describe the medication-taking behaviour, but many physicians prefer the term "adherence", as "compliance" denotes a degree of passivity (on the patient's participation in their therapeutic regimen). Regardless of which word is preferred, the full benefit of the many effective medications that are available will be achieved only if patients accurately follow the prescribed treatment regimen [14–16].

3.2. Patient Adherence to a Medication Regimen

Despite evidence indicating the therapeutic benefit of adhering to a prescribed regimen, many patients do not take medications as prescribed. Studies have shown six general patterns of medication taking among patients with chronic conditions: approximately one-sixth come close to perfect adherence to a regimen; one-sixth take nearly all doses, but with some timing irregularity; one-sixth miss an occasional single day's dose and have some timing inconsistency; one-sixth take drug holidays 3 to 4 times per year, with occasional dose omissions; one-sixth have a drug holiday monthly or more often, with frequent omissions of doses; and one-sixth take few or no doses while giving the impression of good adherence [13].

Adherence with glaucoma medications is a fundamental problem in the care of glaucoma patients as 24–59% fail to receive the intended or full effect of the treatment [17]. The barriers to adherence in glaucoma are complex, and glaucoma patients vary widely in the way they take their topical glaucoma medications. Patients naturally want to please the doctor, which makes them reluctant to admit to nonadherence [13]. The typical glaucoma patients are older adults who have inherent difficulties taking any medications, the most commonly cited being trouble with manual dexterity and inadequate vision, which are reasons for relying on others to administer their drops [18].

Lacey et al. identified multiple obstacles to adherence with anti-glaucomatous therapy: lack of initial education about application techniques, forgetting drops, drop-scheduling, as well as problems with drop supply. Sight preservation appeared to be the major motivation for adherence and thus, it appeared that despite these issues, the majority continued to administer drops due to faith in drop efficacy's preserving their sight or because they already had symptomatic visual loss [19].

Only a few studies have investigated how patients store their prescription drugs at home. One study concluded that more than half of older patients comply with general drug storage recommendations and more than half of the drugs requiring refrigeration were not stored accordingly [20]. To our knowledge, glaucoma medication does not require refrigeration (but we assume that it would have been a reason for a lower adherence to treatment).

The Glaucoma Adherence and Persistency Study most often identified the following factors as possible barriers to compliance: cost (55%), forgetfulness (32%), fear or denial (16%), lack of understanding about glaucoma (16%), and regimen complexity (15%). From the physicians' own perspective, the most important barriers identified were: lack of patient motivation to use drops (50%), lack of patient understanding about glaucoma (41%), inability to communicate why compliance is important (15%), and limited time spent with patients in the context of a brief office encounter (12%). In addition, the study defined 3 groups of physicians on the basis of the attitudinal and behavioural variables: reactive (41%), sceptical (44%), and idealistic (16%) physicians. The reactives were least likely to detect and address nonadherence proactively. The sceptics were least likely to discuss glaucoma or the importance of treatment with the patient when initiating treatment, because they were less likely to believe that they could change medication adherence. The idealists believed in addressing adherence and reported behaviour consistent with that goal, such as discussing a drug's mechanism of action, educating patients on how to use drops, and using telephone appointment reminders, which have been shown to improve adherence. They were more likely to seek to understand and follow concepts that were important to the patient when they suspected nonadherence [21].

Failure to take medication as prescribed increases the risk that patients will not receive the intended benefit, often leading to negative sequelae, such as worsening of disease and higher healthcare costs overall. Thus, understanding factors associated with maintaining one's medication regimen is important to patients and doctors.

3.3. Methods of Measuring Adherence

Before engaging in efforts to change the patient's attitude on glaucoma therapy, the clinician first needs to detect non-adherence (and to realize that the attitude needs to be changed). Patient adherence to medication regimens has been monitored since the time of Hippocrates and, to this day, measurement of patient adherence is essential if management of poor adherence is to be adressed efficiently. The methods available for measuring adherence can be divided into direct and indirect methods, each method having advantages and disadvantages. A gold standard method to measure adherence in patients with glaucoma is required but has not been established yet.

The direct methods of measuring adherence include directly observed therapy, which has the highest accuracy, and measurement of concentrations of a drug in blood. The direct methods require expensive assays, can be burdensome for the ophthalmologist, and are susceptible to distortion by the patient [16].

Indirect methods of measurement of adherence include collecting patient questionnaires or self-reports, asking the patient to keep a medication diary, asking the patient about how easy it is to apply the prescribed medication, assessing clinical response, ascertaining rates of refilling prescriptions, using electronic medication monitors, and assessing children's or elderly patients' adherence by asking the help of a caregiver. Verbal questioning of the patient, questionnaires, and patient diaries are methods that are simple and relatively easy to use, but they can be altered by the patient [16].

Patients do not want to be perceived as misbehaving by their physicians, so they may withhold information about non-adherence. A possible solution is to encourage the patient's participation in a partnership between him or her and the physician, based on valuing the patient's beliefs, concerns, and preferences. Thus, a good patient should be perceived as someone who works with the physician to overcome the inevitable concerns about medication and logistical barriers to adherence [22,23]. To accomplish this, ophthalmologists can use self-reported adherence measures such as glaucoma therapy adherence questionnaires, which assess whether and what the patient understands about her or his medical regimen and the confidence she or he has in medication adherence [23]. Self-reported measures may be the most cost-effective and simple way for providers to evaluate the rate of non-compliance and contribute to a better understanding of the obstacles to, and the motivations for adherence with glaucoma medication and to explore potential methods to improve adherence [19,24].

3.3.1. 24 h Intraocular Pressure Curve

Single-day IOP measurements during office hours can only provide limited information of treatment efficacy as it is widely known that IOP fluctuates during the 24-h period. The most common method for evaluating glaucoma patients' IOP is via a diurnal tension curve, which encompasses multiple IOP readings at different time points during office hours. Mansouri et al. suggested that night-time measurements in the habitual position are very important for the accuracy of the IOP profile since the measurements more closely align with an individual's circadian rhythm and natural body positioning. This intervention shows the impact of adherence to glaucoma treatment by delineating an IOP profile on a 24-h period, and it may be used when inpatient and outpatient IOP measurements differ greatly. In addition, this method may provide a better understanding of the true IOP-lowering effect of treatment by revealing a typical fluctuation of IOP over the circadian cycle, leading to a consequent improvement in adherence and treatment outcomes and the possibility of individualized disease management [25].

3.3.2. Questionnaires

Questionnaires are a useful resource that can expose poor adherence to glaucoma therapy by asking whether the patients know why they are taking their medication, whether they have experienced any side effects to their eye drops, or what their motivations to take the treatment are [16]. Lacey et al. published a qualitative research study based on a patient interview, aiming to identify motivational factors for adhering to glaucoma medication. The interview consisted of questions regarding therapy, memory and routine of taking the eye drops, difficulties experienced with medication, motivations in applying the eye drops, and the patients' ideas to help future adherence. The authors reported barriers to adherence derived directly from participants' experiences, such as the lack of patient instruction and a desire for improved delivery of education, concentrating on drop application techniques and the consequences of poor adherence. Additionally, patients proposed the idea of receiving regular feedback about drop efficacy to strengthen their faith in adherence. Furthermore, the questions on adherence revealed that many patients experienced problems with drop application methods, forgetting drops, or practical difficulties such as being untreated for short periods due to running out of medication, finding a convenient location to apply the drops during the day, or having inadequate time to administer them while at work [19].

This method, however, is susceptible to error with increases in time between visits. Results are easily distorted by the patient, which usually leads to an overestimation of the patient's adherence [16] A few studies evaluated the validity of self-reported measures against more controllable measures such as electronic monitoring devices or pharmacy records in glaucoma patients, and discovered that they tended to overvalue the doses taken and timing (adherence to glaucoma therapy) [24]. Consequently, Sayner et al. advanced the idea that ophthalmologists may need to use a careful and reassuring approach when talking to patients in order to detect pitfalls with applying drops on time, making them feel comfortable, and consequently helping the identification of poor adherence (for example: "I know it must be difficult to take your medication regularly. Tell me about the last time you forgot to take your drops" [16,24].

3.3.3. Rate of Refilling Prescriptions

Rates of refilling prescriptions, as indirect methods of determining adherence, are an accurate measure of adherence in a medical system that uses electronic medical records and a closed pharmacy system as long as the refills are measured occasionally. Pharmacy records can provide the clinician with objective information on rates of refilling prescriptions, which can be used to assess whether a patient is adhering to the glaucoma therapy. Moreover, the records can be confirmed with the patient's responses to direct questions or questionnaires [16]. However, fulfilment of a prescription at the pharmacy does not mean that the patient will apply the medication. The Glaucoma Adherence and Persistency Study analyzed large pharmacy databases to quantify adherence in a cohort of patients with glaucoma. The study highlighted several limitations of using pharmacy records to determine adherence to glaucoma medication. First, it showed that misclassification of added versus switched medication may have occurred, because patients mistakenly believed that the second medication should replace the first or a refill of the first drug was delayed because the patient had a large supply of it. In addition, patients who receive samples will be considered to have poor adherence. The samples given by the ophthalmologist do not appear in the claims data and this implies a difficulty in quantifying them, as well as in identifying the patients who may experience adverse effects or other barriers to adherence while taking the sample drug [26].

3.3.4. Electronic Medication Monitoring

The most accurate indirect method of determining how patients use glaucoma medication is electronic monitoring with a Medication Event Monitoring System (MEMS), which is capable of recording and stamping the time of opening bottles and dispensing drops [16]. This automatic compilation of times of medication intake (dosing history) is an approach widely used in other medical specialities. It provides a thorough characterization of medication adherence, with clear distinctions between initiation, implementation, and discontinuation.

However, electronic monitoring of drop-taking is performed rarely in ophthalmic research, in part because of the technological difficulties involved. On the one hand, it implies a greater difficulty in measuring eyedrop usage compared with measuring pill usage, and on the other hand, alteration of the eyedrop bottle itself is expensive and difficult to achieve [27]. Therefore, an important drawback is the cost, which makes them impractical for monitoring adherence in clinical settings. Additionally, these devices do not document whether the patient actually applied the drop in the conjunctival sac. Thus, patients may open the container but not apply the drop correctly or may waste multiple drops out of the container at the same time [16]. Reports based on pharmacy records concluded that adherence and persistence (duration of continuous treatment with the initially prescribed medication) are higher for prostaglandins than with other drugs. Nevertheless, there has been no direct comparison using electronic monitoring and it will be of great interest to develop a method to compare adherence by electronic monitoring between the once-daily hypotensive agents and other glaucoma drugs that require more frequent dosage [27]. Another limitation of electronic monitoring of glaucoma medication is that patients who know they are monitored may change their behaviour simply because they are observed, a phenomenon called the Hawthorne effect [28].

A disadvantage is that electronic monitoring can only be used with specific medications, for example the Travatan Dosing Aid (DA; Alcon, Fort Worth, TX), which can only provide data on use of travoprost, because no other bottle of glaucoma medication fits within it. A bottle of travoprost is placed in the device and a handle is fully depressed to administer the medication. A built-in memory chip records the date and time of the event and the data is later downloaded to a computer [29].

The Travatan Dosing Aid Study assessed patients' adherence and patterns of usage of topical once-daily therapy with travoprost (for glaucoma) in 196 patients over a 3 month period. The study revealed that, even though they were aware that they were being monitored and that they were provided with free medication, 45% of patients used their drops less than 75% of the time, thus displaying low compliance. In addition, patients reported considerately higher medication use than in reality and those with adherence of less than 50% of expected doses showed far higher dose taking immediately after the office visit and just before the return visit at 3 months. Finally, the study showed the poor ability of the physician to identify non-adherent patients, based on their self-reports, IOP measurements, or other subjective indicators. It concluded that in order to identify the less adherent patients, there is a need for better communication skills, better electronic monitoring, or both [27]. Robin et al. used electronic monitoring to objectively measure patient adherence with once-daily prostaglandin analogues as the sole ocular hypotensive therapy and to compare them with adjunctive medicine to the prostaglandin analogues and concluded that more complex dosing regimens result in poorer adherence, while once-daily drugs in a complex dosing regimen were found to have good adherence [30].

However, the studies we found advanced the idea that electronic monitoring of glaucoma therapy provides the most accurate data on adherence to glaucoma medication and very detailed knowledge regarding patterns of medication-taking behaviour.

3.4. Strategies for Addressing Nonadherence

The interventions to improve non-adherence represent an important goal of glaucoma research and require a complex approach, which is dependent on the patients' needs and lifestyle [31]. Glaucoma is a unique chronic disease since the rates of adherence and compliance in the treatment of the condition are relatively low compared to other chronic conditions which require lifelong therapeutic interventions [32]. Currently, there is a paucity of research examining intervention strategies to enhance glaucoma medication adherence. Methods that can be used to enhance adherence in glaucoma therapy can be grouped into: patient education, improved communication between physicians and patients, simplifying and optimizing treatment regimens, and better patient interaction with the health care system. Budenz published a guide of interventions for improvement of glaucoma therapy adherence based on studies of the treatment of systemic hypertension, which promotes involving or empowering patients in the use of their own treatment and a proactive approach of the physician. Reviews of hypertension adherence studies have shown that three of the most straightforward strategies that improve adherence to therapy are to simplify treatment regimens, to optimize treatments to reduce side effects, and to reduce medication costs [16].

3.4.1. Patient Education

The first step in improving patient adherence to a medication regimen is patient education (as glaucoma medications are effective only if patients use them) [1]. Education should be delivered in the form of both verbal and written instructions, including color-coded medication schedules, pictures, and adapted information for those with poor vision or low literacy. The ophthalmologist must make sure that the patient understands the treatment regimen and for this purpose, didactic presentations on proper drop application are important and should be repeated periodically to ensure that the patient continues to use the proper technique. Patients should be instructed about correct dosing schedules, minimization of waste of medication, and a clear discussion regarding the fact that vision can be irreversibly lost if the medications are not properly applied. Moreover, regular review of drug administration at each visit helps reinforce adherence by providing the physician with information regarding the patient's level of understanding of his treatment regimen. In addition, patients should be encouraged to participate in their own treatment by keeping a daily record of medication dosage. With the availability of cell phones and Internet communication, there are several potential avenues that deserve exploration to improve compliance using continuous reminder systems, such as those available on the telephone (alarms, applications, text-messages, and phone calls) or e-mails, to reduce forgetfulness [16,33].

Situational and environmental factors play a role in adherence of glaucoma patients as there are individual specific daily situations that make it difficult for patients to be compliant [3]. It is very important to incorporate a regimen that is easy to use and easy to integrate into the daily lives of patients. Treatment adherence has been shown to be lower in the younger age groups, in spite of having greater access to electronic devices, often due to a busy lifestyle and work commitments. Therefore, involving patients can take the form of asking them to integrate their treatment into their daily activities. For example, they can take a bottle of drops at work or put the drops next to the bed, desk, or toothbrush. Moreover, physicians may suggest involving a helpful family member to assist with applying drops or reminding the patient to take drops [16]. Even though young patients can manage online information without the physician's advice, it does not seem to improve their adherence. There is evidence showing that adherence with glaucoma treatment is lower in the first year of diagnosis, and improved education about the disease may help patients persevere with their treatment [34].

3.4.2. Patient-Physician Communication

Carpenter et al. studied whether patient–physician communication increases the medication self-efficacy of glaucoma patients and concluded that it can improve the treatment adherence. Thus, providers should adopt a patient-centred approach, taking time to educate patients about their chronic disease and to assess their views on the treatment. The study also indicated that patients who ask more medication-related questions may have less confidence that they can adhere to their glaucoma regimen and should receive more support to address the adherence barriers [2]. A study of 279 patients with glaucoma who were video-recorded during their visit showed that educating patients about their condition occurred during approximately two-thirds of the visits, but was not significantly associated with whether patients took their doses on time during the next period of time after the visit. Instead, education regarding administration of the eye drops was the only provider communication variable that was significantly associated with adherence. Accordingly, thorough understanding of glaucoma must be supported by health professionals by allocating more time to providing information to patients [35].

An observational study investigated an intervention program consisting of education and a reminder system. The adherence rate with glaucoma medication increased from 54% to 73% in patients whose baseline drop-taking was under 75%. Improvement was immediate and sustained over 3 months. The research suggested that using a multifaceted approach improved the probability that the interventions changed medication use. The study could not determine which aspects of the intervention were most valuable and which strategies can be implemented in clinical practice. Additionally, the researchers found that there was greater improvement in adherence among white patients and those with the lowest baseline adherence. Additionally, improvement in adherence did not correlate with the level of IOP measured in the clinic. To this end, the results of the study showed that many nonadherent patients had satisfactory IOP at routine visits and thus, measurement of IOP was considered inadequate for estimating adherence. Finally, it was underlined that further research is needed to distinguish poor adherence in patients to avoid overmedication and to determine which elements of the adherence program were most effective [33].

3.4.3. Simplifying Medication Regimen

Interventions designed to increase patients' medication-related self-efficacy should consider prescribing simpler medication regimens. The importance of simplifying patients' medication regimen has been emphasized by many studies that showed that patients on more complex regimens were less likely to take their doses on time and they were less likely to take the correct number of prescribed doses each day [30,35]. Additionally, it was demonstrated that patients taking once-daily drugs in a complex dosing regimen were found to have good adherence [30]. It was shown that 3 and 4 times-a-day dosing and improper spacing of doses, versus twice-a-day dosing, increase noncompliance; hence, the fewest number of medications, instilled with the least frequency, enhance patient satisfaction and dosing convenience [36].

Shirai et al. evaluated Japanese patients' adherence to fixed and unfixed combination eyedrops and found that patients with fixed combination therapy had a higher adherence to their regimen. The main reason may be that a fixed combination is more convenient for patients. It is easier and faster to apply one drop of an ophthalmic solution than two drops from separate bottles of medication, with no waiting period between the two types of drops, with similar or possibly superior efficacies in daily practice compared with unfixed-combination therapies. Furthermore, it is more advantageous because of the decreased exposure to preservatives and thus decreased risk of developing ocular surface diseases [37].

Possible solutions when patients require multiple medications and doses would be coordinating administration with daily events, such as meals or brushing teeth and using a written schedule for medications [1]. Furthermore, patients' compliance is enhanced when patients are aware of the possible adverse effects of a medication and patient education should include a discussion of treatment alternatives. Research has suggested that individuals receiving preservative-free medication demonstrate lower rates of nonadherence (12.5%) and it has been indicated that switching to preservative-free therapies may be of particular benefit regarding adherence with self-administered treatments [38].

3.4.4. Medication Cost

Many studies have confirmed that the majority of glaucoma office visits do not include a discussion of medication cost. Providers often do not ask if their patients have glaucoma medication cost problems and, in turn, although patients may experience financial dificulties with regard to the treatment regimen, they rarely mention it to their doctors. Therefore, ophthalmologists should consider mentioning medication cost during office visits in order to improve adherence from the beginning of glaucoma treatment [39]. A possible solution to overcome the barriers of cost and the physical burden of drug acquisition would be to provide free eye drops to patients, either by occasionally giving free samples or by rendering the medication reimbursable.

Finally, a cost-utility analysis assessed the societal costs of optimal versus poor adherence to glaucoma medications among people over 40 years of age with newly diagnosed glaucoma on a 60-year time horizon and demonstrated that being adherent to glaucoma medications resulted in improved quality of life for a relatively low increase in lifetime healthcare costs [40].

3.4.5. Self-Measurement of Intraocular Pressure

The measurement of intraocular pressure (IOP) is one of the most important diagnostic methods to determine the effectiveness of glaucoma treatment. However, a single measurement of IOP during office visits does not reveal the true level of intraocular hypertension and of the daily fluctuations in IOP. Astakhov et al. assessed the convenience of patients' self-monitoring their IOP at home using Icare® HOME tonometers and noted an increase in the level of adherence to treatment. The study showed that independent participation of the patient in the diagnostic process improves awareness and understanding of the disease and the importance of following the doctor's instructions [41].

Chen et al. evaluated the reliability of measurements made by patients themselves using iCare tonometers and compared these with Goldmann applanation tonometry measurements. The study showed that patients appreciated the method of self-measuring their IOP at home as it has the advantage of saving time for both the patients themselves and the glaucoma care providers. The iCare One self-tonometer allowed patients to instantly read the results, which made them feel positively toward this possibility. Moreover, patients wished this method could be a part of future glaucoma monitoring. Thus, home IOP monitoring provides valuable information for glaucoma care and might improve adherence to treatment [42].

4. Conclusions

In summary, the body of literature on glaucoma medication adherence shows that it is a challenging problem for ophthalmologists who provide services to patients with this chronic disease and the many tested interventions have had varying degrees of success.

We believe ophthalmologists should suspect a potentially reduced adherence when the IOP level is not congruent with the prescribed regimen, when the patient has not been well educated and does not understand his chronic disease and the importance of treatment on his vision-related outcome, or when the patient has a complicated medication regimen. Additionally, we must take into consideration that most glaucoma patients are older adults who may have physical or cognitive disabilities and limited financial resources as well as impaired visual acuity, which may interfere with the administration of eyedrops. Daily routine measures to detect reduced adherence, which are simple and relatively easy to use, include evaluation of patient diaries and questioning the patient about difficulties encountered with applying the treatment, drops schedule, side effects of the eyedrops, and the patient's opinion regarding the regimen.

Measures to improve adherence, which may have a great effect on boosting the patient's ability to follow a medication regimen are patient education, therapy reminder systems (e.g., alarms, text-messages), simplifying the therapy and tailoring it to the individual's lifestyle with patient participation, preservative-free medication to lower the possible side effects, and better communication between the patient and the health care provider. Integrating a person-centred method may help in treating the patient as a whole by allowing a focus on both the eye disease and quality of life.

Even though there are myriad causes of nonadherence and there remain large gaps in detecting, identifying, and addressing nonadherence, a multifaceted approach seems to be a problem-solving strategy [13,16].

Author Contributions: Conceptualization, A.-C.Z. and R.-E.R.; methodology M.R.; software M.R.; validation, A.-C.Z., R.-E.R. and M.R.; resources, R.-E.R.; data curation, M.R.; writing—original draft preparation, A.-C.Z.; writing—review and editing, O.-M.D. and A.-C.Z.; visualization, A.-C.Z.; supervision, A.-C.Z.; project administration, A.-C.Z. All authors have read and agreed to the published version of the manuscript.

Funding: This research received no external funding.

Institutional Review Board Statement: Not applicable.

Informed Consent Statement: Not applicable.

Conflicts of Interest: The authors declare no conflict of interest.

References

1.   Girkin, C.A.; Bhorade, A.M. Chapter 7: Medical Management of Glaucoma. In *BCSC 2019–2020: Glaucoma*; American Academy of Ophthalmology: San Francisco, CA, USA, 2019; pp. 169, 186.
2.   Carpenter, D.M.; Blalock, S.J.; Sayner, R.; Muir, K.W.; Robin, A.L.; Hartnett, M.E.; Giangiacomo, A.L.; Tudor, G.E.; Sleath, B.L. Communication Predicts Medication Self-Efficacy in Glaucoma Patients. *Optom. Vis. Sci.* **2016**, *93*, 731–737. [CrossRef]
3.   Tsai, J.C. A Comprehensive Perspective on Patient Adherence to Topical Glaucoma Therapy. *Ophthalmology* **2009**, *116*, S30–S36. [CrossRef]
4.   Zemba, M.; Stamate, A.-C.; Tataru, C.P.; Branisteanu, D.C.; Balta, F. Conjunctival flap surgery in the management of ocular surface disease (Review). *Exp. Ther. Med.* **2020**, *20*, 3412–3416. [CrossRef]
5.   Barac, I.R.; Balta, G.; Zemba, M.; Branduse, L.; Mehedintu, C.; Burcea, M.; Barac, D.A.; Branisteanu, D.C.; Balta, F. Accelerated vs. conventional collagen cross-linking for infectious keratitis. *Exp. Ther. Med.* **2021**, *21*, 285. [CrossRef]
6.   Branisteanu, D.C.; Stoleriu, G.; Branisteanu, D.E.; Boda, D.; Branisteanu, C.I.; Maranduca, M.A.; Moraru, A.; Stanca, H.T.; Zemba, M.; Balta, F. Ocular cicatricial pemphigoid (Review). *Exp. Ther. Med.* **2020**, *20*, 3379–3382. [CrossRef]
7.   Tăbăcaru, B.; Stanca, S.; Mocanu, V.; Zemba, M.; Stanca, H.T.; Munteanu, M. Intraoperative flap-related complications in FemtoLASIK surgeries performed with Visumax®femtosecond laser: A ten-year Romanian experience. *Exp. Ther. Med.* **2020**, *20*, 2529–2535. [CrossRef]
8.   Tătaru, C.-I.; Tătaru, C.-P.; Costache, A.; Boruga, O.; Zemba, M.; Ciuluvică, R.C.; Sima, G. Congenital cataract–clinical and morphological aspects. *Rom. J. Morphol. Embryol.* **2020**, *61*, 105–112. [CrossRef]
9.   Branisteanu, D.C.; Branisteanu, D.E.; Feraru, C.I.; Branisteanu, C.I.; Moraru, A.; Zemba, M.; Balta, F. Influence of unilateral intravitreal bevacizumab injection on the incidence of symptomatic choroidal neovascularization in the fellow eye in patients with neovascular age-related macular degeneration (Review). *Exp. Ther. Med.* **2020**, *20*, 182. [CrossRef]
10. Hoevenaars, J.G.M.M.; Schouten, J.S.A.G.; Borne, B.V.D.; Beckers, H.J.M.; Webers, C.A.B.; Schouten, J.S. Will improvement of knowledge lead to improvement of compliance with glaucoma medication? *Acta Ophthalmol.* **2008**, *86*, 849–855. [CrossRef]
11. Quaranta, L.; Riva, I.; Gerardi, C.; Oddone, F.; Floriano, I.; Konstas, A.G.P. Quality of Life in Glaucoma: A Review of the Literature. *Adv. Ther.* **2016**, *33*, 959–981. [CrossRef]
12. Loon, S.C.; Jin, J.; Goh, M.J. The Relationship between Quality of Life and Adherence to Medication in Glaucoma Patients in Singapore. *J. Glaucoma* **2015**, *24*, e36–e42. [CrossRef]
13. Budenz, D.L. A Clinician's Guide to the Assessment and Management of Nonadherence in Glaucoma. *Ophthalmology* **2009**, *116*, S43–S47. [CrossRef]
14. Robin, A.; Grover, D.S. Compliance and adherence in glaucoma management. *Indian J. Ophthalmol.* **2011**, *59*, 93–96. [CrossRef]
15. Ahmed, R.; Aslani, P. What is patient adherence? A terminology overview. *Int. J. Clin. Pharm.* **2014**, *36*, 4–7. [CrossRef]
16. Osterberg, L.; Blaschke, T. Adherence to Medication. *N. Engl. J. Med.* **2005**, *353*, 487–497. [CrossRef]
17. Guven, S.; Koylu, M.T.; Mumcuoglu, T. Adherence to glaucoma medication, illness perceptions, and beliefs about glaucoma: Attitudinal perspectives among Turkish population. *Eur. J. Ophthalmol.* **2021**, *31*, 469–476. [CrossRef]
18. Windham, B.G.; Griswold, M.E.; Fried, L.P.; Rubin, G.S.; Xue, Q.-L.; Carlson, M.C. Impaired Vision and the Ability to Take Medications. *J. Am. Geriatr. Soc.* **2005**, *53*, 1179–1190. [CrossRef]
19. Lacey, J.; Cate, H.T.; Broadway, D.C. Barriers to adherence with glaucoma medications: A qualitative research study. *Eye* **2008**, *23*, 924–932. [CrossRef]
20. Vlieland, N.D.; Bemt, B.J.F.V.D.; Bekker, C.L.; Bouvy, M.L.; Egberts, T.C.G.; Gardarsdottir, H. Older Patients' Compliance with Drug Storage Recommendations. *Drugs Aging* **2018**, *35*, 233–241. [CrossRef]
21. Gelb, L.; Friedman, D.S.; Quigley, H.A.; Lyon, D.W.; Tan, J.; Kim, E.E.; Zimmerman, T.J.; Hahn, S.R. Physician Beliefs and Behaviors Related to Glaucoma Treatment Adherence. *J. Glaucoma* **2008**, *17*, 690–698. [CrossRef]
22. Stevenson, F.A.; Cox, K.; Britten, N.; Dundar, Y. A systematic review of the research on communication between patients and health care professionals about medicines: The consequences for concordance. *Health Expect.* **2004**, *7*, 235–245. [CrossRef] [PubMed]
23. Hahn, S.R. Patient-Centered Communication to Assess and Enhance Patient Adherence to Glaucoma Medication. *Ophthalmology* **2009**, *116*, S37–S42. [CrossRef] [PubMed]
24. Sayner, R.; Carpenter, D.M.; Blalock, S.J.; Robin, A.L.; Muir, K.W.; Hartnett, M.E.; Giangiacomo, A.L.; Tudor, G.; Sleath, B. Accuracy of Patient-reported Adherence to Glaucoma Medications on a Visual Analog Scale Compared With Electronic Monitors. *Clin. Ther.* **2015**, *37*, 1975–1985. [CrossRef] [PubMed]
25. Mansouri, K.; Tanna, A.P.; De Moraes, C.G.; Camp, A.S.; Weinreb, R.N. Review of the measurement and management of 24-hour intraocular pressure in patients with glaucoma. *Surv. Ophthalmol.* **2020**, *65*, 171–186. [CrossRef]
26. Friedman, D.S.; Quigley, H.A.; Gelb, L.; Tan, J.; Margolis, J.; Shah, S.N.; Kim, E.E.; Zimmerman, T.; Hahn, S.R. Using Pharmacy Claims Data to Study Adherence to Glaucoma Medications: Methodology and Findings of the Glaucoma Adherence and Persistency Study (GAPS). *Investig. Ophthalmol. Vis. Sci.* **2007**, *48*, 5052–5057. [CrossRef] [PubMed]
27. Okeke, C.O.; Quigley, H.A.; Jampel, H.D.; Ying, G.-S.; Plyler, R.J.; Jiang, Y.; Friedman, D.S. Adherence with Topical Glaucoma Medication Monitored Electronically: The Travatan Dosing Aid Study. *Ophthalmology* **2009**, *116*, 191–199. [CrossRef]

28. De Amici, D.; Klersy, C.; Ramajoli, F.; Brustia, L.; Politi, P. Impact of the Hawthorne Effect in a Longitudinal Clinical Study: The Case of Anesthesia. *Control Clin. Trials* **2000**, *21*, 103–114. [CrossRef]
29. Friedman, D.S.; Jampel, H.D.; Congdon, N.G.; Miller, R.; Quigley, H.A. The TRAVATAN Dosing Aid Accurately Records When Drops Are Taken. *Am. J. Ophthalmol.* **2007**, *143*, 699–701. [CrossRef]
30. Robin, A.; Novack, G.; Covert, D.W.; Crockett, R.S.; Marcic, T.S. Adherence in Glaucoma: Objective Measurements of Once-Daily and Adjunctive Medication Use. *Am. J. Ophthalmol.* **2007**, *144*, 533–540.e2. [CrossRef]
31. Boland, M.V.; Chang, D.S.; Frazier, T.; Plyler, R.; Friedman, D.S. Electronic Monitoring to Assess Adherence with Once-Daily Glaucoma Medications and Risk Factors for Nonadherence. *JAMA Ophthalmol.* **2014**, *132*, 838–844. [CrossRef]
32. Rajurkar, K.; Dubey, S.; Gupta, P.P.; John, D.; Chauhan, L. Compliance to topical anti-glaucoma medications among patients at a tertiary hospital in North India. *J. Curr. Ophthalmol.* **2017**, *30*, 125–129. [CrossRef] [PubMed]
33. Okeke, C.O.; Quigley, H.A.; Jampel, H.D.; Ying, G.-S.; Plyler, R.J.; Jiang, Y.; Friedman, D.S. Interventions Improve Poor Adherence with Once Daily Glaucoma Medications in Electronically Monitored Patients. *Ophthalmology* **2009**, *116*, 2286–2293. [CrossRef] [PubMed]
34. McClelland, J.; Bodle, L.; Little, J.-A. Investigation of medication adherence and reasons for poor adherence in patients on long-term glaucoma treatment regimes. *Patient Prefer. Adherence* **2019**, *13*, 431–439. [CrossRef] [PubMed]
35. Sleath, B.; Blalock, S.J.; Carpenter, D.; Sayner, R.; Muir, K.W.; Slota, C.; Lawrence, S.D.; Giangiacomo, A.L.; Hartnett, M.E.; Tudor, G.; et al. Ophthalmologist–Patient Communication, Self-efficacy, and Glaucoma Medication Adherence. *Ophthalmology* **2015**, *122*, 748–754. [CrossRef]
36. Stewart, W.C.; Konstas, A.G.; Pfeiffer, N. Patient and Ophthalmologist Attitudes Concerning Compliance and Dosing in Glaucoma Treatment. *J. Ocul. Pharmacol. Ther.* **2004**, *20*, 461–469. [CrossRef]
37. Shirai, C.; Matsuoka, N.; Nakazawa, T. Comparison of adherence between fixed and unfixed topical combination glaucoma therapies using Japanese healthcare/pharmacy claims database: A retrospective non-interventional cohort study. *BMC Ophthalmol.* **2021**, *21*, 52. [CrossRef]
38. Wolfram, C.; Stahlberg, E.; Pfeiffer, N. Patient-Reported Nonadherence with Glaucoma Therapy. *J. Ocul. Pharmacol. Ther.* **2019**, *35*, 223–228. [CrossRef]
39. Slota, C.; Davis, S.A.; Blalock, S.J.; Carpenter, D.; Muir, K.W.; Robin, A.L.; Sleath, B. Patient-Physician Communication on Medication Cost during Glaucoma Visits. *Optom. Vis. Sci.* **2017**, *94*, 1095–1101. [CrossRef]
40. Newman-Casey, P.A.; Salman, M.; Lee, P.; Gatwood, J.D. Cost-Utility Analysis of Glaucoma Medication Adherence. *Ophthalmology* **2020**, *127*, 589–598. [CrossRef]
41. Astakhov, S.Y.; Farikova, E.E.; Konoplianik, K.A. The role of self-dependent tonometry in improving diagnostics and treatment of patients with open angle glaucoma. *Ophthalmol. J.* **2019**, *12*, 41–46. [CrossRef]
42. Chen, E.; Quérat, L.; Åkerstedt, C. Self-tonometry as a complement in the investigation of glaucoma patients. *Acta Ophthalmol.* **2016**, *94*, 788–792. [CrossRef] [PubMed]

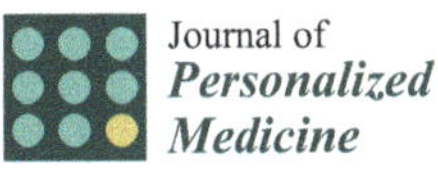

Journal of
*Personalized
Medicine*

Study Protocol

Programs Addressed to Family Caregivers/Informal Caregivers Needs: Systematic Review Protocol

Luís Sousa [1,2,*], Laurência Gemito [1,2], Rogério Ferreira [2,3], Lara Pinho [1,2], César Fonseca [1,2] and Manuel Lopes [1,2]

1 São João de Deus School of Nursing, University of Évora, 7000-811 Évora, Portugal; mlpg@uevora.pt (L.G.); lmgp@uevora.pt (L.P.); cfonseca@uevora.pt (C.F.); mjl@uevora.pt (M.L.)
2 Comprehensive Health Research Centre (CHRC), 7000-811 Évora, Portugal; ferrinho.ferreira@ipbeja.pt
3 School of Health of Beja, Polytechnic Institute of Beja, 7800-111 Beja, Portugal
* Correspondence: lmms@uevora.pt

Abstract: (1) Background: considering the growing increase in informal caregivers or family caregivers, it is critical to identify the unmet care needs of informal caregivers to improve their experiences, health, and well-being, contributing to the achievement of care needs of the elderly or people with adult dependency and promotion of successful transitions from health services to the community/home. (2) Objective: to identify the current state of knowledge about programs addressed to family caregivers/informal caregivers needs. (3) Methods: a systematic review will be undertaken with resource to databases from EBSCOhost Research Platform, Scopus, Web of Science, The Virtual Health Library (VHL). Studies published after January 2011 in English, Spanish, French, Italian and Portuguese will be considered. This review will consider all studies that report on any intervention program targeting family caregivers/informal caregivers who need to improve their experiences, health, and well-being, contributing to the meeting of their needs or those who have dementia and cognitive impairment, mental disorders, impairments in activities of daily living, frailty and/or who need health care and/or promoting successful transitions of community. (4) Discussion: The results of this review could be used to develop an intervention model to meet the needs of the family caregivers/informal caregivers. Furthermore, these findings will help to guide the construction of health policies regarding family caregivers/informal caregivers, as well their needs.

Keywords: caregiver; informal caregiver; needs; intervention; patient-focused care

Citation: Sousa, L.; Gemito, L.; Ferreira, R.; Pinho, L.; Fonseca, C.; Lopes, M. Programs Addressed to Family Caregivers/Informal Caregivers Needs: Systematic Review Protocol. *J. Pers. Med.* **2022**, *12*, 145. https://doi.org/10.3390/jpm12020145

Academic Editors: Júlio Belo Fernandes, Fábio G. Teixeira and Catarina Godinho

Received: 30 December 2021
Accepted: 20 January 2022
Published: 21 January 2022

Publisher's Note: MDPI stays neutral with regard to jurisdictional claims in published maps and institutional affiliations.

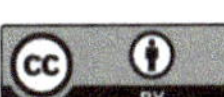

1. Introduction

The aging index of the European population is increasing rapidly, and a more significant increase is expected in the near future. Aging is related to health impairment and an increment in the number of chronic diseases [1]. This implies a significant global increase in the number of people living with chronic diseases [2]. Population aging is expected to increase the need for and consumption of long-term health care [1].

In this sense, many European countries have made significant reforms in the policy and systems of long-term care. In addition, cuts in professional health care are increasing the demand for informal care considerably, both by family and non-family caregivers [3,4].

Most people who need home care are older adults, have dementia and moderate cognitive impairment, dependence on activities of daily living, high degrees of fragility, and complexity in health care [5].

Most of these people remain at home, depending on informal caregivers to provide support to meet their needs [2]. Despite receiving awards associated with care, informal caregivers equally suffer from collateral effects, such as overload, stress, and physical and mental health problems [2]. In addition, family/informal caregivers of older adult residents in the community, specifically their children, reported a greater burden than other caregivers, even when referring to positive aspects in the provision of this care [6].

When older adults have dementia, the informal caregiver is the cornerstone and their suffering is associated with the worsening of various health outcomes of people with dementia, namely, worsening of the behavioral and psychological symptoms of dementia and abuse of the elderly [7].

Informal caregiver´s health suffers from the impact of caring, but its effect may vary according to the needs and expectations of informal caregivers and the support policies that are available to caregivers [4,8].

The causes of physical and psychological problems are related to four types of needs, mainly: (1) information on subjects related to mobility and prevention of falls, information on diseases, death, and dying; (2) social, financial, and e-health support; (3) organizational (balance between family and professional life, breaks, among others); and (4) social recognition [8]. When caring of people with cognitive disorders due to Alzheimer's, the needs of the informal caregiver may evolve with the progression of the disease and the transition from dementia, and are related to information, psychosocial, social, psychoeducational support, among others. These needs should be assessed regularly and considered for the need for new knowledge, ability adjustment, support, and available services [9].

Currently, the support policies available in European countries such as Austria, Germany, Spain, France, Belgium, Czech Republic, Sweden, Netherlands, Denmark, Switzerland, Luxembourg, and Slovenia are the ones that promote better health for people cared for and for informal caregivers by: (1) providing off-duty time, (2) emotionally helping them to deal with care, and (3) teaching skill sets to improve care and deal effectively with these situations [4]. These intervention programs must be framed within a patient- and family-centered care perspective, as they take into account the patient's values in personal care decisions, as well as including the patient´s and family's role as essential counselors and partners in improving practices of care [10].

Patient- and family-centered care, as a set of interventions, aimed to meet the needs not only of the patient, but also of their families. Patient- and family-centered care is defined as mutually beneficial partnerships between healthcare professionals, patients, and families in the planning, delivery, and evaluation of healthcare [11]. Evidence indicates that patient- and family-centered care is considered a fundamental approach to improving the quality of health care through positive patient outcomes and generating a good working environment for healthcare professionals [12].

Bearing in mind the growing increase in informal family or paid caregivers, it is essential to identify the unmet care needs of the elderly and support needs for informal caregivers to improve their experiences, health, and well-being, contributing to achieve the care needs of the elderly and/or promoting successful transitions from health services to the community/home [6]. Knowledge of the unmet needs of informal/family caregivers allows to plan and provide more adjusted, patient- and family-centered care, with reduced gaps and higher quality [13].

1.1. Objective

The main objective of this review is to identify the current state of knowledge about programs addressed to family caregivers/informal caregivers needs.

1.2. Review Questions

This review aims to answer the following questions:

What are the strategies/interventions that address family caregivers/informal caregivers needs?

What are the health gains for the person being cared for, the informal caregiver/family caregivers, and the health system?

What are the facilitators and barriers identified in the implementation of interventions that address family caregivers/informal caregivers needs?

2. Materials and Methods

A systematic review of qualitative and quantitative studies was selected to be carried out, since it contributes to a better understanding of the most recent and available evidence on the topic; in addition, both perspectives are necessary to inform clinical policies or organizational decisions [14].

This protocol will follow the recommendations of the preferred reporting items for systematic reviews and meta-analyses (PRISMA) protocol statement [15].

The data from the included studies will be synthesized using a narrative synthesis approach and analyzed thematically to combine the results of studies that used several methods (qualitative, quantitative, and mixed methods).

This protocol was developed in February 2021 and the respective review will be completed by the end of 2021. PROSPERO registration number CRD42021241297.

2.1. Eligibility Criteria

This systematic review aims to ensure the accuracy and systematization proper to this type of study, and has established eligibility criteria which are presented below.

2.2. Population

Studies will be included whose populations are made up of informal caregivers/family caregivers of adults or elderly people, or who have dementia and cognitive impairment, mental disorders, activities of daily living with a disability, fragility and/or who need health care.

2.3. Types of Intervention(s)/Phenomena of Interest

This literature review will consider studies on any family-centered care program addressed to family caregivers/informal caregivers needs in order to improve their experiences, health, and well-being, contributing to meeting the needs of adults (>18) or elderly people, or who have dementia and cognitive impairment, mental disorders, activities of daily living disability, fragility and/or who need health care and/or promoting successful transitions of community/home health services.

In a Portuguese study, the most prevalent health needs found were food preparation, medication/taking tablets, taking care of the house, using the bathroom, sensory problems, communication/interaction, bladder, intestines, eating and drinking, memory, sleeping, and preventing falls [16].

Some of the interventions targeting informal caregivers are based on the recognition and application of anxiety management interventions, as well as depression and caregiver burden [17]. This includes individualized and high quality interventions, such as psychological and emotional stability [16], and interventions to preserve and enhance social support as a way to reduce depressive symptoms of informal caregivers [18].

2.4. Comparison

This review will include studies with or without a comparative group.

2.5. Phenomena of Interest

The qualitative component of this review will explore the experiences of caregivers who have participated in intervention programs, and the facilitators and barriers identified in the implementation of these programs.

2.6. Study Design

This systematic review should include primary empirical studies. The quantitative component of the review will consider both experimental and epidemiological study designs, including randomized controlled trials, non-randomized controlled trials, quasi experimental, before and after studies, prospective and retrospective cohort studies, case–control studies, and analytical cross-sectional studies.

The qualitative component of the review will contemplate studies that focus on qualitative data including, but not limited to, designs such as phenomenology, grounded theory, ethnography, and action research.

2.7. Context

All studies on programs that address the unmet care needs of informal caregivers/family caregivers of community-dwelling adults or elderly people, or who have dementia and cognitive impairment, mental disorders, activities of daily living with a disability, fragility and/or who need health care, regardless of context (community, culture, or specific environment), will be included in this review. Studies carried out in European countries will be included.

2.8. Primary Outcome

The main outcomes appraised would be indicators of worsening health, well-being and financial; these can be assessed in a general or specific way when applied to informal caregivers/family caregivers of dependent people in the community. The data obtained may be represented quantitatively, such as averages, measures of prevalence or incidence, frequencies, economic indicators concerning evaluations, or they may be of a qualitative essence.

With the analysis of quantitative studies, we expect to find results that incorporate psychosocial or satisfaction indicators, such as stress, anxiety, depression, quality of life, family functioning, family empowerment, or satisfaction with family-centered care.

2.9. Secondary Outcomes

The secondary outcomes considered in this review will be the facilitators and barriers identified in the implementation of patient- and family-centered care programs that address the unmet care needs informal caregivers/family caregivers of community-dwelling dependent people.

2.10. Search Strategy

2.10.1. Data Sources

Given the nature of the research, the strategy to be adopted consists of the conduction of a comprehensive bibliographic search with recourse to the following databases: EBSCOhost Research Platform (CINAHL® Plus with Full Text; Nursing & Allied Health Collection; Cochrane Plus Collection, including Cochrane Central Register of Controlled Trials; Cochrane Database of Systematic Reviews (CDSR) e Database of Abstracts of Reviews of Effects (DARE); MedicLatina; MEDLINE®, including International Nursing Index). PubMed via MEDLINE, CINAHL, Scopus, Web of Science, and The Virtual Health Library (VHL). Open Grey e Grey Literature Report.

2.10.2. Search Terms

Subject headings (MeSH) will be used and according to it, an arrangement of four key concepts will include: Caregiver, Patient-Centered Care, Disabled Persons, Community-Based Distribution in the title, keywords, and abstract. Free terms such as program, intervention, and approach may be used. In this case, the search will be: ((Caregiver) OR (Care Giver*) OR (Caregiver*, Family) OR (Caregiver*, Spouse)) AND ((Disabled Persons) OR (elderly dependent) OR (Aged) OR (dementia) OR (Alzheimer) OR (Disability) AND ((Care, Non-Professional Home) OR (Nonprofessional Home Care) OR (Old Age Assistance) OR (Patient-Centered Care) OR (Patient Centered Nursing) OR (Patient-Focused Care) OR (needs assessment) OR (care management) OR (health care) OR (psychosocial care) OR (community) OR (Community-Based Distribution).

The strategy will be adapted according to each database and will be restricted to the last 10 years, therefore, from 2011 to 2021, in English, Portuguese, Spanish, French, and Italian. The pre-test of the research is found in Table 1.

The studies resulting from the research in each database will be exported to Microsoft Word® (Microsoft, Redmond, WA, USA) and duplicates will be removed.

Table 1. Search Strategy.

Data Base	Search Strategy
CINAHL® Plus with Full Text Nursing & Allied Health Collection; Cochrane Central Register of Controlled Trials; Cochrane Database of Systematic Reviews; Cochrane Methodology Register; Cochrane Clinical Answers; MedicLatina; MEDLINE® with Full Text	((((Caregiver) OR (Care Giver*) OR (Caregiver*, Family) OR (Caregiver*, Spouse)) AND ((Disabled Persons) OR (elderly dependent) OR (Aged) OR (dementia) OR (Alzheimer) OR (Disability)) AND ((Care, Non-Professional Home) OR (Nonprofessional Home Care) OR (Old Age Assistance) OR (Patient-Centered Care) OR (Patient Centered Nursing) OR (Patient-Focused Care) OR (needs assessment) OR (care management) OR (health care) OR (psychosocial care) OR (community) OR (Community-Based Distribution)))
Scopus	TITLE-ABS-KEY ((caregiver*) AND ((disabled AND persons) OR (elderly AND dependent) OR (aged) OR (dementia) OR (Alzheimer) OR (disability)) AND ((nonprofessional AND home AND care) OR (patient-centered AND care)))
Web of Science	3#-660-#2 OR #1 Bases de dados = WOS, CCC, DIIDW, KJD, MEDLINE, RSCI, SCIELO Tempo estipulado = 2011–2021 Idioma da pesquisa = Auto 2#-400–KP = ((((Caregiver) OR (Care Giver*) OR (Caregiver*, Family) OR (Caregiver*, Spouse)) AND ((Disabled Persons) OR (elderly dependent) OR (Aged) OR (dementia) OR (Disability)) AND ((Care, Non-Professional Home) OR (Nonprofessional Home Care) OR (Old Age Assistance) OR (Patient-Centered Care) OR (Patient Centered Nursing) OR (Patient-Focused Care) OR (needs assessment) OR (care management) OR (health care) OR (psychosocial care) OR (community) OR (Community-Based Distribution))) Bases de dados = WOS, CCC, DIIDW, KJD, MEDLINE, RSCI, SCIELO Tempo estipulado = 2011–2021 Idioma da pesquisa = Auto 1#-261–TI = ((((Caregiver) OR (Care Giver*) OR (Caregiver*, Family) OR (Caregiver*, Spouse)) AND ((Disabled Persons) OR (elderly dependent) OR (Aged) OR (dementia) OR (Disability)) AND ((Care, Non-Professional Home) OR (Nonprofessional Home Care) OR (Old Age Assistance) OR (Patient-Centered Care) OR (Patient Centered Nursing) OR (Patient-Focused Care) OR (needs assessment) OR (care management) OR (health care) OR (psychosocial care) OR (community) OR (Community-Based Distribution))) Bases de dados = WOS, CCC, DIIDW, KJD, MEDLINE, RSCI, SCIELO Tempo estipulado = 2011–2021 Idioma da pesquisa = Auto
The Virtual Health Library (VHL)—abstract (MEDLINE; LILACS; IBECS)	((((Caregiver) OR (Care Giver*) OR (Caregiver*, Family) OR (Caregiver*, Spouse)) AND ((Disabled Persons) OR (elderly dependent) OR (Aged) OR (dementia) OR (Alzheimer) OR (Disability)) AND ((Care, Non-Professional Home) OR (Nonprofessional Home Care) OR (Old Age Assistance) OR (Patient-Centered Care) OR (Patient Centered Nursing) OR (Patient-Focused Care) OR (needs assessment) OR (care management) OR (health care) OR (psychosocial care) OR (community) OR (Community-Based Distribution)))

2.11. Data Collection and Analysis

2.11.1. Selection of Studies

The criteria selected for the inclusion of studies in this investigation will consist of the reading of title, abstract, and keywords by two reviewers, and those which do not meet the inclusion criteria established for this review will not be included in it. A third reviewer will be included in case of divergences or doubts. Subsequently, the full texts will also be evaluated by two reviewers independently. For the presentation of this selection process, the PRISMA flowchart, with the results of the screening in the different phases, will be presented.

2.11.2. Quality Appraisal

Prior to the inclusion of any component in this review, the quantitative articles selected from retrieval will be examined by two independent reviewers to validate them methodologically using standardized critical appraisal tools of the Joanna Briggs Institute Review and Statistical Evaluation of Meta-Analysis Instrument (JBI-MAStARI) to validate its inclusion in the review.

Should discrepancies exist between the reviewers' assessments, these will be solved through discussion, or by the intervention of a third reviewer.

The qualitative articles selected from retrieval will be examined by two independent reviewers in order to validate them methodologically using standardized critical appraisal tools of the Joanna Briggs Institute Qualitative Assessment and Review Instrument (JBI-QARI) to validate its inclusion in the review.

Should discrepancies exist between the reviewers' assessments, these will be solved through discussion, or by the intervention of a third reviewer.

The process of results exposure of the critical appraisal will consist of a narrative form and in a table.

Regardless of the outcome of the methodological quality assessment, all studies will be part of the data synthesis phases of the review.

2.11.3. Data Extraction

With regard to data extraction, at the initial stage, an individual descriptive analysis of each case will be carried out, considering the new research questions, and using extraction tools designed for the purpose.

Using JBI-MAStARI data extraction tools, quantitative data will be extracted from the articles to be included in the analysis.

Exhaustive details of the data extracted will be set out, including the purpose of the study, participants, assessment tools, intervention, significant outcomes and key findings, and study design. Standardized JBI data extraction tools will be used to extract data from the articles to be included in the review and to identify facilitators and barriers associated with program implementation.

Two independent reviewers will perform the extraction of the data and should discrepancies exist between the reviewers' assessments, these will be solved by the intervention of a third reviewer.

2.12. Strategy for Data Synthesis

The intention is to synthesize the results and present them using a table and the help of text and figures.

Whenever possible, the qualitative research findings will be gathered with the meta-aggregation approach. This will involve aggregating or synthesizing the findings to generate a set of statements that represent that same aggregation, bringing the findings together and categorizing them based on similarity of meaning.

These categories will then be synthesized to produce a range of integrated conclusions than can be used as a standard for evidence-based practice.

The narrative form of presenting results will be considered whenever the textual pooling is not feasible.

2.13. Patient and Public Involvement

During the construction or development of this review, there will be no involvement of patients or persons.

2.14. Ethics and Dissemination

Only secondary data will be considered and, therefore, no ethical approval is required to implement this study. This study consists of a systematic review protocol, that being, the results have not been extracted or analyzed yet, and will only be published through a publication after peer-review.

3. Discussion

Caregivers of adults with dementia or disabilities presented as the largest number of the whole group of caregivers. These caregivers, like caregivers of people with dementia or disability, delivered a broad spectrum of health-related tasks and experienced negative emotions, including mainly anxiety, depression, caregiver burden, and restrictions on social participation [17–20].

The unmet needs of informal caregivers may be one of the main areas for improvement in policy and service delivery [21]. Although the circumstances and conditions of informal caregivers/family caregivers have generally improved in recent years, longitudinal monitoring in family care in old age is extremely important [22].

With this review, we intend to summarize the main intervention programs to address the needs of family/informal caregivers, not only for those identified as high risk, but also those at medium and low risk. In this sense, the identification and implementation of interventions focused on informal caregivers/family caregivers of community-dwelling adults or the elderly, or who have dementia and cognitive impairment, mental disorders, impairment of activities of daily living, fragility and/or who need health care, must reduce anxiety, depression, and caregiver burden, prevent disease conditions, and improve quality of life.

The programs and services most often offered to caregivers are dementia management education and training services through the course of work, specific psychosocial support service, respite services, and information or advice on legal rights issues. In the context of the coronavirus disease 2019 (COVID-19), many caregivers experience an increase in social isolation, a greater burden of care, and deteriorating physical and mental health. Programs such as the World Health Organization iSupport, mDementia, and e-mhGAP (Mental Health Gap Action Programme) play an important role in supporting the caregiver, as they provide the opportunity to overcome obstacles related to access and care, as well as the interruption of services due to COVID-19 [23].

4. Strengths and Limitations of This Study

This review protocol may have important implications for teaching in the health field, especially in nursing education, because if family care is almost absent from nursing education curricula and practice standards, nurses will not have the knowledge needed to enhance the role of family caregivers in patient-centered care teams and will not be able to meet the health needs of caregivers themselves.

The results of this review could be used to develop an intervention model to answer the needs of the informal caregiver. These findings will also help to guide the construction of health policies regarding informal caregivers taking in account their needs.

Regarding the limitations of this study, the research strategy will be adapted according to each data base and will be restricted to the last 10 years, i.e., from 2011 to 2021 in the English, Spanish, French, Italian, and Portuguese languages.

Author Contributions: Conceptualization, L.S., M.L., L.P. and C.F.; methodology, all authors; investigation, L.S., L.P., R.F. and L.G. writing—original draft preparation, L.S. and L.P.; writing—review and editing all authors.; supervision, M.L. and C.F.; project administration, M.L.; funding acquisition, M.L. and C.F. All authors have read and agreed to the published version of the manuscript.

Funding: This research was funded by FEDER. Programa Interreg VA España-Portugal (POCTEP), grant number 0499_4IE_PLUS_4_E.

Institutional Review Board Statement: Not applicable.

Informed Consent Statement: Not applicable.

Data Availability Statement: Not applicable.

Conflicts of Interest: The authors declare no conflict of interest.

References

1. Willemse, E.; Anthierens, S.; Farfan-Portet, M.I.; Schmitz, O.; Macq, J.; Bastiaens, H.; Dilles, T.; Remmen, R. Do informal caregivers for elderly in the community use support measures? A qualitative study in five European countries. *BMC Health Serv. Res.* **2016**, *16*, 270. [CrossRef] [PubMed]
2. Ploeg, J.; Markle-Reid, M.; Valaitis, R.; McAiney, C.; Duggleby, W.; Bartholomew, A.; Sherifali, D. Web-Based Interventions to Improve Mental Health, General Caregiving Outcomes, and General Health for Informal Caregivers of Adults With Chronic Conditions Living in the Community: Rapid Evidence Review. *J. Med. Internet Res.* **2017**, *19*, e263. [CrossRef] [PubMed]
3. Van Groenou, M.I.B.; De Boer, A. Providing informal care in a changing society. *Eur. J. Ageing* **2016**, *13*, 271–279. [CrossRef] [PubMed]
4. Calvó-Perxas, L.; Vilalta-Franch, J.; Litwin, H.; Turro-Garriga, O.; Mira, P.; Garre-Olmo, J. What seems to matter in public policy and the health of informal caregivers? A cross-sectional study in 12 European countries. *PLoS ONE* **2018**, *13*, e0194232. [CrossRef] [PubMed]
5. Poss, J.W.; Sinn, C.-L.J.; Grinchenko, G.; Blums, J.; Peirce, T.; Hirdes, J. Location, Location, Location: Characteristics and Services of Long-Stay Home Care Recipients in Retirement Homes Compared to Others in Private Homes and Long-Term Care Homes. *Healtc. Policy.* **2017**, *12*, 80–93. [CrossRef]
6. Kristof, L.; Fortinsky, R.H.; Kellett, K.; Porter, M.; Robison, J. Experiences of Informal Caregivers of Older Adults Transitioned From Nursing Homes to the Community Through the Money Follows the Person Demonstration. *J. Aging Soc. Policy* **2016**, *29*, 20–34. [CrossRef] [PubMed]
7. Stall, N.M.; Kim, S.J.; Hardacre, K.A.; Shah, P.S.; Straus, S.E.; Bronskill, S.E.; Lix, L.M.; Bell, C.M.; Rochon, P.A. Association of Informal Caregiver Distress with Health Outcomes of Community-Dwelling Dementia Care Recipients: A Systematic Review. *J. Am. Geriatr. Soc.* **2018**, *67*, 609–617. [CrossRef]
8. Plöthner, M.; Schmidt, K.; De Jong, L.; Zeidler, J.; Damm, K. Needs and preferences of informal caregivers regarding outpatient care for the elderly: A systematic literature review. *BMC Geriatr.* **2019**, *19*, 82. [CrossRef]
9. Novais, T.; Dauphinot, V.; Krolak-Salmon, P.; Mouchoux, C. How to explore the needs of informal caregivers of individuals with cognitive impairment in Alzheimer's disease or related diseases? A systematic review of quantitative and qualitative studies. *BMC Geriatr.* **2017**, *17*, 86. [CrossRef]
10. Millenson, M.L.; Shapiro, E.; Greenhouse, P.K.; DiGioia, A.M., III. Patient- and Family-Centered Care: A Systematic Approach to Better Ethics and Care. *AMA J. Ethic.* **2016**, *18*, 49–55. [CrossRef]
11. Kokorelias, K.M.; Gignac, M.A.M.; Naglie, G.; Cameron, J.I. Towards a universal model of family centered care: A scoping review. *BMC Health Serv. Res.* **2019**, *19*, 564. [CrossRef] [PubMed]
12. Park, M.; Giap, T.-T.; Lee, M.; Jeong, H.; Jeong, M.; Go, Y. Patient- and family-centered care interventions for improving the quality of health care: A review of systematic reviews. *Int. J. Nurs. Stud.* **2018**, *87*, 69–83. [CrossRef] [PubMed]
13. Cloyes, K.G.; Hart, S.E.; Jones, A.K.; Ellington, L. Where are the family caregivers? Finding family caregiver-related content in foundational nursing documents. *J. Prof. Nurs.* **2019**, *36*, 76–84. [CrossRef] [PubMed]
14. Stern, C.; Lizarondo, L.; Carrier, J.; Godfrey, C.; Rieger, R.K.L.; Salmond, S.; Apóstolo, J.; Kirkpatrick, P.; Loveday, H. Methodological guidance for the conduct of mixed methods systematic reviews. *JBI Evid. Synth.* **2020**, *18*, 2108–2118. [CrossRef]
15. Moher, D.; Shamseer, L.; Clarke, M.; Ghersi, D.; Liberati, A.; Petticrew, M.; Shekelle, P.; Stewart, L.A.; PRISMA-P Group. Preferred reporting items for systematic review and meta-analysis protocols (PRISMA-P) 2015 statement. *Syst. Rev.* **2015**, *4*, 1. [CrossRef]
16. Abreu, W.; Tolson, D.; Jackson, G.A.; Staines, H.; Costa, N. The relationship between frailty, functional dependence, and healthcare needs among community-dwelling people with moderate to severe dementia. *Health Soc. Care Community* **2018**, *27*, 642–653. [CrossRef]
17. Mei, Y.; Wilson, S.; Lin, B.; Li, Y.; Zhang, Z. Benefit finding for Chinese family caregivers of community-dwelling stroke survivors: A cross-sectional study. *J. Clin. Nurs.* **2017**, *27*, e1419–e1428. [CrossRef]
18. Sandoval, F.; Tamiya, N.; Lloyd-Sherlock, P.; Noguchi, H. The relationship between perceived social support and depressive symptoms in informal caregivers of community-dwelling older persons in Chile. *Psychogeriatrics* **2019**, *19*, 547–556. [CrossRef]
19. Riffin, C.; Van Ness, P.H.; Wolff, J.L.; Fried, T. Family and Other Unpaid Caregivers and Older Adults with and without Dementia and Disability. *J. Am. Geriatr. Soc.* **2017**, *65*, 1821–1828. [CrossRef]

20. Shi, J.; Huang, A.; Jia, Y.; Yang, X. Perceived stress and social support influence anxiety symptoms of Chinese family caregivers of community-dwelling older adults: A cross-sectional study. *Psychogeriatrics* **2020**, *20*, 377–384. [CrossRef]
21. Diwan, S.; Hougham, G.W.; Sachs, G.A. Strain Experienced by Caregivers of Dementia Patients Receiving Palliative Care: Findings from the Palliative Excellence in Alzheimer Care Efforts (PEACE) Program. *J. Palliat. Med.* **2004**, *7*, 797–807. [CrossRef] [PubMed]
22. Wolff, J.L.; Mulcahy, J.; Huang, J.; Roth, D.L.; Covinsky, K.; Kasper, J.D. Family Caregivers of Older Adults, 1999–2015: Trends in Characteristics, Circumstances, and Role-Related Appraisal. *Gerontologist* **2017**, *58*, 1021–1032. [CrossRef] [PubMed]
23. World Health Organization (WHO). Global Status Report on the Public Health Response to Dementia. Available online: https://digitalcommons.fiu.edu/srhreports/health/health/65/ (accessed on 18 January 2022).

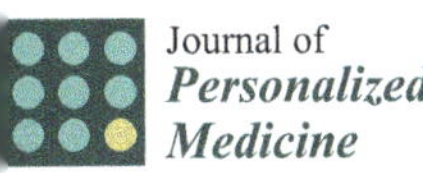

Journal of
*Personalized
Medicine*

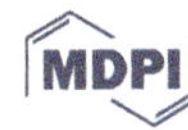

Protocol

Safety-Promoting Interventions for the Older Person with Hip Fracture on Returning Home: A Protocol for a Systematic Review

Paula Rocha [1,2,3,*], Cristina Lavareda Baixinho [3,4,5], Andréa Marques [6,7] and Adriana Henriques [3,5]

1 Local Health Unit of Guarda, 6300-749 Guarda, Portugal
2 PhD Student of University of Lisbon, 1649-004 Lisboa, Portugal
3 Nursing Research, Innovation and Development Centre of Lisbon (CIDNUR), 1900-160 Lisboa, Portugal; crbaixinho@esel.pt (C.L.B.); ahenriques@esel.pt (A.H.)
4 Center for Innovative Care and Health Technology (ciTechCare), Polytechnic of Leiria, 2411-901 Leiria, Portugal
5 Nursing School of Lisbon, 1900-160 Lisboa, Portugal
6 Nursing School of Coimbra, Health Sciences Research Unit: Nursing (UICISA:E), 3000-232 Coimbra, Portugal; andreamarques23@esenfc.pt
7 Department of Rheumatology, Centro Hospitalar e Universitário de Coimbra, 3000-071 Coimbra, Portugal
* Correspondence: rochapinhel@gmail.com

Abstract: Ageing and physical frailty associated with decrease in muscle and bone mass lead to the older persons' vulnerability and increased risk of falling. It is estimated that one in every ten falls in this age group results in a fracture, leading to a downward spiral in their health status, causing greater dependence, with a progressive functional decline that makes it difficult to return to their functional and social status prior to the fracture. The aim of this study is to identify the available evidence on the interventions that promote the safety of older people with hip fracture after hospital discharge. A search will be performed in MEDLINE and CINAHL databases. Randomised and controlled studies that focus on functional assessment, performance in activities of daily living, level of concern about falls, risk and prevalence of falls, injuries secondary to falls, re-fracture rate and health-related quality of life in hip fracture patients will be included. Two authors will perform the study selection, data extraction, and quality assessment independently. Any disagreements will be resolved through discussion with a third researcher. Methodological quality of the included trials will be evaluated by the Cochrane risk-of-bias criteria, and the Standards for Reporting Interventions in Controlled Trials.

Keywords: hip fracture; hospital discharge; older person; returning home; safety

Citation: Rocha, P.; Baixinho, C.L.; Marques, A.; Henriques, A. Safety-Promoting Interventions for the Older Person with Hip Fracture on Returning Home: A Protocol for a Systematic Review. *J. Pers. Med.* **2022**, *12*, 654. https://doi.org/10.3390/jpm12050654

Academic Editors: Fábio G. Teixeira, Angela Renee Starkweather, Catarina Godinho and Júlio Belo Fernandes

Received: 25 February 2022
Accepted: 13 April 2022
Published: 19 April 2022

Publisher's Note: MDPI stays neutral with regard to jurisdictional claims in published maps and institutional affiliations.

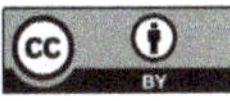

1. Introduction

Fractures resulting from falls trigger a downward spiral in the health status of older persons, causing greater dependence and disability, and may lead to long-term complications [1]. This condition is also associated with an increase in mortality when compared to the general population, a marked decline in quality of life, and consequently represents a notable burden on health systems [2].

Osteoporosis, characterized by a reduction in bone mineral density and micro-structural deterioration of bone tissue, increases bone fragility, inducing greater susceptibility to fragility fractures [3–5]. With the increase in life expectancy and the ageing of the population, the occurrence of fragility fractures, and more specifically of hip fractures (HF), has been increasing [2,4]. Most fragility fractures occur in people aged over 65 years, and result from low-impact trauma to osteoporotic and, therefore, more fragile bone, often associated with a fall [6,7]. Women are the most affected by this situation, at a ratio of 3:1 compared to man [2].

This clinical condition, more prevalent in older people [4], is asymptomatic until the moment when the first manifestation associated with a low impact trauma appears, often causing a fragility fracture [8], so reducing the risk of falls is crucial. Approximately 1/3 of the elderly aged 65 years suffer at least one fall per year; above 85 years this risk increases to 50% [9,10]. The fracture that occurs in 5–10% of fall events leads to difficulty in returning to the person's functional and social state prior to the fracture [11]. This leads to a need for care, with the main goal being unequivocally to maximize functional potential and provide the quickest possible return to the previous level of functionality [12]. This objective is achieved not only through surgical intervention, which provides the necessary stability to allow early mobilization and locomotion, but also through patient rehabilitation in the post-surgical context, with the aim of maximizing functional potential [12].

The significant impact that these fractures have in terms of public health is related to their high prevalence, the medical consequences that they entail, and also the reduction in the quality of life of the patient and their caregivers [6]. In this respect, it is estimated that 20–30% of patients with these fractures die in the following year; 50–60% of cases present some type of functional and/or motor loss, and only 30–40% of patients achieve a level of functional recovery similar to that before the HF [13]. Most of these patients require continued care for a long period, and 20% of them are institutionalised during the year following the fracture, which is the main reason for the loss of self-care in carrying out the activities of daily living [10,14].

Several studies have shown the importance of transitional care in the process of rehabilitation and readaptation of the elderly person during the process of discharge from hospital to home [15–17]. Transitional care should start at the time of admission, continue during hospitalisation and remain after discharge, which implies changing the ways of providing continuity of care to these people, since hospital environments only address biological aspects, and are not operationally designed to help older people recover or improve their functionality and return to their activities after hospitalisation [17,18].

In a study analysing the transition care of elderly patients with hip fracture, eight relevant domains were identified, including the complexity of the patient and system constraints, which, as inherent factors to the context, tend to hinder transition care. Others include patient involvement and choice, the role of the family caregiver, strong relationships, role coordination, documentation and information sharing are areas with the potential to support and improve transition care [19].

Involving patients in their care process by encouraging their participation may result in better outcomes [20]. The implementation of interventions that integrate exercises should include strategies to motivate and adhere to exercise, as well as contents related to components of the home care programme [21].

In view of the above, the aim of this systematic review is to identify the available evidence on interventions that promote the safety of older people with hip fracture after hospital discharge.

2. Materials and Methods

2.1. Type of Study

The protocol for this systematic review was designed according to the recommendations of the Preferred Reporting Items for Systematic Review and Meta-Analysis (PRISMA) Protocols checklist [22], PRISMA-P (Preferred Reporting Items for Systematic review and Meta-Analysis Protocols) [23] and the Cochrane Guidelines for Systematic Reviews of Interventions [24].

To answer the research question, which interventions promote the safety of older people returning home after a HF? the option was the use of a systematic method that enables reliable results to be obtained, from which conclusions can be drawn and decisions made, minimizing the risk of bias [22,24], and to guide clinics and health policies on the basis of research results.

2.2. Eligibility Criteria

All randomised controlled trials (RCT's) addressing interventions promoting the safety of the elderly person with proximal femur fracture in returning home will be included.

The target population will be people with hip fracture (including trochanteric, neck and subtrochanteric fractures) aged over 65 years, who had been admitted to hospital and had undergone orthopaedic surgery.

The types of interventions that promote the safety of the elderly person with HF, after hospital discharge, in returning home, are described below and grouped into categories that emerged from the literature review. As this is an incipient field of global research, this list is not exhaustive, providing only a few examples of the diverse interventions that have been carried out:

- Health literacy activities targeting the patient and caregiver to reduce complications associated with fracture.
- Follow-up programmes and monitoring of the functional assessment and performance in the activities of daily living.
- Programmes to reduce/control the risk and prevalence of falls and/or the occurrence of new falls.
- Interventions to monitor and improve health-related quality of life after HF.
- Environmental modification interventions to promote accessibility and mobility indoors.
- Transitional care interventions to promote adherence to the rehabilitation programme upon return home.
- Action plans that include strategies to improve the quality of care and follow-up of older people with fractures on their return home [1,7,11,12,15–21,25].

Exclusion criteria will be established for studies addressing interventions related to conventional treatment, considering a conventional treatment as that in which the person does not receive any additional intervention beyond verbal advice and/or medication optimisation, and interventions for the adult population with fragility fractures.

The review enables the identification and organisation of interventions with evidence for promoting safety after hospital discharge.

2.3. Research Strategy

Taking into account the nature of the research carried out, the strategy adopted will consist of conducting a bibliographical search in the following electronic databases: MEDLINE, and CINAHL. A list of references of the previously selected relevant articles will be compiled, and a search made for possible additional studies that may be relevant, with the aim of increasing the sensitivity of the research.

The search strategy will be developed using the medical subject headings (MeSH) and, in line with them, was based on the following key concepts: "Safety", "Functional Independence", "Elderly", "Hip fracture". The search in the CINAHL database will use the Subject Headings.

The search strategy adopted according to the respective database (Table 1) will be limited to the last 10 years and to the English and Portuguese languages.

Table 1. Search Strategy. Lisbon, 2022.

	Search Strategy	Number of Articles
#1	Elderl*""[Title/Abstract] OR ""aged""[Title/Abstract] OR Age* *""[Title/Abstract] OR Older Person *""[Title/Abstract] OR Older Adult *""[Title/Abstract] OR ((""Aged""[Mesh]) OR ""Frail Elderly""[Mesh])) OR Frail Older Adults ""[Mesh] OR Frail Older Adult ""[Mesh] NOT ""animals""[Mesh]))	395,080
#2	hip fracture*""[Title/Abstract] OR ""fragility""[Title/Abstract] OR ""fragility fracture""[Title/Abstract] OR ""osteoporos*""[Title/Abstract]) OR (""Hip Fractures""[Mesh])) OR Hip injuries [Title/Abstract]) OR hip joint [Title/Abstract])((((((""Osteoporosis""[Mesh])) OR ""Osteoporotic Fractures""[Mesh])	45,597
#3	(""Rehabilitation""[Title/Abstract] OR ""Rehabilitation exercise""""[Title/Abstract] "OR(""Rehabilitation program ""[Title/Abstract] OR"(""Rehabilitation intervention "[Title/Abstract] OR ""Education program*""[Title/Abstract] OR ""Educational programme*"" ""Education intervention""[Title/Abstract] OR ""Educational strateg*""[Title/Abstract] OR ""Educational tool*""[Title/Abstract] OR ""Healthy-interactions""[Title/Abstract] OR ""Educational therapy""[Title/Abstract] OR ""Health literature""[Title/Abstract] OR ""Activities of daily living programs""[Title/Abstract] OR ""Safety promot*""[Title/Abstract] OR ""Patient education""[Title/Abstract] OR ""Program*""[Title/Abstract] OR ""Tool*""[Title/Abstract] OR ""training""[Title/Abstract]) OR (((((((""Rehabilitation""[Mesh]) OR ""rehabilitation"" [Subheading]) OR ""Rehabilitation Nursing""[Mesh]) OR ""Orthopedic Procedures""[Mesh]) OR ""Exercise Therapy""[Mesh])) OR (""Patient Education as Topic""[Mesh])) OR rehabilitation/education ""[Mesh]) OR ""mobilization""[Title/Abstract] OR ""Early Ambulation""[Mesh])) OR ""exercise training""[Title/Abstract] OR ""exercise""[Mesh])) ""gait training""[Title/Abstract] OR ""Walking Speed""[Mesh])) OR "" environmental risk control""[Title/Abstract] OR "" daily living activity""[Title/Abstract] OR ""Activities of Daily Living""[Mesh]))	116,945
#4	""risk of falling""[Title/Abstract] OR ""prevalence of falls""[Title/Abstract] OR ""re-fracture""[Title/Abstract] OR ""Injuries secondary to the fall""[Title/Abstract] OR ""quality of life""[Title/Abstract] OR ""health-related quality of life""[Title/Abstract] OR ""security""[Title/Abstract] OR ""functional independence""[Title/Abstract]) OR Readmissions ""[Title/Abstract] OR Gait Ability OR (""Quality of Life""[Mesh])) OR (""Quality Indicators, Health Care""[Mesh])) OR (""Functional Status""[Mesh])))	494,110
#5	((""randomized controlled trial""[Title/Abstract] OR ""controlled clinical trial""[Title/Abstract] OR ""randomized""[Title/Abstract]) OR (""Randomized Controlled Trial"" [Publication Type]))"	861,759
#1 AND #2 AND #3 AND #4 AND #5		4860

2.4. Selection Process

Two reviewers will independently select, extract and code the data. In turn, a third reviewer will mediate any discrepancies in the selection of studies [22,24].

The results of the research will be inserted in the Rayyan® platform, facilitating collaboration between the three reviewers in the process of study selection.

Thus, all the titles and abstracts obtained in the research will be analysed in relation to the established inclusion criteria, with the aim of assessing the eligibility of the studies. Studies considered relevant will be selected for further reading and then included in the review. The reasons for exclusion of the studies will be documented.

For each of the studies that fulfil the inclusion criteria, data extraction and codification will be carried out by two reviewers (independently), using a previously prepared, simple and standardised form that describes the characteristics of the study. The data extraction form will include:

- Study design, title, authors' names, publication date, country, sample size, funding source.
- Characteristics of the population (number of participants, average age, proportion of each sex).
- Method (sampling, instruments and randomisation method).
- Characteristics of the intervention (type and period of intervention).
- Results.

2.5. Assessment of Methodological Quality and Risk of Bias

Two reviewers will perform the quality assessment of the included studies independently. A third reviewer may clarify any discrepancy that may arise. If the reviewers are co-authors of some studies, they will not evaluate the risk of bias in these studies [22].

The assessment of the risk of bias of the included studies will take into account the potential sources of bias and may determine a low risk of bias (if all criteria were fulfilled), moderate risk of bias (one or more criteria were partially fulfilled), high risk of bias (one or more criteria were not fulfilled) and unclear (not enough information is available to assess the study with regard to the risk of bias). The Cochrane Risk of Bias Assessment Tool [22,24] will be applied.

2.6. Data Synthesis

The synthesis of the information regarding the characteristics and results of the included studies will be presented in a table and complemented with a narrative summary, which will assess the methods used, and the results of the studies.

If there are sufficient RCTs, a meta-analysis will be produced, in which synthesis of the data will be carried out using the Review Manager software® (version 5.3, Cochrane Collaboration, London, UK). If it is not possible to perform meta-analysis, the results will be presented descriptively [22]. The strength of the body of evidence will be assessed using the GRADE framework [22–24].

The results of the systematic review will be reported according to the PRISMA guidelines [22].

3. Discussion

It is estimated that around 50–60% of people that have suffered a HF have some type of functional and/or motor loss, and that in only 30–40% of cases is a level of functional recovery attained similar to that which existed before the fracture, thus requiring continued care for a long period of time to reduce the loss of independence to perform activities of daily living [13,17].

On returning home, associated with the restriction of self-imposed and hetero-imposed mobility and loss of gait capacity, these people frequently present a functional decline, unable to recover to pre-fracture functional levels. Sometimes, it is also associated with an increased risk of falling and difficulties in accessing healthcare [11,13,26–28], which, together, represent serious problems, with a great impact on people and health services.

After the occurrence of a fragility fracture there is a high risk of a subsequent one, so the prevention of a new fall is a key aspect, requiring the development of strategies to increase safety at home [17]. The development of post-discharge transition programmes has proved to be successful in contributing to reduce readmissions and disability [25]. However, there is no systematisation of many of the interventions implemented in these programmes, nor indication of their effectiveness in maintaining the person's safety in his/her home environment, enabling recovery and avoiding postoperative complications.

Other authors have observed that despite the growing increase in scientific knowledge, there have been some gaps in the description of interventions, which have consequently made the assessment of results and their replication and implementation in practice difficult [7,21], with an important impact on the process of transition from hospital to home.

After the occurrence of this type of fracture, rehabilitation carried out in the post-acute phase aims to rescue as much autonomy as possible for patients affected by such pathological situations; however, its duration is sometimes clearly insufficient to ensure an effective and lasting result on the return home [11]. In this context, home-based rehabilitation is recommended, producing considerable positive effects on physical functioning after a femur fracture, and contributing towards a significant improvement in mobility, daily activity, instrumental activity and balance [8].

Thus, this systematic review will strengthen the evidence base on safety-promoting interventions for older people with proximal femur fracture upon return home, exploring potential outcomes regarding functional assessment, performance in activities of daily living, level of concern about falls, risk and prevalence of falls, injuries secondary to falls, fracture rate, and health-related quality of life. It could potentially benefit health professionals and researchers by facilitating the design and implementation of interventions to improve the care of these people. It will also provide information that may make an important contribution to policymaking regarding the development of strategies to improve the quality of care and follow-up of older people after HF.

This review has potential limitations related to the fact that the search strategy did not include sources of information available in languages other than English and Portuguese.

4. Conclusions

This systematic review protocol will allow identification of the available evidence on the interventions that promote the safety of the elderly person with proximal femur fracture upon returning home, thus contributing to the systematisation of transitional care interventions that promote rehabilitation, prevent the recurrence of falls, the immobility syndrome and other postoperative complications associated with this type of surgery, which translate into loss of quality of life and decreased life expectancy.

The systematisation of these interventions will make it possible to guide the clinic and contribute to the training of health professionals in this area.

Author Contributions: Conceptualization, P.R., A.H. and C.L.B.; methodology, P.R., A.H., A.M. and C.L.B.; formal analysis, P.R., A.H., A.M. and C.L.B.; investigation, P.R., A.H., A.M. and C.L.B.; resources, P.R., A.H., A.M. and C.L.B.; writing—original draft preparation, P.R., A.H., A.M. and C.L.B.; writing—review and editing, P.R., A.H., A.M. and C.L.B.; supervision, A.H.; project administration, A.H. and C.L.B.; funding acquisition: A.H. and C.L.B. All authors have read and agreed to the published version of the manuscript.

Funding: The present study was funded by the Center for Research, Innovation, and Development in Nursing, in Portugal, by means of grants provided to some of the authors (CIDNUR_Less#Falls_2021).

Institutional Review Board Statement: The present study was carried out according to the guidelines of the Declaration of Helsinki and approved by an Ethics Committee.

Informed Consent Statement: Not applicable.

Data Availability Statement: Data are available only upon request to the authors.

Acknowledgments: The authors express their gratitude to CIDNUR.

Conflicts of Interest: The authors declare no conflict of interest.

References

1. Cunha, L.C.; Baixinho, C.L.; Henriques, M.A.; Sousa, L.M.M.; Dixe, M.A. Evaluation of the effectiveness of an intervention in a health team to prevent falls in hospitalized elderly people. *Rev. Esc. Enferm. USP* **2021**, *55*, 03695. [CrossRef] [PubMed]
2. Marques, A.; Lourenço, Ó.; da Silva, J.A. Portuguese Working Group for the Study of the Burden of Hip Fractures in Portugal. The burden of osteoporotic hip fractures in Portugal: Costs, health related quality of life and mortality. *Osteoporos. Int.* **2015**, *26*, 2623–2630. [CrossRef] [PubMed]

3. Abtahi, S.; Driessen JH, M.; Vestergaard, P.; van den Bergh, J.; Boonen, A.; de Vries, F.; Burden, A.M. Secular trends in major osteoporotic fractures among 50+ adults in Denmark between 1995 and 2010. *Osteoporos. Int.* **2019**, *30*, 2217–2223. [CrossRef] [PubMed]
4. Rodrigues, A.M.; Canhao, H.; Marques, A.; Ambrósio, C.; Borges, J.; Coelho, P.; Costa, L.; Fernandes, S.; Gonçalves, I.; Goncalves, M.J.; et al. Portuguese recommendations for the prevention, diagnosis and management of primary osteoporosis—2018 update. *Acta Reumatol. Port.* **2018**, *43*, 10–31. [PubMed]
5. Marques, A.; Rodrigues, A.M.; Romeu, J.C.; Ruano, A.; Barbosa, A.P.; Simões, E.; Águas, F.; Canhão, H.; Alves, J.D.; Lucas, R.; et al. Multidisciplinary Portuguese recommendations on DXA request and indication to treat in the prevention of fragility fractures. *Acta Reumatol. Port.* **2016**, *41*, 305–321. [PubMed]
6. Paiva, S. Incidência de Fratura da Extremidade Proximal do Fémur em Mulheres Pós-Menopáusicas e a Mortalidade Pós-Evento. Master's Dissertation, Universidade da Beira Interior, Covilhã, Portugal, 2017. Available online: https://ubibliorum.ubi.pt/bitstream/10400.6/8086/1/5450_10952.pdf (accessed on 23 January 2022).
7. Keene, D.J.; Forde, C.; Sugavanam, T.; Williams, M.A.; Lamb, S.E. Exercise for people with a fragility fracture of the pelvis or lower limb: A systematic review of interventions evaluated in clinical trials and reporting quality. *BMC Musculoskelet. Disord.* **2020**, *21*, 435. [CrossRef]
8. Wu, C.-H.; Tu, S.-T.; Chang, Y.-F.; Chan, D.-C.; Chien, J.-T.; Lin, C.-H.; Singh, S.; Dasari, M.; Chen, J.-F.; Tsai, K.-S. Fracture liaison services improve outcomes of patients with osteoporosis-related fractures: A systematic literature review and meta-analysis. *Bone* **2018**, *111*, 92–100. [CrossRef]
9. Buckinx, F.; Rolland, Y.; Reginster, J.Y.; Ricour, C.; Petermans, J.; Bruyère, O. Burden of frailty in the elderly population: Perspectives for a public health challenge. *Arch. Public Health* **2015**, *73*, 19. [CrossRef]
10. Baixinho, C.L.; Dixe, M.A.; Madeira, C.; Alves, S.; Henriques, M.A. Falls in institutionalized elderly with and without cognitive decline A study of some factors. *Dement. Neuropsychol.* **2019**, *13*, 116–121. [CrossRef]
11. Contro, D.; Elli, S.; Castaldi, S.; Formili, M.; Ardoino, I.; Caserta, A.V.; Panella, L. Continuity of care for patients with hip fracture after discharge from rehabilitation facility. *Acta Bio-Med. Atenei Parm.* **2019**, *90*, 385–393. [CrossRef]
12. Direção-geral da saúde. *Fracturas da Extremidade Proximal do Fémur no Idoso, Recomendações para Intervenção Terapêutica*; Orientações Técnicas; Ministério da Saúde: Lisboa, Portugal, 2003.
13. Laires, P.A.; Perelman, J.; Consciência, J.G.; Monteiro, J.; Branco, J.C. Epidemiology of hip fractures and its social and economic impact. *Acta Reum. Port.* **2015**, *40*, 223–230. Available online: http://hdl.handle.net/10362/21964 (accessed on 24 January 2022).
14. Lavareda Baixinho, C.; Dixe, M.A. ¿Cuáles son las prácticas y comportamientos de los mayores institucionalizados para prevenir las caídas? *Index Enferm.* **2017**, *26*, 255–259. Available online: https://scielo.isciii.es/scielo.php?script=sci_arttext&pid=S1132-12 962017000300004 (accessed on 9 December 2021).
15. Flesch, D.L.; Araújo, T.C.C.F. Hospital discharge of elderly patients: Needs and challenges of continuity of care. *Estud. Psicol.* **2014**, *19*, 227–236. [CrossRef]
16. Hakkarainen, T.W.; Arbabi, S.; Willis, M.M.; Davidson, G.H.; Flum, D.R. Outcomes of Patients Discharged to Skilled Nursing Facilities After Acute Care Hospitalizations. *Ann. Surg.* **2016**, *263*, 280–285. [CrossRef] [PubMed]
17. Ferreira, E.M.; Lourenço, O.M.; Da Costa, P.V.; Pinto, S.C.; Gomes, C.; Oliveira, A.P.; Ferreira, Ó.; Baixinho, C.L. Active Life: A project for a safe hospital-community transition after arthroplasty. *Rev. Bras. Enferm.* **2019**, *72*, 147–153. [CrossRef] [PubMed]
18. Mudge, A.M.; Shakhovskoy, R.; Karrasch, A. Quality of transitions in older medical patients with frequent readmissions: Opportunities for improvement. *Eur. J. Intern. Med.* **2013**, *24*, 779–783. [CrossRef] [PubMed]
19. Stolee, P.; Elliott, J.; Byrne, K.; Gould, J.S.; Tong, C.; Chesworth, B.; Egan, M.; Ceci, C.; Forbes, D. A Framework for Supporting Post-acute Care Transitions of Older Patients with Hip Fracture. *J. Am. Med. Dir. Assoc.* **2019**, *20*, 414–419.e1. [CrossRef]
20. Asplin, G.; Carlsson, G.; Zidén, L.; Kjellby-Wendt, G. Early coordinated rehabilitation in acute phase after hip fracture—A model for increased patient participation. *BMC Geriatr.* **2017**, *17*, 240. [CrossRef]
21. Slade, S.C.; Dionne, C.; Underwood, M.; Buchbinder, R.; Beck, B.; Bennell, K.; Brosseau, L.; Costa, L.; Cramp, F.; Cup, E.; et al. Consensus on Exercise Reporting Template (CERT): Modified Delphi Study. *Phys. Ther.* **2016**, *96*, 1514–1524. [CrossRef]
22. Page, M.J.; Moher, D.; Bossuyt, P.M.; Boutron, I.; Hoffmann, T.C.; Mulrow, C.D.; Shamseer, L.; Tetzlaff, J.M.; Akl, E.A.; Brennan, S.E.; et al. PRISMA 2020 explanation and elaboration: Updated guidance and exemplars for reporting systematic reviews. *BMJ* **2021**, *3*, 160. Available online: https://www.bmj.com/content/372/bmj.n160 (accessed on 7 January 2022). [CrossRef]
23. Shamseer, L.; Moher, D.; Clarke, M.; Ghersi, D.; Liberati, A.; Petticrew, M.; Shekelle, P.; Stewart, L.; PRISMA-P Group. Preferred reporting items for systematic review and meta-analysis protocols (PRISMA-P) 2015: Elaboration and explanation. *BMJ* **2015**, *349*, g7647. [CrossRef] [PubMed]
24. Higgins, J.; Thomas, J.; Chandler, J.; Cumpston, M.; Li, T.; Page, M.; Welcht, V. *Cochrane Handbook for Systematic Reviews of Interventions*, 2nd ed.; John Wiley & Sons: Chichester, UK, 2019.
25. Gilboa, Y.; Maeir, T.; Karni, S.; Eisenberg, M.E.; Liebergall, M.; Schwartz, I.; Kaufman, Y. Effectiveness of a tele-rehabilitation intervention to improve performance and reduce morbidity for people post hip fracture—Study protocol for a randomized controlled trial. *BMC Geriatr.* **2019**, *19*, 135. [CrossRef] [PubMed]
26. Hertz, K.; Santy-Tomlinson, J. *Fragility Fracture Nursing*; Springer International Publishing: Berlin/Heidelberg, Germany, 2018; 158p. [CrossRef]

---

27. Orwig, D.; Mangione, K.K.; Baumgarten, M.; Terrin, M.; Fortinsky, R.; Kenny, A.M.; Gruber-Baldini, A.L.; Beamer, B.; Tosteson, A.; Shardell, M.; et al. Improving community ambulation after hip fracture: Protocol for a randomised, controlled trial. *J. Physiother.* **2017**, *63*, 45–46. [CrossRef]
28. Baixinho, C.L.; Bernardes, R.A.; Henriques, M.A. How to evaluate the risk of falls in institutionalized elderly people? *Rev. Baiana Enferm.* **2020**, *34*, e34861. [CrossRef]

MDPI

St. Alban-Anlage 66

4052 Basel

Switzerland

Tel. +41 61 683 77 34

Fax +41 61 302 89 18

www.mdpi.com

Journal of Personalized Medicine Editorial Office

E-mail: jpm@mdpi.com

www.mdpi.com/journal/jpm

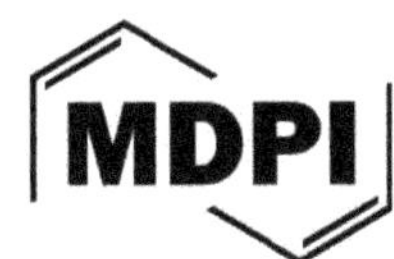

www.ingramcontent.com/pod-product-compliance
Lightning Source LLC
LaVergne TN
LVHW070013070726
842759LV00012B/66